# Caring for Women
# Cross-Culturally

# Caring for Women Cross-Culturally

**PATRICIA F. ST. HILL, PhD, MPH, RN**
**JULIENE G. LIPSON, PhD, RN, FAAN**
**AFAF IBRAHIM MELEIS, PhD, RN, FAAN**

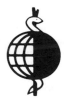

F.A. DAVIS COMPANY
Philadelphia

F. A. Davis Company
1915 Arch Street
Philadelphia, PA 19103
*www.fadavis.com*

Printed in the United States of America

Last digit indicates print number: 10 9 8 7 6 5 4 3 2 1

*Acquisitions Editor*: Robert G. Martone
*Developmental Editor*: Melanie Freely
*Cover Designer*: Louis J. Forgione
*Editor-in-Chief Nursing*: Patti L. Cleary

As new scientific information becomes available through basic and clinical research, recommended treatments and drug therapies undergo changes. The author(s) and publisher have done everything possible to make this book accurate, up to date, and in accord with accepted standards at the time of publication. The author(s), editors, and publisher are not responsible for errors or omissions or for consequences from application of the book, and make no warranty, expressed or implied, in regard to the contents of the book. Any practice described in this book should be applied by the reader in accordance with professional standards of care used in regard to the unique circumstances that may apply in each situation. The reader is advised always to check product information (package inserts) for changes and new information regarding dose and contraindications before administering any drug. Caution is especially urged when using new or infrequently ordered drugs.

**Library of Congress Cataloging-in-Publication Data**

Caring for women cross-culturally / [edited by] Patricia F. St. Hill, Juliene G. Lipson, Afaf Ibrahim Meleis.
    p.;cm.
Includes bibliographical references and index.
ISBN 0-8036-1004-1
    1. Transcultural nursing–United States. 2. Women immigrants–United States–Cross-cultural studies. 3. Women refugees–United States–Cross-cultural studies. 4. Minority women–United States–Cross-cultural studies. I. St. Hill, Patricia F. II. Lipson, Juliene G., 1944- III. Meleis, Afaf Ibrahim.
    [DNLM: 1. Transcultural Nursing–methods. 2. Cross-Cultural Comparison: 3. Women's Health Services. WY 107 C277 2002]
RT86.54. C365 2002
362.1'73–dc21
                                                                                        2002073915

This book was written to honor women who are voiced or silenced, integrated or marginalized. May it help in facilitating their life transitions; eliminating the effects of sexism, racism and nationalism; and empowering them and their health care providers in the pursuit of quality care.

# BRIEF
# BIOGRAPHICAL SKETCHES

## Authors

PATRICIA F. ST. HILL, PhD, MPH, RN

received her PhD from the University of California, San Francisco, School of Nursing, where her degree and research focus has been in community and cross-cultural health nursing. She has completed a post-doctoral fellowship at the University of Washington, Seattle, and taught in nursing programs both in the United States and the Caribbean, where she was born. Presently Dr. St. Hill is an Associate Professor at Texas Women's University, Dallas, Texas.

JULIENE G. LIPSON, PhD, FAAN

a nurse-anthropologist, is a professor in the Department of Community Health Systems, School of Nursing, University of California, San Francisco, where she teaches graduate students in community health and cross-cultural nursing, with an emphasis on culturally competent care and research. Her books include *Self-Care Nursing in a Multicultural Context*, Sage, Thousand Oaks, CA, 1996 and *Nursing Care: A Pocket Guide*, UCSF Nursing Press, San Francisco. Since 1982, Dr. Lipson has done research on the health and adjustment of immigrant and refugees to the United States from several Arab countries, Iran, Afghanistan, Bosnia and the Former Soviet Union. She is active in the Society for Applied Anthropology as well as the Council on Nursing and Anthropology and the Council on Refugees and Immigrants in the American Anthropological Association.

AFAF IBRAHIM MELEIS, PhD, RN, FAAN

is a nurse and a medical sociologist who received her BS in nursing at the University of Alexandria, Egypt, and her MS in nursing, MA in sociology, and PhD in medical and social psychology at the University of California, Los Angeles. She has been a professor at the University of California since 1968 and taught in the Department of Community Health Systems at the University of California, San Francisco from 1971 to 2001. Afaf Meleis is presently Dean of the School of Nursing at the University of Pennsylvania. She has taught nursing theory in numerous countries and has published extensively on nursing theory, cross-cultural care, and women's health. Her research has focused on the relationships between women's multiple roles; on their life transitions and their health; and on immigration, transitions, marginalization, and health. She has conducted collaborative research projects in the United States, Brazil, Colombia, Mexico, Egypt and Kuwait. She established the Mid-East S.I.H.A. Project (study of Middle Eastern Immigrants Health and Adjustment) in the University of California, San Francisco, School of Nursing. She is the president of the International Council on Women's Health Issues.

# CONTRIBUTORS

## AMERICAN INDIAN

**Lillian Tom-Orme, PhD, MPH, RN, FAAN,** is Research Assistant Professor, Department of Family and Preventive Medicine, Health Research Center, University of Utah School of Medicine. She teaches in the Masters in Public Health Program, conducts research in American Indian populations, and mentors American Indian/Alaska Native/Native Hawaiian students. She serves on such committees as the American Diabetes Association, the National Institutes of Health National Center for Health Disparity and Minority Health, American Public Health Association's American Indian/Alaska Native/Native Hawaiian Caucus, National Alaska Native American Indian Nurses Association (NANAINA), the Public Health Service Office on Women's Health Panel of Experts, and the Ethnic Minority Nurses Fellowship Program. She is a fellow in the American Academy of Nursing and President-elect of the NANAINA. Born and raised on the Navajo reservation, she remains fluent in her Diné language.

## ARAB

**Marianne Hattar-Pollara, DNSc, RN, FAAN,** is a graduate from University of California, San Francisco. She is a professor at Azusa Pacific University, School of Nursing. Her research and publications focus on cross-cultural and global women's health issues and international nursing. She is recognized in her native Jordan, the Middle East, and the United States for her expertise, research, and innovations in women's health, particularly that of immigrant women. She has been serving as a consultant on several international USAID women's health projects and health programs.

## BRAZILIAN

**DeAnne K. Hilfinger Messias, PhD, RN,** is an Associate Professor of Nursing and Women's Studies at the University of South Carolina, Columbia. She lived in Brazil for over two decades, working in primary health care, women's health, and nursing education. Her research has focused on various aspects of Brazilian women's health and work, immigrant health, and transition experiences in women's lives. Her dissertation research explored the transnational migration, work, and health experiences of Brazilian immigrant women in the United States.

## CAMBODIAN

**Judith C. Kulig, DNSc, RN,** is an Associate Professor at the School of Health Sciences, University of Lethbridge, Alberta, Canada, an Academic Consultant at the Chinook Health Region, and an Adjunct Assistant Professor within the Faculty of Nursing, University of Alberta. She began working with Cambodian refugees during her master's program and continued as a public health nurse. While completing her dissertation research with Cambodians, she lived with a family and undertook Khmer language classes. She currently teaches in an undergraduate nursing program and continues to work with multicultural populations in Southern Alberta, Canada.

## CHINESE

**Betty L. Chang, DNSc, RN, FNP-C, FAAN,** is a professor in the University of California, Los Angeles, School of Nursing. She has a BS and MA from Columbia Teachers' College, New York, and is a nurse practitioner. Her DNSc is from the University of California, San Francisco. She emigrated from Shantung, China, at 10 years of age. Her research is on the care of the elderly and their family members and the quality of nursing care for persons with chronic illnesses. Dr. Chang edits the "Nursing Informatics Department" for the *Western Journal of Nursing Research*, is Associate Editor of *On-line Journal of Nursing Informatics* (OJNI), and is treasurer of the National Asian American and Pacific Islanders Nurses' Association.

**Lin Zhan, PhD, RN,** is an Associate Professor and Co-Director, College of Nursing, University of Massachusetts, Boston, and The Norton Long Center for Urban Democracy, Asian American Studies Program. Her BS is from the West China University of Medical Science, an MS from Boston University School of Nursing, and a PhD from Boston College School of Nursing. Born in Chengdu, Sichuan, China, she immigrated to the United States at the age of 29. She was editor of the award-winning book *Asian Voices: Asian and Asian American Health Educators Speak out* (1999).

## COLOMBIAN

**Pilar Bernal de Pheils, MS, RN,** is a Family Nurse Practitioner who was born and raised in Cali, Colombia. She received her nursing degree and nurse midwifery specialization in 1972 and 1974 from the Universidad del Valle in Cali, Colombia. She received her master's degree (1986) from the University of California, San Francisco, and teaches in the Family Health Department of the UCSF School of Nursing. She is also a nurse practitioner in the area of reproductive and primary care at a clinic serving primarily Latina women.

**Diva Jaramillo, MPH, RN,** born and raised in Medellín, Colombia, received her nursing degree in 1972 and her master's degree in 1980 from the Universidad de Antioquia in Medellín, Colombia. She is on the faculty of the School of Nursing, Graduate Department, at the Universidad de Antioquia. She has diverse research expertise and has conducted several studies in women's health, specifically on the topic of domestic violence.

## ETHIOPIAN/ERITREAN

**Yewoubdar Beyene, PhD,** is a Medical Anthropologist, born and raised in Addis Ababa, Ethiopia. She received her PhD in 1985 in Medical Anthropology from the Case Western Reserve University, Cleveland. She is currently on the faculty of the Institute for Health and Aging, and the Department of Anthropology, History, and Social Medicine at the University of California, San Francisco. She has diverse research expertise and has conducted cross-cultural research in a variety of settings, both within and outside of the United States. Her primary research interests are women's reproductive health (both in developing and developed nations), immigrant and refugee health, and cultural beliefs and practices of traditional societies.

## FILIPINO

**Judith A. Berg, PhD, RNC, WHNP** is an Assistant Professor at the University of Arizona College of Nursing, where she teaches women's health in the masters and doctoral programs. She received her doctorate in nursing at the University of California, San Francisco. Her research focuses on women's health promotion and symptom management strategies across the lifespan, with special interest in cross cultural variations. Dr. Berg is currently President of the Society for Menstrual Cycle Research, an interdisciplinary international research society dedicated to understanding the role of the menstrual cycle in women's health.

**Carolina P. de Guzman, MSN, CPAN, RN,** is a trainer for the National Asian Women's Health Organization (NAWHO). She obtained her BSN from the University of the Philippines and a MSN from Sonoma State University. She taught at the Philippine General Hospital School of Nursing before migrating to the United States. She is newly retired after 32 years of nursing practice and has served as president of both the Philippine Nurses Association of Northern California and the University of the Philippines Nursing Alumni Association of Northern California, which she founded. She has coordinated numerous health and research events for Filipino Americans in the San Francisco Bay Area, has been active in Sigma Theta Tau and the Peri-Anesthesia Nurses Association of California, and, until her retirement, was an affiliate faculty member at Samuel Merritt College.

**Daisy M. Rodriguez, MN, MPA, RN,** is an Administrative Nursing Supervisor at the San Ramon Regional Medical Center. She received her basic and master's degrees in nursing from the University of the Philippines and has lived in the United States for the past 30 years. Her master's degree in Public Administration-Health Services is from the University of San Francisco, California. She has taught in nursing programs both in the Philippines and in California and received a fellowship in Ethnogeriatrics at the Stanford Geriatric Education Center. She is active in the local and national chapters of the Philippine Nurses Association.

## HAITIAN

**Jessie M. Colin, PhD, RN,** is an Assistant Professor of Nursing at Barry University in Miami Shores, Florida, where she teaches in both undergraduate and graduate programs. She received her BSN and MSN from Hunter College, New York, and her doctorate from Adelphi University, Long Island, NY. Dr. Colin is the immediate past president of the Haitian American Nurses Association (HANA) and has served on national committees and task forces with the American Nurses Association. She is a management consultant with expertise in home care and home infusion, quality improvement, Joint Commission on Accreditation of Healthcare Organizations (JCAHO) certification, culture, and ethnicity. Her research interests are in global health and the role of nursing. Dr. Colin migrated to New York from Haiti at the age of 14.

**Ghislaine Paperwalla, BSN, RN,** is a registered nurse (retired). She has studied both in the United States and Canada and received her Bachelor of Science in Nursing from Florida International University in 1975. She was born and raised in Haiti and migrated to the U.S. in 1960. She has been very actively engaged in health education programs geared for the Haitian community in Miami, focusing mainly on women's health. She has been president of the Haitian American Nurses Association of South Florida Inc from 1989–1997.

## JAPANESE

**Yuko Matsumoto Leong, MS, CNS, RN,** is a public health nurse for City of Berkeley, CA. She was a nurse-midwife and an instructor of maternal nursing in Shizuoka, Japan. She received her master's degree (1998) in community health nursing from

University of California, San Francisco. Her primary interests are the transitional experiences of immigrant women who married American men and the experience of their children in such households.

## KOREAN

**Eun-Ok Im, PhD, MPH, RN, CNS,** is an Assistant Professor at the University of Wisconsin-Milwaukee. She was born and raised in South Korea and moved to the United States to study. Dr. Im received her PhD (1997) in nursing from the University of California, San Francisco, and did postdoctoral study at the same institution. She has expertise in feminist and international and cross-cultural approaches to women's health issues. Her primary research interests include menopause, cancer pain, and breast cancer; and the development of computer programs supporting health care with diverse cultural groups of women.

## MEXICAN

**Kathleen Laganá, PhD, RN,** is Assistant Professor of Nursing and nurse researcher at Oregon Health Sciences University, Ashland, Oregon. Her research interest is cultural determinants of social support and women's health. As a Perinatal Clinical Nurse Specialist she has a special interest in Mexican American women's health during pregnancy. She has conducted field research with Mexican American women in Central California and Southern Colorado. She received her PhD in Nursing at the University of California, San Francisco.

**Leticia Gonzalez-Ramirez, BSN, RN,** is a public health nurse working in California's Salinas Valley. She also works in the Home Health Division for Community Hospital of the Monterey Peninsula. She has written and conducted research on Mexican American health issues.

## PUERTO RICAN

**Maria E. Rosa, PhD, DrPH, MS, MPH,** is the Dean of the Graduate Department and Professor, School of Nursing, Medical Sciences Campus, University of Puerto Rico, San Juan. She received a BS and MS in nursing from the University of Puerto Rico, an MPH (Public Health Administration) and a DrPH (Public Health Education) from Loma Linda University, California, and a PhD in nursing (neuropsychiatry) from the University of California, Los Angeles. Her research has been in community health in the area of nutrition and building a healthy community, as well as on patients with dual diagnoses of substance dependence and chronic mental illness.

## RUSSIAN

**Karen J. Aroian, PhD, RN, CS, FAAN,** is the Katherine E. Faville Professor of Nursing Research, College of Nursing, and Adjunct Professor, Department of Anthropology, Wayne State University, Detroit, Michigan. She received her PhD in Nursing Science from the University of Washington, Seattle, Washington. Research areas are immigrant and minority health, cross-cultural research methods, instrument development, and qualitative research, and she has been funded by the National Institutes of Health and private foundations. Dr. Aroian has 20 data-based articles in peer reviewed journals and three book chapters on research methods and instrument development. Her research on Polish, Irish, Filipino, Vietnamese, and Soviet immigrants and African Americans has focused on immigrant stress, coping and mental health, health care utilization, and symptom self-care.

## SOUTH ASIAN

**Rachel Zachariah, DNSc., RN,** is an Associate Professor, Bouve College of Health Sciences School of Nursing, Northeastern University, Boston, Massachusetts. She has a BSc in Nursing and Midwifery diploma from the Christian Medical College and Hospital, College of Nursing, Vellore, South India (University of Madras), an MS in nursing from the University of California, Los Angeles, and a DNSc from the University of California, San Francisco. Dr. Zachariah's practice and research focus on women's health. She teaches her students to collaborate with providers and residents of Boston neighborhoods and, previously, other rural and urban health centers in the United States and Canada. Dr. Zachariah planned and provided health care for rural and urban populations in South India. She currently conducts federally funded research on predictors of pregnancy outcomes of low-income women.

## VIETNAMESE

**Thu T. Nowak, MS RN,** is a public health nurse with the Fairfax County, Virginia, Health Department. She was born and raised in southern Vietnam and migrated to the United States in 1970. She received a BS in nursing from George Mason University in 1981. Her work involves extensive contact with diverse ethnic groups, including the Vietnamese community of northern Virginia. She also is an authority on meditation therapy and relaxation exercises.

# REVIEWER LIST

MARY BEAR, EdD, MSN
Associate Professor
Brenau University School of Nursing
One Centennial Circle
Gainesville, Georgia 30501

DONNA BRANDMEYER, EdD, RN
Professor and Chair
Division of Nursing
Lewis-Clark State College
Lewiston, Idaho 83501

CYNTHIA CAMERON, PhD
Professor of Nursing
University of South Alabama
1504 Springhill Avenue
Mobile, Alabama 36688

JANE ESHLEMAN, MA, MS, RN
Associate Professor
Bethel College
1001 W. McKinley Avenue
Mishawaka, Indiana 46545-5591

ANDREA KOEPKE, DNS, MA
Director, School of Nursing
Anderson University
1100 E. 5th Street
Anderson, Indiana 46012

EVELYN LABUN, DNSc, MScN
Assistant Professor
University of North Dakota
College of Nursing
Box 9025 University Station
Grand Forks, North Dakota 58202-9025

DEBRA FLOYD LETT, MSN, MPA
Instructor
Auburn University Montgomery
P. O. Box 244023
Montgomery, Alabama 36124-4023

CORA C. MUNOZ, PhD, RN
Associate Professor
Capital University
2199 E. Main Street
Columbus, Ohio 43209

DONNA L. WADDELL, EdD, RN, CS
Professor of Nursing
North Georgia College and State University
Department of Nursing
Dahlonega, Georgia 30597

LYNNE B. WELCH, EdD, MSN
Post Master's Certificate–Family Nurse Practitioner
Dean, College of Nursing and Health Professions
Marshall University
400 Hal Greer Boulevard
Prichard Hall Room 426
Huntington, West Virginia 25755-9500

YU XU, PhD, MSN, MEd
Assistant Professor of Nursing
University of South Alabama
1504 Springhill Avenue,
Mobile, Alabama 36688

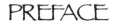

**Caring for Women Cross-Culturally** is a comprehensive source of culturally relevant information for those who provide services to immigrant and minority women. It can benefit professional and student health care providers, social workers, counselors, chaplains, educators, as well as others interested in better understanding the implications of cultural phenomena in immigrant and minority women's health care.

The uniqueness of this book is based on its format. Each chapter is organized according to the same framework, facilitating quick and easy retrieval of information on a specific topic. Each of the 19 chapters represents a separate ethnic/cultural or regional immigrant population. Interspersed through each chapter are *Notes to the Health Care Provider*, intended to alert the provider to potential problems that he or she may encounter at certain developmental stages or when dealing with a particularly sensitive topic, including suggestions of ways to approach these issues.

Except for African American and American Indian/Alaskan Native women, the chapters describe women who came to North America in the last half of the 20th Century. The 1951 United Nations policy on refugees allowed people to enter other countries outside of normal quota restrictions grounded on a well-founded fear of persecution based on race, religion, nationality, social group, or political opinion. The 1965 immigration law of the United States loosened the quota system so that people from all continents could immigrate. Similarly, the Canadian Immigration Act of 1976 advocated a broad basis of selection and eliminated residual "preferred" immigrant barriers. Despite the large number of immigrant/refugee women and the migration stressors that can be threatening to health (Meleis, Lipson, Muecke & Smith, 1998), much of the literature, until recently, limited descriptions of immigrant women's experiences to their reproductive role (Kulig, 1990). This book is an attempt to address this gap.

We selected the chapters based on population size; representation from Asia, Europe, Africa, and South America; how recently the women immigrated; and the relative lack of published cultural and health information on the topics in each chapter to guide providers who work with these women. Chapter authors were selected on the basis of their familiarity with the population, having either been born and/or lived in the country from which immigrants came or having extensive clinical or research experience with the ethnic or immigrant group.

## PRECAUTIONARY NOTE TO THE READER

It is very difficult to describe both common characteristics of a cultural/national group and the diversity within it and still limit the chapter to a reasonable length. In this book, chapters range in scope from less *heterogeneous* groups, such as Cambodian women, to American Indians or immigrants from an enormous and diverse region such as South Asia, in which tribes or ethnic groups should probably be described in separate chapters. Sources of diversity, in addition to how recently they immigrated, include urban/rural origin, socioeconomic status, educational level and source, religion, strength of ethnic identity, family style, and personal characteristics. We respectfully ask you to *avoid* using this book as a cookbook or to stereotype the women described in each chapter. Please use it as a starting point from which to think about and ask whether this particular family, client, or student is similar to or different from what the chapter describes on the topic of interest.

Patricia St. Hill, PhD, MPH, RN
Juliene G. Lipson, PhD, RN, FAAN
Afaf Ibrahim Meleis, PhD, RN, FAAN,

# TABLE OF CONTENTS

# CHAPTER 1

# Theoretical Considerations of Health Care for Immigrant and Minority Women

## AFAF MELEIS, PhD, RN, FAAN

With the increase of migration worldwide, most health care systems must adapt to the increasingly multicultural character of both clients and the health and social service providers who staff these systems. In North America, many women from long-established ethnic groups, or the Indians who first peopled the continent, have migrated from rural to urban areas or to very different regions. Although several comments in this chapter are specific to immigrants, ethnic minority women who are not immigrants also experience many of the issues described here. To understand the health care needs of immigrant or ethnic minority women, to provide them with culturally sensitive care, and to promote their access to the health care system, it is vital to view them within the context of their life histories and to uncover the cultural and structural facilitators and constraints that they may have encountered in their country of origin or current place of residence.

Existing models of women's health tend to neglect the integration between cultural values and norms and structural facilitators and constraints in women's lives that shape their responses and experiences. These models include, among others, the biomedical model, the reproductive and maternal model, and the cultural model. Each of these models will be briefly described before the model proposed in this chapter is presented.

## ⊕ EXISTING MODELS

### The Biomedical Model

The biomedical model assumes that advances in biomedicine that include multiple factors in health and disease are all that are needed to cure any disease of women. Although there are many indications that biomedicine has reduced morbidity and mortality rates for many diseases, its disease orientation ignores gender differences and gender-specific issues, and it rarely includes social, historical, and cultural aspects of health-illness experience. There is very limited research that shows that biomedical models have made a substantive contribution to the quality of life of the population (Hall & Allen, 1995). In women's health care, however, biomedical models fall short in three major ways. First, they tend to explain women's responses to health and illness by reducing them to biomedical processes. For example, in this orientation menopause is seen as a metabolic or endocrine disorder (Abrams & Berkow, 1990), and so women who are experiencing the menopausal transition are defined as patients who have a hormone deficiency syndrome (Coney, 1994). This view of the menopausal transition is distorted and limited because it does not account for women's own experiences in this phase of their lives.

Second, biomedical models fail to incorporate another important aspect of women's health: gender sensitivity and gendered explanations of health and illness. Most of the research on diseases or system dysfunctions has relied on men as subjects, and male attributes are considered to be the norm against which women's health care needs are judged (Davis & Youngkin, 1995). An example is cardiac disease in women that either has been ignored or misdiagnosed or its management has been delayed (O'Toole, 1989; Wenger, et al, 1993; Harris & Weissfeld, 1991). Many examples of neglect of other disease conditions have been documented (Rossner, 1994).

Third, the biomedical model presents the assumption that physicians are in control; this fosters dependency on physicians rather than encouraging women to maintain control of their health (Gannon & Ekstrom, 1993). In other words, the biomedical model medicalizes women's normal health-illness experiences, tends to make them feel helpless, and underlies the loss of women's own ways of managing health and illness experiences, which their grandmothers formerly managed well.

## The Reproductive and Maternal Model

Considerable international evidence has shown that health care systems tend to limit women's health issues to reproductive health. When women's health is debated internationally, the discussion usually focuses on how mortality and morbidity rates can be reduced, how many children need to be planned for, and how and why children need to be spaced. The maternal model has certainly contributed to the reduction of maternal mortality and morbidity, as well as women's morbidity and mortality in general; however, it tends to minimize a lifespan view of women's health issues only to pregnancy and reproductive health. Furthermore, it has made women in nonreproductive life stages invisible in health care systems. For example, elderly women's health care needs have been neglected or ignored.

This model also de-emphasizes many other needs of women, including work, caregiving, the spousal/partner role, and community roles. This model supports the myth that only women can care for children, and it promulgates assumptions about women's limited spheres of functioning and influence. Patriarchal societies support and promote the maternal model. This model also drives policies that exclude women from important clinical trials under the assumption that they must be protected because of their reproductive functions, embryos, or both. Consequently, knowledge of the interaction of drugs and hormones and their effect on women at different stages in their lives is limited (Dubois & Burris, 1994; Weisman, 1998).

## The Cultural Model

While the cultural model improves on the biomedical and reproductive models because it views women throughout the lifespan and within their context, a potential limitation of relying only on a cultural perspective is neglecting to recognize women's individuality in how they conform to traditional values and norms. This model is predicated on the assumption that women's responses and explanatory frameworks of health and illness are products of the norms and values of their society. Cultural models of health care often stereotype women who share the same cultural heritage, and they may also immobilize providers who attempt to change adverse health care situations in the name of protection of this cultural heritage. In other words, cultural relativism has been used to absolve health care professionals from their moral responsibility to develop creative strategies to help women make necessary changes in their lives.

## ● PROPOSED THEORETICAL MODEL

Each of the models previously discussed provides a limited view of health care for women and limited goals for meeting their needs. A more integrative, coherent, and gender-sensitive model that encompasses women's diverse roles and health care needs is needed. Such a model is proposed here. This theoretical framework can be used to drive both research and clinical practice for immigrant and ethnic minority women (Figure 1–1).

Providing quality care for women requires a framework that is driven by well-examined assumptions and careful attention to several necessary components. The following framework is guided by assumptions derived from symbolic interactionism and reflects the capacity of women to define and be defined by their interactions with their environment. According to this framework, the labels, symbols, expectations, and meanings assigned by women and their significant others shape worldview, experiences, and responses (Blumer, 1969). Therefore, how women experience, respond, behave, or interpret their health or illness reflects their individual experiences, the reaction of others to them, and the roles and images that a society assigns to them (Turner, 1978).

How and why women seek and receive care, where they choose to receive care, and under what circumstances they comply with care strategies is shaped by health care providers' assumptions about them as well as their own explanatory models of health, illness, and care. While women's cultural values may play an important role in shaping their worldview, cultural heritage is only one part of what shapes their health and illness experiences and responses. To understand women's health care experiences and responses, this proposed integrated model includes several components: diversity, previous models of care, and development—all of which interact to affect the process of care. In the process, women's transition experiences and the nature of their work affect whether and how they are marginalized in their environment. The dynamic interaction and integration of all these components shape the nature of their interactions with the health care system. Each component is described in the following discussions.

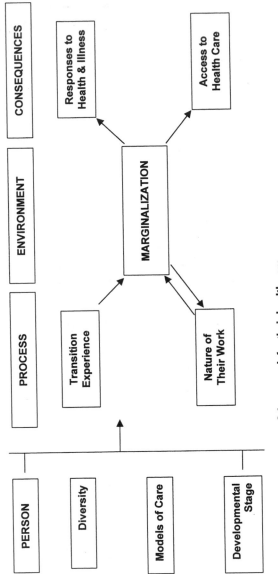

**FIGURE 1–1. Immigrant women. A framework for their health care**

# Person

## Diversity

Immigrant and ethnic minority women share many attributes and experiences related to their gender and migration. Gender is unifying, and shapes women's responses. Much evidence shows that women tend to respond differently than men do to pain, life-threatening diseases, and medication. Evidence, too, shows that women use different cognitive styles, decision-making strategies, and health care providers. Similarly, women who emigrated from the same country or are of the same ethnicity share many historical events, values, and norms driven by their heritage.

Despite shared experiences, however, a great deal of diversity is found among women of any ethnic group. Using "immigrant" or ethnic minority chapters to structure this book may give readers a false impression that women's responses are uniform within one cultural or immigrant group. Considering gender and heritage as one-dimensional variables in shaping experiences leads to stereotyping, an undesirable attitude.

Culturally competent care for immigrant and ethnic minority women requires a delicate balance in assumptions that drive the assessment process and the care plans. For example, assuming that women who emigrated from one country or region share certain values, beliefs, attitudes, and experiences that influence how they will respond to illness, treatment, caring, and recovery must simultaneously be balanced by assuming diversity among those who emigrated from the same place. Women's lived experiences that profoundly influence their health and illness experiences include educational background, family heritage, social class, economic factors, work/occupational experience, urban/rural origin, length of time in the United States (or place of migration), and a variety of individual characteristics or choices such as sexual orientation, disability, and strength of ethnic identity. Therefore, the descriptions of the various "populations" in this volume must be reviewed within a context of diversity within each group.

## Previously Experienced Models of Care

Immigrant and ethnic minority women may have experienced vastly different models of care in their home country, town, reservation, or family of origin. How they interact with the dominant North American health care systems is strongly influenced by their previous experiences with health care and is best understood within that context. While their experience in biomedical health care systems evolves over time, continued interface with different models of care also shapes and reflects their current experiences with mainstream health care, with varying intensity at different times.

One of the earliest models for health care was based on the insights of elderly members of the family. The insights and caring practices of grandmothers have profoundly influenced health care for girls and women in many countries around the world, as well as in North America. In many Asian countries, grandmothers earn respect, wisdom, and power by sacrificing their lives for their families and by gaining significantly increased status when they become grandmothers (Lock, 1994). Members of their families heed their advice and wisdom and accept their authority, especially in matters related to health. Grandmothers may influence the most important decisions in their family's lives, including circumcision of granddaughters, preventive programs, and birth control measures.

The grandmother model of women's health, significant in many parts of the world, is driven by heavy doses of caring, nurturing, and supporting. Grandmothers, knowingly or unknowingly, provide their offspring with the first framework of how families view and deal with women's health. To fully understand and explain health care needs of women requires uncovering the process that grandmothers use to influence health care of girls and women in their families and the goals for health as viewed from their perspective.

The biomedical model of care has dominated health care for women in many countries, and women have come to associate it with better and more modern care. It is reinforced in the media and in public policy as the model of choice for all health care (Ruzek et al., 1997). Therefore, many immigrant women or ethnic minority women prefer it to folk, alternative, or complementary care models.

Yet another women's health and health care model that many immigrant and ethnic minority women experience is the morality model. The premise is that moral values provide a framework within which women should be cared for and designate healthy and unhealthy behaviors. Health beliefs, attitudes, behaviors, and health care practices that are morally unacceptable within a particular society are considered unhealthy. The morality model's health care goals include reforming people and providing need-based health care only to those who are reformed and changing "unhealthy" behaviors in women who do not meet the society's moral standards. For example, a society may question why it should waste money on health care for prostitutes without first reforming them. How women respond to certain health and illness issues or conditions related to sexuality, sexual preferences, and orientation is guided by their perceptions and the interpretations of the morality model. For example, homosexuality may be regarded as a sin by theologians, a legal problem or crime by legislators, a biological anomaly by medical entrepreneurs, and a mental disturbance by psychiatrists or psychologists because of value systems that consider homosexuality a deviance that needs to be corrected (Rossner, 1994). Many Christian societies have placed taboos on homosexuality; and many regard it as a disease, unhealthy condition, or both. Female genital surgery, another example long regarded as normal or healthy in many cultures, explains within a morality model why the practice has endured and why many societies support clitoridectomy/circumcision of females (Ebong, 1997; Wright, 1996).

The morality model is socially and culturally value-laden and frames how women interpret their health and what they accept and reject from health care providers. Many immigrant or ethnic minority women use it to explain or designate what is stigmatizing; what should be kept a secret; and what can be disclosed by whom, to whom, and under what circumstances. Because a morality model of health care shapes the services women seek or the decisions they make in health care systems, health providers must understand the extent to which it is part of women's explanatory models in order to guide appropriate interventions.

## Developmental Stage

A third component of the model is a developmental perspective. Whether considering age, work, transition, or other identifiers in women's lives, a static view limits understanding of women's experiences and responses. A dynamic interrelated and integrated approach to age at immigration —for example, current age, the meaning of age, and experiences perceived to be related to age —needs to be uncovered for a full understanding of women's responses and experiences. In this book, women's issues are described within a developmental perspective that spans infancy to senescence.

## Process

### Transition Experience

To fully understand women's responses, particularly those of women who have immigrated, health providers must pay careful attention to their transition experience. Although women from all backgrounds undergo developmental transitions and the experience of moving from home to other, sometimes vastly different, places, the transition experiences of immigrant women are particularly acute. This multidimensional experience can be differentiated by length of time in transition from country of birth to host country, the number of transitions until settling in the host country, and the reasons for uprooting and rerooting.

Immigrant women face multiple challenges in the transition process, such as loss of familiar networks, support systems, known symbols, and identifiable resources. They also face the stress associated with such losses. New demands are placed on women immigrants, and these demands are different at different stages and phases of an immigration transition. Friends and support systems are frequently their relatives. If the relatives live in another city or country, the women suffer because support is limited. While women in many countries consider their adult children a source of support (Meleis & Bernal, 1996; Meleis et al., 1996), it is important to consider that many immigrants do not think of their children as their support system. Having a social network does not always provide support. It is important to assess the nature of the network and the ways it provides or does not provide support during the many phases of the immigration transition.

Immigrant women face a new society, new values, new norms, and new sets of expectations; and to be confronted with so much that is new, tends to create a sense of disequilibrium and uncertainty. Transitions may also evoke fear of identity loss or changes in roles, patterns of behavior, and dynamics of interaction (Schumacher & Meleis, 1994). Feelings of uprootedness, coupled with the need to function in an unfamiliar environment in which the symbols must be constantly interpreted, lead to feelings of distress manifested as depression and somatic complaints (Mirdal, 1984). This distress adds to women's feelings of isolation and the perception that they are not well understood. A theme of persistent grief may influence everything in the lives of immigrant women (Anderson, 1991).

In general, transitions generate stress; and with the immigration transition, additional stressors occur. Aroian's (1990) study of Polish immigrants in the United States identified such immigration-based stressors as adjusting to the new environment, occupation, and language; not "feeling at home"; and the feeling of being subordinate in the host society. Stressors experienced by Iranian women include occupational and financial difficulties, loss of status, reduced social support, ethnic bias, and differences in values and child rearing styles (Lipson, 1992). A major stressor experienced by a Lao community in Seattle was the threat of persecution by an evil spirit from the home country for having fled home, kind, and country (Muecke, 1987). Such conditions as language proficiency, socioeconomic status, availability of network, and nature of support will influence the progress toward the healthy resolution of stress, fear, and the uncertainty inherent in the immigration transition.

The effects of life transitions may be cumulative. If issues related to one transition are not resolved, they may be aggravated when another transition arises. This cumulative effect results in a different experience for immigrant women than for women who have not immigrated. The postpartum transition, for example, added to an immigration transition, results in changes in social roles, lifestyle, interaction, and support system. Women going through both transitions simultaneously have distinct issues; for example, a constant appraisal of uncertainties, conflicts between traditional and modern systems of birth, and postpartum strain (El Sayed, 1986).

Therefore, health care for immigrant women must take into account all their transitions as a context for the total assessment of their needs and for developing knowledge on which to base intervention strategies.

### Nature of Immigrant Women's Work

Work has invariably been defined as employment, and understanding the nature of women's work has been constrained by economically driven models. While the definition of what constitutes work tends to be problematic for all women, it is particularly problematic for immigrant and ethnic minority women. Among the reasons are the high demands on their time, the complexity and number of roles they are expected to play, the conflict of cultural demands, the participation in family-run businesses, and the low-income, service-oriented jobs. When work is defined as employment for pay and out of the house, most immigrant women's work tends to be invisible and excluded. When their work is invisible, devalued, and unacknowledged, their access to health care may be constrained; and the relationship between their work, stress, and health status may not be considered.

Getting settled in a new country is mostly women's work. At different periods during the settling-in period, women experience such work-related transitions as loss of familiar work, care-giving activities, and lack of support in performing each role. They are expected to be culture brokers and family mediators. They become responsible for maintaining ethnic continuity when immediate and extended families typically expect them to maintain and help family members maintain their culture of origin and, at the same time, integrate into the educational and social systems of society (Hattar-Pollara & Meleis, 1995a; Hattar-Pollara & Meleis, 1995b). This double burden is added to the role overload of other responsibilities that include taking care of extended family locally and abroad (Meleis, 1991).

In sum, the nature of immigrant women's work needs to be carefully assessed to fully understand the experiences and responses of women to their health and illness events and to that of their families.

### Environment

#### Marginalization

Many immigrant and ethnic minority women stand out from dominant cultures because of their clothes, accents, mannerisms, or responses. These differences may set them apart, at the periphery, and may engender prejudice in and discrimination from others. Immigrant women in particular encounter situations in which they are reminded about their foreignness and lack of belonging, which tends to marginalize them and increase their vulnerability.

Marginalization is defined as being different in the sense of being negatively distinguished from the norm. Margins are defined as "the peripheral, boundary-determining aspects of persons, social networks, communities, and environments" (Hall et al, 1994, pp. 24–25). Marginalized people react and respond to situations in ways mainstream people consider unique or odd. Their dress, language, religious practices, food preferences, or other characteristics may distinguish them. Marginalization increases as the person or group moves farther away from practices of those at the center. The center is determined by the majority and populated by more powerful mainstream people. The majority of people tend to allow marginalized people little power and tend not to understand them. Therefore, marginalized people learn to be secretive and to guard information that may expose or further compound their marginalization. They learn to disclose personal information only to those with whom they have developed trust and feel safe. Although they tend to be more reflective about their own and others' behavior and often have profound insights, they may appear silent and voiceless. All these characteristics set them apart and thus marginalize them even more.

Understanding the situation of immigrants requires giving careful attention to the extent to which they experience marginalizing experiences in their new country. These marginalizing experiences may exacerbate the fragmentation in the care they receive. Caregivers need to be aware that institutional barriers and stereotyping tend to marginalize immigrants and ethnic minority women and that these marginalizing experiences define such women's responses and experiences.

In conclusion, immigrant women tend to be more vulnerable than immigrant men and nonimmigrants to illness and barriers in health care. To uncover their experiences (Aroian, in press) and to effectively decrease their vulnerability and enhance their access to care, we suggest that their responses should be considered within a framework that acknowledges their cultural heritage, as well as their diversity. The model also includes women's explanatory frameworks of health and health care, the nature of their transitions, the developmental life stage, and the nature of their work. In addition, the framework acknowledges that immigrant and ethnic minority women experience marginalization, which profoundly influences how they respond to illness, manage their own care, and interact with health care providers, as well as their access to care. Each of these components independently adds insight about women's responses to health and illness and to the health care system; together, these components provide a more holistic approach to viewing women's lives and health. It is with this theoretical framework that health care for immigrant and ethnic minority women can be elucidated and improved.

## BIBLIOGRAPHY

Abrams, W. B., & Berkow, R. (1990). *The Merck manual of geriatrics.* Rahway, NJ: Merck Sharp & Dohme Research Labs.

Anderson, J. M. (1991). Immigrant women speak of chronic illness: The social construction of the devalued self. *Journal of Advanced Nursing, 16,* 710–717.

Aroian, K. J. (2001). Immigrant women and their health. *Annual Review of Nursing Research, 19,* 179–226.

Aroian, K. J. (1990). A model of psychological adaptation to migration and resettlement. *Nursing Research, 39,* 5–10.

Blumer, H. (1969). *Symbolic interactionism: Perspective and method.* Englewood Cliffs, NJ: Prentice-Hall.

Coney, S. (1994). *The menopause industry: How the medical establishment exploits women.* Alameda, CA: Hunter House.

Davis, M. S., & Youngkin, E. Q. (1995). Health and development through life cycle. In E. Q. Youngkin & M. S. Davis (Eds.), *Women's health: A primary care clinical guide* (2nd ed.). Stamford, CT: Appleton & Lange.

Dubois, M. Y., & Burris, J. F. (1994). Inclusion of women in clinical research. *Academic Medicine, 69,* 693–694.

Ebong, R. D. (1997). Female circumcision and its health implications: A study of the urban local government area of Akwa Ibom Stae, Nigeria. *Journal of the Royal Society of Health, 117*(2), 95–99.

El Sayed, Y. A. (1986). *The successive-unsettled transitions of migration and their impact on postpartum concerns of Arab immigrant women.* Unpublished doctoral dissertation, University of San Francisco, California.

Gannon, L., & Ekstrom, B. (1993). Attitudes toward menopause: The influence of sociocultural paradigms. *Psychology of Women Quarterly, 17,* 275–288.

Hall, E., & Allen, M. (1995). The challenge of reform. *Nursing Outlook, 43*(1), 42.

Hall, J. M., Stevens, P. E., & Meleis, A. I. (1994). Marginalization: A guiding concept for valuing diversity in nursing knowledge development. *Advances in Nursing Science, 16*(4), 23–41.

Harris, R., & Weissfeld, L. (1991). Gender differences in the reliability of reporting symptoms of angina pectoris. *Journal of Clinical Epidemiology, 44,* 1071–1107.

Hattar-Pollara, M., & Meleis, A. I. (1995a). Stress of immigration and the daily lived experiences of Jordanian immigrant women in the United States. *Western Journal of Nursing Research, 17,* 521–538.

Hattar-Pollara, M., & Meleis, A. I. (1995b). Parenting their adolescents: The experiences of Jordanian immigrant women in California. *Health Care for Women International, 16,* 195–211.

Lipson, J. G. (1992). Iranian immigrants: Health and adjustment. *Western Journal of Nursing Research, 14,* 10–29.

Lock, M. (1994). Menopause in cultural context. *Experimental Gerontology, 29,* 307–317.

Meleis, A. I. (1991) Between two cultures: Identity, roles, and health. *Health Care for Women International, 12,* 365–378.

Meleis, A. I., & Bernal, P. (1996). The paradoxical world of daily domestic workers in Cali, Colombia. *Human Organization, 55,* 393–400.

Meleis, A. I., Douglas, M. K., Eribes, C., Shih, F., & Messias, D. K. (1996). Employed Mexican women as mothers and partners: Valued, empowered, and overloaded. *Journal of Advanced Nursing, 23,* 82–90.

Meleis, A. I., Lipson, J. G., Muecke, M., & Smith, G. (1998). *Immigrant women and their health: An olive paper.* Indianapolis, IN: Center for Nursing Press, Sigma Theta Tau.

Mirdal, G.M. (1984). Stress and distress in migration: Problems and resources of Turkish women in Denmark. *International Migration Review, 18,* 984–1003.

Muecke, M. (1987). Resettled refugees' reconstruction of identity: Lao in Seattle. *Urban Anthropology and Studies of Cultural Systems and World Economic Development, 16,* 273–289.

O'Toole, M. (1989). Gender differences in the cardiovascular response to exercise. In P. Douglas (Ed.), *Heart disease in women* (pp.17–33). Philadelphia: F. A. Davis.

Rossner, S. V. (1994). *Women's health—Missing from US medicine.* Bloomington: Indiana University Press.

Ruzek, S. B., Olesen, V. L., & Clarke, A. E. (1997). *Women's health: Complexities and differences.* Columbus, OH: Ohio State University Press.

Schumacher, K. L., & Meleis, A. I. (1994). Transitions: A central concept in nursing. *The Journal of Nursing Scholarship, 26*(2), 119–127.

Turner, R. H. (1978). The role and the person. *American Journal of Sociology, 84,* 1–22.

Weisman, C. S. (1998). *Women's health care: Activist traditions and institutional change.* Baltimore: The Johns Hopkins University Press.

Wenger, N. K., Speroff, L., & Packard, B. (1993). Cardiovascular health and disease in women. *New England Journal of Medicine, 324,* 247–256.

Wright, J. (1996). Female genital mutilation: An overview. *Journal of Advanced Nursing, 24*(2), 251–259.

# CHAPTER 2

# African Americans

## PATRICIA F. ST. HILL, PhD, MPH, RN

### 🌐 INTRODUCTION

#### Who are the African-American People?

African Americans (AAs) are not a monolithic group. There are various subcultures within this population, and people may be differentiated on the basis of geographic location, educational level, and socioeconomic status. In terms of appearance, AAs are tremendously diverse, displaying many different skin tones, facial features, and hair textures. The varying physical characteristics observed within the population can be traced back to the early history of the AA people, who were involuntary migrants brought as slaves to the Unites States from Africa. They were sold as beasts of burden to work on Southern plantations, and many illicit liaisons occurred between the slave masters and their black female slaves. All AAs speak English, however, an unofficial second language, generally referred to as Ebonics or Black English, is also spoken within AA communities. Some AAs and some AA communities speak this dialect more frequently than Standard English. Although there is a tendency to associate the use of a dialect with lower educational attainment, care should be taken to avoid this type of stereotyping because within AA culture, one's use of a dialect to communicate with one's peers is often an expression of kinship or camaraderie rather than evidence of a lack of education. Although AAs ascribe to a variety of religious belief systems, the Baptist religion, with its roots deeply embedded in the South, appears to be the most predominant religion.

#### African Americans in North America

As a distinct minority population in North America, the AA people have, over the years, been identified by several terms. Historically, the terms were colored, Negro, black, Afro-Americans, black Americans and, more recently, African Americans.

**ACKNOWLEDGMENT**
Constance Smith Hendricks, PhD, RN and Ruth Johnson, EdD, RN, were consultants on this chapter.

African Americans represent the largest minority population in the United States. Census 2000 reports place the number of AAs in the United States at 36.4 million or 12.9 % of the total U.S. population (U.S. Census Bureau 2001). These figures, in accordance with census data for the period 1990–2000, represent substantial growth in the AA population for that decade—an estimated growth of 4.7 million or 15.6% in the total AA population. Compared with a total U.S. population growth of 248.7 million in 1990 to 281.4 million in 2000, the AA population growth for that decade was greater than that of the general U.S. population. The "ethnic origins" portion of the 1996 Canadian Census lists 233,455 people of African origin and 47,340 blacks.

The Civil War and World War II caused the migration of many AAs from the southern rural areas, where they had historically been enslaved and worked as sharecroppers and unskilled laborers, to northern urban areas such as Chicago, New York City, and Detroit. The reasons for this migration included a search for equality, better living conditions, and better occupational opportunities for themselves and their children.

Most AAs, according to recent census figures, still live in the South (54%), followed by the Northeast (19%), Midwest (19%), and West (8%). The states with the largest AA populations are New York, California, Texas, Florida, and Georgia. The District of Columbia leads all states with the largest percentage of AAs in its population (81%). Other states having large percentages of AAs are Mississippi (37%), Louisiana (32%), South Carolina (30%), and Georgia (29%).

In Canada, people of African or black origin live mainly in Toronto, Montreal, and Vancouver.

## BEING FEMALE IN AFRICAN AMERICAN SOCIETY

Historically, AA women have largely been single parents and heads of households charged with the care of small children. As such, the role of these women has and continues to be one of leadership and strength within the family. Data from the U.S. Commerce Department Census Bureau indicate that out of the 8.4 million AA families in the United States during 1999, 45% were maintained by women with no spouse present. This matriarchal family arrangement can be traced back to the days of slavery, when the males were sold off to other plantations, leaving the females behind to care for their families and the families of the "master." Later, the matriarchal family system was further promoted with the implementation of the welfare system, which forbids males to live in the home if the family is to remain eligible for welfare benefits.

## At Birth

### Preference for Sons

In AA culture, although sons are perceived as a means of keeping the family's bloodline going by passing on the family's last name, all children, regardless of gender, are accepted and viewed as a special blessing or gift from God. It is not unusual, however, for a family to try again and again for a son. Failure to give birth to a male child does not necessarily mean that the husband or male partner will abandon the woman, but it does lead to an increased risk of multiple unspaced pregnancies. As the education level of the parents increases, the need to "continue trying until a son is produced" appears to decrease.

### Birth Rituals

Birth rituals in the AA culture vary based on region and religious affiliation. Baptism of the infant into the religion of his or her parents is customary with some religious groups, while other religious groups refer to this process as dedication of the infant. Male circumcision is routinely practiced, as is true in the majority population.

## Childhood and Youth

### Stages

Childhood developmental stages in the AA culture are fairly consistent with those of the dominant culture. The period between birth and age two is considered the infancy stage. By ages 10 to 12, the child is perceived as a youth or pre-teen. At this stage sex role differentiation becomes very evident. The young girl is expected to assist with the care of younger siblings and carry out domestic chores, while the young boy is typically assigned the task of taking out the trash, cleaning the yard, and feeding and walking the family's dog. By ages 13 through 18, these youngsters are recognized as young adults. As such, they are expected to assume even greater responsibilities within the family unit. However, as young adults they are afforded much greater freedoms, including staying out later with their friends and dating. Sexual activity and childbearing at this developmental stage is still strongly discouraged.

### Family Expectations

Children are expected to respect their parents and older members of the community. This is especially true in the close-knit communities of the deep South, where most members of the community know the children and their parents.

In most families, especially middle-class ones, the expectations are that children will have more opportunities to create a better and more financially secure life for themselves than did their parents. Also, most AA parents see it as their responsibility to give their children "what they never had." Many will work two or more jobs and sacrifice financially to be able to move to a "better" section of town, remove their children from high-crime areas and gangs, and into better school systems.

### Social Expectations

Prevailing expectations for male and female children do not vary significantly. The hope is that all children will grow up to become responsible and productive adults capable of contributing positively to the community. Given the large number of AAs making up the prison population, it is an ongoing challenge for most single and inner city parents to keep their children on the right path.

### Importance of Education

Over the years, AAs have become increasingly aware of the importance of advanced education and training if one is to be successful. For many AA youngsters, however, the cost of a higher education is beyond the financial capability of their families. As a result, most (both boys and girls) are forced to compete for sport scholarships to the university or college of their choice. The number of young AA women going on to college continues, nonetheless, to surpass that of their male counterparts. Statistical data from the U.S. Census Bureau showed that as of 1999 black women were more likely than black men to have completed at least a bachelor's degree (16.4% versus 14.2%, respectively).

# Pubescence

## Psychosexual Development

Most AA females achieve menarche between the ages of 10 and 12. Males, on the other hand, tend to experience initial pubescence, evidenced by deepening of their voice, between the ages of 13 and 15. For many parents, this developmental stage is marked by heightened conflict with the young girl whose physical maturity often precedes her emotional maturity. Her sudden interest in boys and attempts to draw attention to her developing body by wearing tight and revealing clothing is often unsettling to many parents.

## Rituals and Rites of Passage

In African-American society no prevailing rituals or rites of passage are recognized at this developmental stage in a child's life.

## Teen Sexuality

**Social Restrictions and Pressures.**  Although national data indicate that teenagers in the United States are engaging in sexual activity at an earlier age and in larger numbers, teen sex is generally not condoned in the AA community. At the same time, it is not a common practice for AA mothers to discuss "the birds and the bees" with their teenage daughters. Much of what the young girls learn about sex, including the importance of practicing safe sex, is from their friends or sex education classes at school, if such classes are offered. Homosexual teens face far greater conflicts and pressures from their peer group and family members as they begin to demonstrate their sexual preferences

**Teen Pregnancy.**  African-American teenagers demonstrate higher rates of pregnancy and out-of-wedlock births than do their white and Hispanic peers, according to census data. Most mothers, however, dread the prospect of their teen daughters becoming pregnant. At the same time, it is often a financial necessity for many single AA mothers to work a second job, leaving their teen daughters at home and unsupervised for long periods, potentially increasing the prospects of sexual involvement and pregnancy. In the event a pregnancy occurs, it is customary in many families for the girl's mother or an older relative to raise the child, permitting the girl to finish school.

Typically, a family's socioeconomic status and/ or religious beliefs dictate its acceptance of single motherhood or a teenage daughter's decision to live with a man outside of marriage. Middle-class families, in which the parents have themselves achieved a better education and a higher standard of living, generally place greater pressures on their daughters to attend college and postpone childbearing.

Menstruation

**Relationship to Health.** The menstruating woman is not perceived as being ill; nonetheless, during the menstrual period, AA women often will refrain from washing their hair, taking baths, or exposing themselves to the cold ambient temperature. Many women will attempt to keep themselves warm by drinking warm teas and wearing extra clothing, including socks or sweaters around the house and to bed. It is also not uncommon for some women to avoid strenuous activity at this time, fearing excessive bleeding. No social restrictions are placed on the menstruating woman's activities but most refrain from sexual intercourse while bleeding.

**Relationship to Fertility.** Regular menstrual cycles and menstrual flows are perceived as demonstrable signs of a woman's health and fertility. Although the infertile woman is generally not ostracized nor abandoned in this culture, having a baby or babies is nonetheless the woman's perceived responsibility to her husband or partner. Several menopause studies note that at the cessation of the menstrual cycle, several AA women interviewed spoke about their inability to have more babies as a loss.

**Dysmenorrhea.** Dysmenorrhea, experienced by many AA women, is viewed as more of a monthly annoyance rather than a health threat. Most often it is treated with hot herbal teas and soups, but some women may also apply an electric heating pad or hot water bottle to the abdomen in an attempt to ease the cramping. In this culture it is also acceptable practice for a woman to take the day off from school or work and stay in bed if the bleeding (menstrual flow) and cramping are substantial.. If severe cramping persists over time most women will seek medical attention.

## Female Modesty and Touching

The concepts of self-respect and of respecting one's body are themes that deeply permeate the AA people's belief system. Accordingly, women are expected to wear appropriately fitting clothing, not "too tight" or "too short." Women who fail to observe this norm will often be perceived as "loose" or "Hoochie Mammas," seeking inappropriate sexual attention from men. Furthermore, AA culture does not endorse the public display of affection by couples or the touching or embracing of women by men other than their spouses/partners or close relatives.

**Relationship to Health Care.** There are no restrictions or observed taboos against AA women being treated or examined by male practitioners. If there is a choice, however, most AA women will prefer to be treated by a female practitioner, especially if the examinations and tests require exposure of their "private parts." African American women, especially older ones, also shy away from annual pelvic examinations and Papanicolaou smears (Pap smears) and mammograms. In the clinical setting, practitioners can expect to encounter a few AA women in their 30s and 40s who have never had a mammogram or pelvic examination outside of labor and delivery.

---

**NOTE TO THE HEALTH CARE PROVIDER**

Be tolerant and nonjudgmental of women who fail to obtain routine gynecological check-ups. Explain the benefits of early diagnosis and treatment of diseases, especially cancer. African Americans are at a much greater risk of dying from cancer than are Caucasians because of late diagnosis and treatment of the disease. Also, the practitioner needs to be extremely careful about preserving the young woman's privacy during the course of the physical or gynecological examination.

---

# Adulthood

### Transition Rites and Rituals

There are no culturally recognized rites or rituals to mark a young woman's transition into adulthood. Although the dominant society considers young women to be adults at the age of majority (18 or 21, depending on the state), in AA society a young woman is generally considered an adult when she marries, moves out of the house, or is financially capable of providing for herself.

### Social Expectations

Consistent with the many recent and rapid changes to the norms and values long observed in this culture, AA girls, especially those of the upper and middle classes, face increasing family and social pressure to complete high school, go on to college, and seek out successful careers. The same is not true, however, for girls from poor neighborhoods and inner-city areas, where day- to-day survival is paramount. For these girls, there is far less family and social pressure to excel in academics. Being successful, for them, has more to do with staying out of trouble and avoiding early motherhood.

### Union Formation

**Union Types.**   Monogamous marriage unions are the prevailing norm. It is not unusual, however, to find large numbers of single or never-married mothers among the poor. As of 1999, U.S. Census reports indicate that fewer black families were married-couple families than was true of other cultures. According to these reports, less than one-half (47%) of all black families were married-couple families in 1999, and 45% of black families were maintained by women with no spouse present.

**Social Sanctions for Failing to Enter into Union.**   Marriage and the family are very important in AA culture. With few exceptions, young women by their late 20s are expected to be married and have started a family. Women who fail to enter into union, although not publicly ridiculed, often feel pressured to meet these social expectations and may feel "out of place" around their married peers.

Traditionally, AA women looked primarily within the church community when seeking out a compatible mate. Today, this is not as true. Women now have a variety of places, including the work place, in which to seek out that special someone. In the majority population, the internet/computer dating and dating services has enjoyed growing popularity in recent years; however, these are not attractive options for most AA women contemplating a serious, long-term relationship.

### Domestic Violence

African-American women are reportedly victims of deadly violence from family members at rates decidedly higher than those from other racial groups in the United States. Because of the failure of many battered victims to report this crime to the authorities or seek help, the precise number of AA households affected by this epidemic of violence remains unknown. Figures from the Justice Department's 1994 National Crime Victimization Survey indicates that only about one-half of the women who were victims of domestic violence between 1987 and 1991 reported the abuse to law enforcement authorities.

The stigma, shame, and self-blame often associated with domestic violence cause many women to "suffer in silence." Additionally, for AA women, the lack of viable options forces many to remain in a battering relationship. Notably, most AA women have lower income levels than white women; at the same time, they also tend to have more dependent children. These economic constraints force many to remain in battering relationships, despite the abuse. Additionally, available community support systems, including shelters, safe houses, and other service programs are often viewed by AA women as programs designed for white women, unable to understand or meet their special needs.

---

**NOTE TO THE HEALTH CARE PROVIDER**

Because of the AA woman's reluctance to report domestic violence, providers need to be particularly vigilant in screening for signs of battering, especially in emergency room settings. Assist and support the woman with her immediate needs for security, and make the appropriate referrals.

---

### Rape

Most AAs think of rape and sexual abuse of young children as white crimes. The reality is that these unspeakable crimes exist within the AA community as well. Because of the stigma and shame frequently surrounding these acts of sexual violence, few outside the home ever hear about their occurrence. And if the rape results in a pregnancy, the decision to terminate the pregnancy becomes a family secret that remains strictly within the family.

### Divorce

**Sociocultural Views.** The divorce rate for AA couples is decidedly high despite the traditional cultural view of marriage as being for "keeps," and the religious advocacy of the notion of "till death do us part." Some reports claim that as many as two out of three AA marriages end in divorce and that 60% of AA children live with only one parent. The high incidence of divorce and parental estrangement afflicting this community may be directly linked to the pervasive poverty, unemployment and underemployment, as well as the illicit use of drugs and alcohol found in many spheres of the AA community.

**Women and Divorce.** Divorce, although not stigmatized in the AA community, is often quite devastating to the divorced woman. First, if she is closely associated with the church she may struggle with feelings of guilt and shame for having failed to keep her marriage vows, which she has made before God. Second, if she has small children from the failed marriage, she may have feelings of insecurity and self-doubts about her ability to make ends meet financially and still be an effective single parent. Third, finding a new spouse or male companion can also be a challenge, particularly if she is a middle-aged woman or a woman with minor children from the failed marriage.

**Child Custody Practices.** Upon the dissolution of a marriage or consensual union, it is customary for the children resulting from that union to live with their mothers. This arrangement accounts, in large part, for the high number of single-parent households headed by women found in the AA population. Following the divorce mothers and their children generally suffer economically more than fathers.

Although the law mandates child support payments, these monies are often very difficult for AA women to collect because of the high levels of incarceration, unemployment, underemployment and unwillingness on the part of some men to pay child support. Rather than being financially and emotionally available to their dependent children, many men simply move on and start new families when their marriages or consensual unions end, forcing their former partners to seek public assistance for the dependent children or to work two or even three jobs to meet the needs of the family.

---

**NOTE TO THE HEALTH CARE PROVIDER**

Since the economic impact of divorce is generally devastating to the single parent left to care for the minor children, providers must first consider making referrals to social service programs to address the family's immediate financial needs. Then consider job training programs to help the woman acquire or improve her job skills and earning potential.

---

### Fertility and Childbearing

**Family Size.** Historically, African Americans have maintained large households. In past years, especially in the deep South, it was not unusual for a woman to have 10 or more children, many of whom were needed to assist the family with picking cotton and working on the plantations and farms. Today, although there is no need for that type of child labor, AA family size remains large relative to other groups, although smaller than in the past. As of 1999, AA married-couple families were more likely than their non-Hispanic white counterparts to have five or more members, according to the U.S. Census Bureau.

**Contraceptive Practices.** African American women, although not bound by any social or religious mandates prohibiting contraceptive use, lag behind other ethnic groups when it comes to the acceptance and use of a reliable form of modern contraception. Sexually active adolescent girls are reportedly the least likely users of contraception and are the ones most likely to have multiple sex partners. This risky behavior may, in part, explain the high incidence of sexually transmitted diseases (STDs), adolescent pregnancy, and the large number of AA households headed by single or never-married mothers.

---

**NOTE TO THE HEALTH CARE PROVIDER**

Health care providers should take every opportunity to provide health education sessions that include information on contraceptive use, the various methods of modern contraception available, advantages and disadvantages associated with each method, and the importance of safe sex to protect against pregnancy and STDs, including human immunodeficiency virus (HIV).

---

**Role of the Male in the Couple's Fertility Decision-Making.** The use and choice of contraception generally is left up to the female. Many AA males dislike condoms and often avoid using them, believing that they decrease sensation and sexual pleasure. Given the high incidence of STDs reported in the AA community, however, health care professionals must emphasize the importance of condom use.

## Abortion

**Cultural Attitudes.**  Abortion is a topic few AAs openly and freely discuss, even with their health care provider. Given the choice of abortion or carrying a pregnancy to term and assuming the role of single parent, most AA women will choose the latter option. Religious influences plus the willingness of family members to assist with childcare may be influential in this decision making process.

**Teen Abortion.**  Pregnancy rates among AA teenagers are known to be extremely high; nonetheless, the extent to which teen abortions occur in the AA community is not well known. The veil of secrecy surrounding the abortion issue, plus issues of confidentiality, obscures these statistics.

---

**NOTE TO THE HEALTH CARE PROVIDER**
Given the high number of teenagers having early unprotected sex, multiple partners, multiple pregnancies, and increased risk for contracting STDs, providers must take every opportunity to educate both teenage boys and girls (with parental consent) about the spread of STDs and responsible sexual behavior.

---

### Miscarriage

Miscarriage or "loss of the pregnancy" is a source of considerable grief and suffering for the woman. Seldom are supernatural explanations given for the occurrence of a miscarriage; however, many "at risk" women rely heavily on prayer for favorable pregnancy outcomes and some women resist acquiring baby clothing prior to the delivery, fearing that something bad will happen to the baby. Because heavy lifting, stress, standing for long periods of time, and poor nutrition during pregnancy are thought capable of causing a woman to miscarry, most women, especially those with past histories of miscarriage, typically take the necessary precautions beginning early in the pregnancy.

---

**NOTE TO THE HEALTH CARE PROVIDER**
Be supportive and permit the woman and her partner (if involved in the pregnancy) to grieve their loss. Reassure the woman that miscarriages occur for a variety of reasons, some of which are unknown, hence she need not feel guilty or responsible for the pregnancy loss. The practitioner also needs to carefully assess the couples' need for grief and/or spiritual counseling and make the necessary referrals.

---

### Infertility

Childbearing is a very important aspect of the woman's role as a wife and member of the community. Given the importance ascribed to the roles of wife and mother in this community, the infertile woman risks not only "losing face" among her peers and in the community, but conceivably her marriage as well.

## Pregnancy

**Activity Restrictions and Taboos.** Both pregnancy and childbearing are highly valued in this culture. Accordingly, the pregnant woman is treated with a great deal of respect, and if the pregnancy is her first, she is likely to receive a great deal of unsolicited advice and information from female relatives, friends, and co-workers about what she is likely to experience as her pregnancy progresses. Advice against heavy lifting, bending, standing for long periods, reaching over her head, and exercising vigorously are typical. Pica, the craving /eating of non-food items such as chalk, clay, and dirt is common during pregnancy.

**Prenatal Care.** The importance of early and sustained prenatal care cannot be over-emphasized; nonetheless, far too often prenatal care is sought at later stages in the pregnancy and frequently not at all by pregnant teens who need it most because of their high risk status. Adherence to prenatal instructions and keeping follow-up prenatal appointments tend to vary with level of educational attainment and socioeconomic status. This is also a good time to begin teaching about breastfeeding and its benefits to the newborn.

## Birthing Process

**Home Versus Hospital Delivery.** Most deliveries occur in the hospital setting. Typically, the woman presents at the hospital during the later stages of labor, accompanied by relatives. Today it is common for the father of the baby (if involved with the pregnancy) to be present during labor and delivery, although he is not likely to be the one actively engaged in coaching and comforting the laboring woman. This task is typically left to her female relatives or close friends.

**Cesarean Section Versus Vaginal Delivery.** Vaginal deliveries are preferred, except in the event of an emergency or complications presenting a threat to the baby's well-being. Typically, cesarean delivery, with the potential complications and risks that accompany abdominal surgery, is viewed as serious and avoided as much as possible.

**Labor Management.**   During the early stages of labor, the laboring woman (with membranes intact) is encouraged take long walks to "help the baby down the birth canal." As labor contractions increase in intensity and frequency some women are likely to be vocal and express their pain.

As a group, AA women are receptive to the use of analgesics, including spinal blocks, for pain management.

**Placenta.**   The placenta holds no special cultural significance; medical staff may discard it unless the patient or family make a special request.

### Postpartum

During the recuperation period, which generally lasts from 7 to 10 days, the woman is encouraged to rest. Typically, a female relative (generally the maternal grandmother) will stay with the new mother to help care for the baby and permit the woman to regain her strength. During this period, the woman's nutritional intake is judged very important. Hence, she is fed nourishing soups and drinks. The use of herbal teas to help with the contraction of the uterus is also quite common. To further protect the health of the mother, exposure to cold air and drafts, which are believed to cause thickening and premature stoppage of the bloody discharge, is avoided.

### Newborn and Infant Care

**Breastfeeding Versus Bottle-Feeding.**   The convenience, economy, and health benefits associated with breastfeeding, including enhancement of mother-child bonding, makes breastfeeding a superior choice over bottle-feeding. Fewer and fewer AA women, however, are choosing to breastfeed. The number of women breastfeeding has and continues to shown steady declines over the past several years. Recent statistics from the Ross Formula Company shows that while still in the hospital only 41.3% of AA women attempted to breastfeed, and 6 months later a mere 14% were still breastfeeding. The increasing number of AA women who are single mothers and employed outside the home, with jobs requiring them to return to work shortly after delivery, may partly explain the noted declines in breastfeeding.

**Infant Protection.** Protecting the newborn from exposure to drafts and cold air is customary. During the first few days of life most parents avoid taking their infants outdoors unless it is absolutely necessary and then he/she is wrapped in several blankets to be kept warm. As further protection for their offspring, AA parents, with few exceptions, comply in meeting the immunization requirements for their infants and toddlers. By school age, most children have had the immunizations required for school enrollment. Major reasons for children falling behind with their scheduled shots is the lack of transportation to the clinic and clinic hours that are incompatible with the work schedule for mothers employed outside the home.

**Primary Caregiver.** Typically, mothers are the primary care providers for their children. Few fathers assume a major role in childcare, although this is changing as more women enter the work force on a fulltime basis.

## Middle Age

### Cultural Attitudes and Expectations

African American women are considered middle-aged between the ages of 40 and 55. By this time, their children are generally grown and have moved out of the home. For most women, this is seen as an ideal time to focus on self and to do the things that were impossible during the earlier childbearing and childrearing years, when caring for the children was a priority. At this stage it is not unusual to find many women returning to school to further their education or to acquire new job skills that will increase their salaries.

### Psychological Response

Most AA women respond to the middle years with a sense of relief and accomplishment, having completed both their childbearing and childrearing roles. It is not unusual to hear middle age women say, "It is now my time to do what I want to do." Ironically, however, more and more AA grandparents are, today, finding themselves charged with the responsibility of raising their grandchildren because of their adult children's inability to assume the parenting role. The "empty nest" phenomenon associated with midlife is, in actuality, a non-event for many AA women.

### Menopause

**Onset and Duration.** The onset of menopause for most AA women occurs between their mid-40s to about age 52. With some women symptoms of menopause, especially hot flashes, have known to begin as early as their mid-30s. Genetic factors as well as nutritional and health status are heavily determinant factors as to the age of onset of menopause

**Sexual Activity.** Menopause physiologically represents the end of a woman's childbearing years; however, for many women in this culture, it also marks the beginning of another stage in their life. Sexual activity during the peri- and postmenopausal periods is fully accepted and very much the norm for AA women. With the threat of unwanted pregnancy gone, many women feel a new sense of freedom and the ability to express themselves sexually. To compensate for the typical menopausal discomforts of vaginal dryness, hot flashes, and lowered libido, herbal teas and vaginal lubricants are widely used. Far less frequently is hormone replacement therapy (HRT) used.

**Coping.** Menopause, viewed as a "natural" developmental stage in a woman's life, is generally well accepted and coped with by most AA women. The use of HRT, thought of as a "synthetic" drug used to treat a "natural" biological occurrence, is unacceptable to many. Fear of breast and uterine cancer associated with the use of HRT is another reason given for the limited and non-use of this drug. Lastly, a significant number of AA women still think of HRT as a "white women's drug," not intended for them. The use of herbal teas are, on the other hand, widely embraced.

Some of the teas most often used to control hot flashes are lemon and water and the Chinese herbal tea dong quai.

---

**NOTE TO THE HEALTH CARE PROVIDER**

Acknowledge the woman's ambivalence about HRT use. Also, provide factual information (including printed literature) regarding the risks and benefits associated with this drug. Allow client to discuss herbal treatments used, and advise about potential drug interaction with prescription medication.

---

# Old Age

## Cultural Attitudes

Over the past few decades the life expectancy for all North Americans, including AAs, has steadily increased. Life expectancy rates for AAs, however, continue to lag behind those in whites. As of 1999, the Department of Health and Human Services showed the life expectancy rate for white females is 79.9 years, compared to 75.0 for AA females. The elderly are highly respected in the AA culture and abuse or neglect of the elderly is judged harshly. In the past it was customary for families to care for their elderly relatives. This trend is changing. Because of increasing economic pressures to work outside the home, more adult children are finding it necessary to place their aging parents in extended care facilities, board and care assisted living, or nursing homes.

# Death and Dying

## Cultural Attitudes and Beliefs

As a deeply spiritual people, death, especially of the elderly or a terminally ill person, is fairly well accepted and thought of as "God's will" for that person. It is not unusual to hear the death of an individual referred to as "God having called that person home" or that the individual is "gone to be with the Lord." Another component of

Christianity or the Christian belief system, adhered to by most AAs, is the faith and belief that the deceased person is on his or her way to heaven to be rewarded for the good works done on earth. Even though there is sadness, there is the expressed hope and an understanding that the ways of the Lord are simply not questioned. Death, from this perspective, is not the end of life. Rather, death is viewed as the beginning, a beginning where there is only joy for the many faithful who are reunited with the Lord.

### Rites and Rituals

The funeral service provides both an occasion for family members and friends to gather together to "pay their last respects to the deceased" and a forum for sharing grief. Before and after the funeral service, female relatives and friends serve to those in attendance the large quantities of traditional ethnic and soul foods prepared for the occasion. At this gathering it is not uncommon for the guests to tell anecdotal stories laced with humor about the deceased person's life. The gathering also serves as a time for crying and expressing sadness, as well as for updating everyone on what has occurred in the family since the last gathering.

### Mourning

Despite the AA community's seeming acceptance of death, grief is a normal reaction to the loss. It is culturally acceptable for family members and close friends of the deceased to openly express their grief by crying out loudly during the wake or funeral service. At this time they will generally be embraced and comforted by mourners in their immediate vicinity.

Following the funeral, family members generally mourn the passing of the individual by wearing dark or black clothing and little makeup and by refraining from social gatherings, such as parties. There is no prescribed time frame for mourning, the belief being that each person grieves differently and will require a different timeframe for the healing process.

**Coping.** The support of family and friends, plus the spiritual hope and belief that the deceased person is in a "better place," provide much solace to the surviving spouse.

---

**NOTE TO THE HEALTH CARE PROVIDER**
Provide privacy for family members to grieve their loss. Since most AAs prefer burying the body intact, practitioners should be extremely tactful in any discussion of organ donations.

---

 IMPORTANT POINTS FOR PROVIDERS CARING FOR AFRICAN-AMERICAN WOMEN

## The Medical Intake

### Literacy and English Proficiency

Although literacy levels vary, clients are proficient in English and are capable, for the most part, of understanding simple explanations, devoid of medical terminology, concerning their medical condition and required tests. To reinforce medical instructions and information provided in the clinic setting, it may be prudent to provide clients (especially older adults) with educational materials written in simple, easy-to-understand language.

### Status of the Provider

Health care providers are generally recognized and respected for their medical expertise. Because of the history of past medical and research atrocities committed against AAs, however, health care providers are still often viewed suspiciously and are not trusted. Poor and less educated AAs receiving care in public clinics and hospital facilities feel particularly vulnerable to medical misconduct and experimentation. It is not unusual to hear these clients voice complaints about feeling disrespected or "talked down to" by health care providers of different ethnicities.

### Communicating Illness and Symptoms

Elderly AA women are more inclined to provide elaborate explanations regarding their medical histories, including signs and symptoms of current ailments, than are their younger counterparts. Asking direct, pertinent questions is more likely to yield the needed information. Practitioners should pose questions of a sensitive nature, such as those pertaining to the woman's sexual activity and sexually transmitted diseases, only after they have established a dialogue and rapport with the client.

---

**NOTE TO THE HEALTH CARE PROVIDER**
To effectively provide care for AA clients, it is important to first establish a trusting relationship. Doing so may require taking extra time to listen to their voiced concerns about their illness, providing clear explanations as to why certain questions were asked and why a certain course of treatment or medical procedure was decided on. Demonstrating concern for the client's needs and well being by setting follow-up appointments and referrals as indicated will also be effective.

---

## The Physical Examination

### Modesty and Touching

There are no cultural restraints against male providers caring for females. It is, however, important to maintain the female's privacy at all times. This includes limiting the number of medical and nursing students allowed to view procedures done on the client, especially if such procedures require the client's private parts to be exposed. Also, touching by persons not directly involved in providing patient care should be avoided; appropriate touching is that which is limited to medical treatment and care.

### Expressing Pain

Neither physical nor emotional pain is readily expressed by many AA woman. The belief that the black woman needs to be "strong," expressions of weakness, or the inability to cope are not viewed favorably. This belief system may be may be tie to the fact that AAs typically seek medical care at advanced stages in the disease process, resulting in poor health outcomes. Mental illness in women, particularly depression, often dismissed as a simple case of "the blues" is a typical example of the group's reluctance to express pain and seek appropriate care.

## Prescribing Medications

### Drug Interaction

African Americans often use over-the-counter medications, home remedies, and herbal teas to treat ailments they perceive to be minor. There is a real possibility of negative drug interactions if the patient continues to use home remedies concurrently with prescription drugs. It will be beneficial for the clinician to inquire about both prescription and non-prescription medications that the client may be taking.

### Medication Sharing

Medication sharing between friends and family members is very common, especially among the elderly and less-educated members of the AA community. Antibiotics and pain medications are among the medications most often shared.

### Compliance

Compliance with prescription medication, dose, frequency, and duration is a persistent problem. When signs and symptoms of the disease subside, clients tend to feel that they are cured and no longer need to complete the full course of medication or treatment. This occurs most commonly with the use of antibiotics. The importance of completing the full course of all prescription medications should be emphasized.

## Follow-up Appointments

A lack of transportation, lack of childcare, or the inability to take time off from work, cause many women to miss their follow-up clinic appointments. Scheduling clients for follow-up care in clinics closest to their homes, staggering clinic hours to include evening clinics that accommodate working women, and sending a reminder card in the mail or leaving a phone message the day before the appointment are likely to improve client compliance with follow-up appointments.

### Orientation to Time

Time orientation is largely a present orientation. Planning for future events, including follow-up medical appointments, often assumes a lower priority in the day-to-day struggle to meet immediate needs. Consequently, missing or arriving late for appointments is seldom viewed as a major infraction.

## Prevalent Diseases

A combination of genetic factors, dietary patterns, obesity, and sedentary lifestyles contribute to the high prevalence of heart disease, diabetes, cancer, and cerebrovascular disease (including stroke)—the four leading causes of death in AA women. The major health conditions affecting AA women include the following:

1. Hypertension/ high blood pressure prevalence is believed to be among the highest in the world. Compared with whites, AAs develop hypertension at an earlier age, are more prone to substantially elevated blood pressure, and receive treatment at later stages in the disease process, when major organs such as the kidneys, heart, and blood vessels are already affected.
2. Diabetes, attributed to lifestyle and lack of exercise, dietary patterns, obesity, and genetic predisposition, is 60% more common in AA women than in their white counterparts.
3. Lupus, an autoimmune disease in which the individual's immune system attacks "self," is twice as common in AA women as in white women.
4. HIV/AIDS is the leading cause of death for AA women aged 25 to 44.
5. Breast cancer contributes to high mortality rates in the AA community. Although the prevalence of breast cancer is higher among white women, disease outcomes and quality of life following surgery are far worse in the AA population because of later diagnosis and treatment.

## Health-Seeking Behaviors

Preventive testing and care are seldom sought. In the event of illness, clients generally enter the health care system at later stages in the disease process. This practice contributes in large part to the higher mortality rates reported for AAs. Likewise, this group's failure to incorporate health promotion activities, such as healthy food choices, an exercise regimen, and avoidance of cigarette smoking, further contribute to the high morbidity and mortality rates noted for AAs.

## ⊕ REFERENCES

Lipson, J.G., Dibble, S.L. & Minarik, P.A. (1996). *Culture & Nursing Care: A Pocket Guide.* San Francisco, CA: UCSF Press, pp 37–43.

Purnell, L.D., & Paulanka, B.J. (1998). *Transcultural Health Care: A Culturally Competent Approach.* Philadelphia, PA: F.A. Davis, pp 53–73.

Spector, R.(2000). *Cultural diversity in health & illness.* New Jersey: Prentice Hall Health.

U.S. Census Bureau. (1999). The black population in the United States (March, 1999). U.S. Department of Commerce Economics and Statistics Administration, Washington, D.C.

U.S. Census Bureau. (2001). Census Bureau Release Update on Country's African American Population., Washington, D.C.

# CHAPTER 3

# American Indians and Alaska Natives

## LILLIAN TOM-ORME, PhD, MPH, RN, FAAN

### INTRODUCTION

### Who are the American Indian and Alaska Native People?

American Indians and Alaska Natives (AI/AN) tribes have a government-to-government relationship with the U.S. government and prefer AI/AN to "Native American." The word "Aboriginal" is used in the Canadian Census to include different tribes in Canada, the largest number of people designating themselves as North American Indian. Although most examples in this chapter are of Navajo or Diné people, because of the author's membership in this tribal nation, lack of other tribal examples in no way means lack of importance, and some require approval for use of the name.

The AI/AN people are indigenous to North America. Although this chapter provides a broad overview of general AI/AN cultural beliefs and practices, readers are cautioned to be very careful not to generalize and stereotype this diverse and heterogeneous population, which is composed of more than 560 tribes and who speak at least 100 languages. One should ask about tribally specific beliefs and practices and also be aware of diversity based on educational level, socioeconomic status, place of residence, and acculturation to the dominant society. Many AI/AN people speak their own language exclusively, others have lost it, and some are conscientiously relearning their native languages.

For centuries, AI/AN tribes lived harmoniously within their environment, refining subsistence methods and unique cultural systems that worked for them. For example, the Ojibwa built summer bark homes close to rice lands and lived in teepees during winter and early spring; although the **Diné** (Navajo for "the People") usually lived in dirt-covered structures, they lived in arbors during the summer; and the Cherokee lived in mud huts in the winter. Coastal peoples fished, and northern Plains tribes hunted buffalo. The Great Lakes and other woodland tribes harvested rice and hunted. The O'odham and other desert people used natural rivers to develop sophisticated irrigation techniques.

As the U.S. colonial population grew and the need for resources increased, AI/AN often were removed to unfamiliar territories or were forced to exchange their lands for federal treaty rights that promised education, health care, employment, housing, and continued protection; many of these promises were broken. Since the early colonial period, treaties have recognized tribes as individual nations with unique constitutions and governments. Not until 1924, however, did the United States formally recognize American Indians as U.S. citizens. Congressional legislation and the Constitution have mandated AI/AN rights. Honoring Indian tribal sovereignty ensures that federal programs include direct consultation with tribes and increased self-government and self-determination.

## American Indians and Alaska Natives in North America

Today, AI/AN live in rural, reservation, or urban settings. According to the 2000 U.S. Census, 2,475,998 AI/AN people are in the United States, about 0.9% of the population. The largest numbers are in California, Oklahoma, and Arizona, but they are frequently excluded from national or state statistics. American Indians comprise 8% or more of the population in Alaska (15%), New Mexico (9.5%), and South Dakota (8.3%). As of the 1996 census, 1,101,955 people of Aboriginal heritage lived in Canada, the largest numbers in Winnipeg, Vancouver, and Edmonton.

AI/AN adapt to their environment, and some attempt to maintain traditional patterns of living. For example, the Southwest Diné herd sheep and maintain their traditional hogans. Some Northern Plains tribes manage buffalo herds for economic, spiritual, and cultural reasons. Many reservations lack electricity, running water, and sanitary systems. Recently, some tribes have used casino income for housing, schools, health centers, and college education. Although each tribe has unique traditions and legends, there are many similarities. Tribes and tribal communities greatly respect their ancestors and elders, who experienced hardship and fought for cultural integrity. Traditional lands are valued, and native people perceive themselves to be caretakers of "Mother Earth." They deeply respect traditional stories, songs, and dances that are perceived to be gifts from the Great Spirits passed on through generations through oral traditions, recordings, or writings.

AI/AN women comprise about 50% of the population. In general, AI/AN populations are younger than the national average, undereducated, and have a median income of under $20,000. The average life expectancy of AI/AN females is 74.7 years, in contrast to the national average of 78.9 years. Employment rates vary across AI/AN groups, but unemployment among women is 13.4%, more than twice the national average. Almost one-third of those residing in reservation states have incomes below the poverty level, ranging from 24% in Alaska to 50% in the Northern Plains.

---

**NOTE TO THE HEALTH CARE PROVIDER**

Young parents who migrate from reservations to urban areas for employment often have poor or no access to health care. They often do not realize that the Indian Health Service (HIS) may not be available to them once they leave the reservation. These families may live in the poorer sections of towns, with limited transportation. They also may suffer from loneliness, isolation, and depression, or may be easily targeted as crime victims. Particularly vulnerable are urban families that are female-headed or lack health coverage. It is important to help the family locate an Indian resource center to assist with social, cultural, and economic needs.

---

While differences exist among the various tribes, many groups are matrilineal, and grandmothers and mothers are at the center of many Indian societies. For example, the grandmother of the house may make the important family or health decisions, a new husband may move into the wife's family home, and property may be passed down along maternal lines. Tribal traditional stories and history help health providers understand the status and role of AI/AN women. Examples include respect and honor given the roles of the Onandaga clan mothers and faith keepers, the Lakota story of White Buffalo Girl, and the Diné Changing Woman.

## At Birth

All AI/AN peoples value and welcome children. Gender preference is not typical of most AI/AN societies. Traditional teachings always valued both sexes as both contributed equally to the life of the tribe or village.

### Response to the Birth of a Female

Today, AI/AN peoples continue to value female infants, as women play a major part in tribal worldview and mythology. Females represent fertility in both humankind and nature, and tribes value them for their future roles in childrearing, home-based subsistence, health matters, and caring; they also expect females to maintain the lifeways of the culture. Some groups regard the birth of twins, however, cautiously.

In the United States, the AI/AN infant mortality rate is 9.3 per 1000 live births compared with the national average of 7.6 per 1000. Several factors that may contribute to AI/AN infant mortality rates include later prenatal care, higher tobacco and alcohol use among pregnant women, poor nutrition, and congenital anomalies.

### Birth Rituals

Birth rituals vary with the tribe; for example, the father may follow some ritual avoidances from the birth process until the baby's umbilical cord falls off. Shortly before or after delivery, many tribes expect the father or another family member to prepare a cradleboard that functions as a carrier, provides comfort, and is thought to assist in shaping the baby's future. The cradleboard is blessed and carefully decorated with beads, feathers, or other items that represent all positive things bestowed on the baby. Some traditional families are reluctant for an infant to be born in the hospital, seeing the hospital as a place where people die. Perhaps because of the higher infant mortality, many tribes do not prepare a nursery or hold baby showers until after the child's birth.

## Childhood and Youth

### Stages

No known studies have described the social stages of AI/AN children and youth, but some tribes celebrate developmental milestones. Thirty days after the baby's birth, Hopis "introduce" the baby to the sun. A public naming ceremony in which the baby or child receives an Indian name integrates him or her into the larger community. Some, like the Diné, hold a "first laugh" celebration to welcome the baby's first responsiveness to others. These activities recognize the baby's maturation and becoming aware of surroundings, including recognizing family members. Parents, grandparents, or godparents may give the child moccasins, beadwork, baskets, jewelry, blankets, or other cultural objects. The Crow of Montana celebrate the baby's first walk.

Until they enter school, children have much freedom; this period is generally known as an age of innocence and exploration. Entering school definitely marks a new phase of life for AI/AN children because it is the child's first separation from the family.

---

**NOTE TO THE HEALTH CARE PROVIDER**

In making well-child assessments, providers should include culturally appropriate questions, such as tribe-specific growth and development questions, in addition to general questions about what age the baby is expected to teethe, to sit or walk, and to make eye contact. If parents are using a cradleboard, the practitioner should ask how frequently they allow the baby to stretch and have some freedom of movement. The provider also should ask whether the baby or child is properly restrained, just as he or she was restrained and kept safe in the cradleboard. A major concern is tooth loss from periodontal disease in young children because mothers tend to bottle feed soda or fruit drinks at an early age. Thus, asking specific questions about feeding and oral hygiene is very important.

---

### Family Expectations

Children are expected to respect their elders. Female roles are taught by role modeling and demonstration and through stories. For example, the Diné tell creation stories during the winter season; stories provide lessons to guide young women's values and conduct. Young girls are expected to learn their roles by participating in daily subsistence activities. Older children typically are taught responsibility for younger children and others, which is done by their assuming care of siblings.

Children are disciplined through storytelling or being allowed to learn from their mistakes. Spanking may be observed occasionally; however, those outside the AI/AN cultures may view AI/AN children as having a generous amount of freedom and minimal discipline.

### Social Expectations

Children learn that they are a part of nature and, as such, expected to respect their place within this larger environment. They are also expected to be responsible to the community and to seek help within the family.

### Importance of Education

Formal education is valued; however, mainstream education methods are commonly perceived as not matching the learning modes of native people. AI/AN students are taught to treat one another as equals who all belong to their tribe or society. To boast or compete is considered antisocial behavior and is admonished, which partially explains students' reluctance to be outspoken or dwell on academic excellence. Consequently, many AI/AN students leave school early, explaining that they have been "pushed out" rather than having "dropped out." In 1990, 65.3% percent of AI/AN were high school graduates or higher compared with 75.2% nationally. Only 9% percent of AI/AN have a bachelor's or higher degree compared with the national average of 20.3%.

## Pubescence

### Psychosexual Development

Onset of menses means that a girl has reached adulthood. AI youth, however, are encouraged to socially mature early; thus, social maturity may precede physical development. The onset of menses marks entrance into the world of womanhood.

---

**NOTE TO THE HEALTH CARE PROVIDER**

Parents do not always inform adolescent girls about changes associated with puberty; thus, some girls become alarmed about breast development, body hair, and their first menses. Some families leave this topic to the school, books, or others. Young girls may seem shy initially, but they usually open up once they have established familiarity and trust with outsiders, such as health professionals.

The suicide rate among AI/AN teens is high. Providers should ask mothers about how their adolescents are doing and ensure that adolescents who come in for health care have enough time to talk. Practitioners need to assure teen clients that they can talk about any issues of concern during this challenging period.

---

### Teen Sexuality

Teen sexual activities and relationships are accepted as a fact of life; however, different families handle them in various ways. Some families monitor their daughters very closely, while others tend to allow them greater freedom. Teens' freedom and activities vary by urban and rural living conditions, after-school supervision, socioeconomic status of the family, residence in housing developments, and accessibility to outside entertainment influences (which some describe as "ruining" children).

The teen pregnancy rate of AI/AN is among the highest of all ethnic groups; approximately 45% of AI/AN are younger than age 20 years when they give birth for the first time. Lack of birth control education and age-specific and culture-specific family planning, as well as cultural beliefs, may account for this trend.

Traditionally, young women were considered to be marriageable at 14 years of age, old enough to have children. Contemporary AI/AN women with more education tend to postpone pregnancy until later, when they are more economically secure or when they have achieved their educational goals.

### Menstruation

**Relationship to Health.**   Menstruation is definitely linked to fertility and health. Amenorrhea leads to a concern that a woman may not be fertile.

**Taboos and Restrictions During Menstruation.**   Dietary restrictions during menstruation include moderate use of salt, sugar, and fat in the diet, and women avoid laziness and sleeping too much. Women avoid sexual activity during this time. Women are taught to dispose of soiled clothes and toiletries properly.

**Dysmenorrhea.** Excessive blood loss and severe dysmenorrhea are considered unhealthy and require medical attention. Some women seek treatment from herbalists for cramps or discomfort; others seek help from traditional practitioners or biomedical providers.

### Female Modesty and Touching

Modesty norms vary by tribe or region as well as by education level. In general, older women are more modest than younger women. Many believe that the only person who is allowed to see or touch a nude woman is the woman's partner.

## Adulthood

### Transition Rites and Rituals

Tribes and communities that are matrilineal, matrilocal, or matriarchal hold elaborate celebrations to mark the transition to womanhood. For example, the Diné and Apache hold four-day celebrations to honor the young woman and her family through community recognition of the **Kinaalda,** during which all the good things representing womanhood are brought forth and celebrated. Attendees bestow good thoughts and teachings on the novitiate. They teach the young woman about her role as an adult and the creation story; they offer many songs and prayers to reinforce her role in the traditions and culture. Family and clan members offer support for the future.

### Social Expectations

Matrilineal or matriarchal groups expect women to carry on the clan lineage. Traditional teachings revolved around chastity and sexual loyalty, but as women become more acculturated to dominant American norms, these values are also changing. Women of childbearing age are expected to have the basic knowledge required to operate a household, mother, teach the young, and be a strong role model. Many native women are strong leaders within the family, village, clans, and community. Today, various external influences such as urban living and peer pressure pose challenges to the lives of both children and their parents. As a result, traditional childbearing practices are rapidly being modified and replaced.

### Union Formation

Unions are monogamous; however, they are not necessarily publicly sanctioned. Common-law unions may last for varying periods before they are legalized or dissolved. Very traditional people may continue to practice arranged marriage based on clan systems, while urban women may follow the practices of the dominant society as to variety and choice, including interracial and intertribal marriages.

While union is desired, single women are neither admonished nor pressured into seeking a mate. Today, many marriages are extremely brittle as a result of the ever-changing nature of society; thus, tribal societies are more understanding and tolerant of single women.

### Domestic Violence

Traditional practices strongly discourage domestic violence, seeing it as an obstacle to harmony among kin and clans. The recent increase in domestic violence must be viewed within the context of current societal conditions. Pressures on people to compete, support their families, and be independent, along with the loss of traditional extended family support, have broken down the well-defined roles of men and women and have negatively affected relationships. Middle-aged to older tribal members who, as children, were forced into boarding schools and severely punished for breaking school policies, describe domestic violence as "posttraumatic stress syndrome." Some explain that being removed from loving homes in early childhood and socialized to abandon their native traditions have made them unloving and incapable of passing on native values to their children and grandchildren. Others attribute loss of traditions and changing values to assimilation and acculturation influenced by the wage economy.

Culturally appropriate resources for victims of domestic violence are scarce. Abused women tend not to seek immediate help from authorities. No accurate statistics are found because programs and surveillance are poorly funded. Most tribes, however, are beginning to address the increase in domestic violence by seeking resources and holding community discussions. The Diné use the traditional peacemaking process to negotiate between the involved parties, with an authority providing consultation. This practice is based on the tradition that a union of two parties is really a union of two families, the joining of which requires talk; thus, disputes necessitate talk.

---

**NOTE TO THE HEALTH CARE PROVIDER**

Practitioners should include in women's health assessments a question or two about possible domestic violence. The client may not be vocal or welcome attention to this matter. If a provider suspects domestic violence, he or she should mention it and offer the client appropriate help, such as available community resources and referral to a counselor or traditional practitioner. Being discrete and providing support can help the client feel sufficiently comfortable to talk about abusive relationships. The client may want to keep the topic private because of fear of reprisal; thus, the practitioner must reassure the woman of protection and confidentiality.

---

### Rape

No accurate statistics about rape are available because of inconsistency in asking questions during assessments and health care program reporting. Women may not report rape because of shame and the stigma associated with this type of attack and its violation of human dignity. If someone else finds out, however, those who support the woman will encourage her to report it to proper officials.

### Divorce

Divorce has become more common. Divorced women with children may seek refuge with and support from family members; childless women may remain independent or seek support from friends. Women are especially apt to receive support in cases where they might have been abused. Stigmatization is not a major problem unless the community or family thinks the woman was "at fault" for causing a divorce from a respectable man. Nevertheless, divorce is difficult for women, and providers should always offer counseling.

Traditional marriages not only brought couples together but also served to unify families and the community. As more AI/AN people adopt marriage practices of the dominant culture, relationships have become more vulnerable to divorce. And as domestic violence increases, children may be removed under the provisions of the Indian Child Welfare Act from families who cannot provide appropriate care. Relatives or another AI/AN family may adopt these children; a non-Indian family adopts such children only as a last resort.

## Fertility and Childbearing

**Family Size.** The AI/AN birth rate is reportedly 24.1 per 1000, in contrast to the U.S. national average of 14.8 per 1000. AI/AN value and have more children than many other groups. Traditional families preferred larger family units for purposes of distribution of labor. For example, Diné children assisted adults on farms and with sheep-herding tasks. As traditional lifestyles are less practiced, the need for large family units has lessened, and families are smaller, typically two to four children.

**Contraceptive Practices.** Family planning rates and practices vary widely across AI/AN populations. Women in Alaska make the highest number of clinic visits, while those in California make the fewest (781 vs. 338 visits per 1000 women aged 15 to 45 years). Family planning clinics are available in many communities today. Although it is an individual choice, women who have completed their families tend to favor tubal ligation as the most convenient method of birth control. Depo-Provera is popular among younger women. Women use intrauterine devices infrequently because of a high rate of associated infections.

---

**NOTE TO THE HEALTH CARE PROVIDER**
Counseling and stressing regular appointments for women who are using Depo-Provera is very important because regular injections are required. The provider must advise the woman not to miss appointments. If the woman must miss an appointment, she should be encouraged to use an additional means of contraception.

---

**Role of the Male Partner in the Couple's Fertility Decision-Making.** Both partners tend to discuss and make decisions about the method when they decide to use contraception. In many cases, particularly among young couples, there is no discussion about contraception, resulting in an above-average rate of out-of-wedlock births.

## Abortion

**Cultural Attitudes.** In their early history, some tribes might have practiced infanticide in cases of illness or congenital malformations. As in the general North American societies, abortion has its proponents and opponents among AI/AN, although it is not a topic for public discussion. Rather, it is a private matter that is decided by the immediate family and through legal means in the case of incest or rape. No tribe practices abortion for population control. A woman who attends a Christian church may believe that abortion is a sin.

**Sources of Abortions.** Given the high birth rate among AI/AN, abortion is obviously not the norm. Those seeking abortions use professional rather than lay services. Since the U.S. Indian Health Service does not cover abortions, women use services in towns and cities and pay for them out of their own pockets.

**Teen Abortion.** Statistics on teen abortion are not available, and federal family planning programs that teens use do not cover abortions. Teens who seek abortions may, depending on family values, use private family resources. Those without such access or who do not qualify for any available resources often are left on their own. A young woman who might still be in high school and in no position to afford or care for children might decide to get an abortion; she makes this decision jointly with her boyfriend, parents, or both.

---

**NOTE TO THE HEALTH CARE PROVIDER**
Providers should discuss current information with teens and parents who inquire about abortion and its possible complications so that they can make a well-informed decision. They need to always emphasize confidentiality since abortion is a very private matter.

---

## Miscarriage

AI/AN people desire and cherish children; thus, they avoid miscarriages at all cost. More traditional families may attribute a miscarriage to a parental taboo violation or excessive physical activity. Some tribes teach parents to avoid contact with death, such as attending funerals or seeing dead animals, or to correct "bad" dreams by taking part in various ceremonies.

Miscarriages or congenital malformations may be attributed to alcohol use. Pregnant women are told not to abuse illicit drugs, but they may be prescribed a traditional medicine or ceremony to ensure a healthy baby.

## Infertility

Although American Indian populations prefer to increase their numbers, they recognize infertility as a fact of life. Some couples take herbs or have ceremonies performed in an effort to ensure a pregnancy whenever there might be a question of infertility. Although fertility is valued, infertility is also accepted. Women are not shunned or in any way mistreated if they are infertile. Many tribes, particularly matrilineal ones, believe that women are capable of mothering in spite of their infertility. The role of mother does not necessarily require having given birth because motherhood extends through kinship and clan relations, which are highly regarded. Other women may use modern methods to treat infertility.

## Pregnancy

Pregnancy is a special time, a sacred period endowed with many traditional rituals and taboos for the woman and her partner to observe. In particular, Diné believe that pregnancy is a very normal but special life phase, and all actions and thoughts should be as positive as possible. The health provider should ask the expectant family how closely they observe their native traditions and how the provider might support those beliefs and practices.

**Activity Restrictions and Taboos.** During pregnancy, women may be admonished to refrain from looking at dead animals, thinking negative thoughts, sleeping too much, being physically inactive, attending funerals, eating fatty or sweet foods, or using too much salt or sugar.

**Prenatal Care.**  Women tend to view pregnancy as a normal process that does not require early medical intervention. Compared with the 81% national rate of women beginning prenatal care in the first trimester, only about 66% of AI/AN women have their first appointment in the first trimester. This rate ranged from 53.5% of women from the Diné area to 77.4% of native women in Alaska. Women may not keep regular prenatal appointments because of problems with transportation, long waiting times, or employment, or as a result of diabetes or other health problems.

---

**NOTE TO THE HEALTH CARE PROVIDER**

AI/AN women have pregnancy risks related to diabetes, drinking, and smoking. Low birth weights are less a concern than high birth weights because of diabetes; approximately 45 per 1000 live births were to mothers with diabetes compared with 25 per 1000 in the general population. Drinking during pregnancy is three times more frequent than in the general population (4.5 vs. 1.5 per 1000), and fetal alcohol syndrome (FAS) has had devastating effects on an increasing number of families. The AI/AN smoking rate is 20.4% in contrast to 13.9% in the general population. Low birth-weight births associated with smoking occur in 29% of all AI/AN births. Diné women have the lowest rate of smoking, and women from Alaska and the Northern Plains reported the highest rates.

---

Birthing Process

**Home Versus Hospital Delivery.**  Childbirth practices vary among tribes. Childbirth now takes place in modern facilities, primarily in hospital settings and occasionally in childbirth centers. Home births are no longer common because of many years of teaching against home birth by health care practitioners. In the past, a birth attendant, medicine person, or both were called in to assist, and some people may request these attendants even in modern facilities.

**Cesarean Section Versus Vaginal Delivery.**  As in other populations, AI/AN women prefer vaginal delivery. They have a very high vaginal delivery rate as compared with other populations. Specifically, women from the Navajo nation and Alaska have the highest rate of vaginal deliveries.

**Labor Management.**  The male partner or a female family member (either mother or sister) may attend the delivery. Women are allowed to move in early labor. Couples who have participated in childbirth classes may use breathing techniques. In facilities staffed by certified nurse midwives, active breathing and other natural methods are strongly emphasized, and labor is closely monitored.

**Placenta.**  People in many tribes believe in preserving human body parts, including the placenta and umbilical cord. The placenta nourished and protected the fetus during pregnancy; therefore, it should not be disposed of without proper respect and burial. Some AI/AN have heard of human tissue being used by the cosmetic industry for profit, which is unthinkable to many. Others, however, no longer save and bury the placenta for practical reasons, especially if they live in a city. Instead, they may wish to save the umbilical cord. Practitioners should ask their preference for saving one or both. The Diné believe that the placenta and umbilical cord symbolically represent home; and if they are discarded, children will not know their ties to home and will have wandering and unsettled spirits.

## Postpartum

The time of mother-child bonding is typically the first month or so. The Ute and Hopi observe a fairly strict 30-day period for mother and baby to remain home. A single woman might observe a shorter "maternity leave" before she returns to work. Many traditional practices are increasingly being abandoned as more AI/AN women and their partners enter the workforce, a modern necessity that interferes with continuation of traditions. In many traditional societies a *doula* (mothering person) helped the new mother adjust to her new role and provided the needed attention and pampering of both mother and baby.

## Newborn and Infant Care

**Breastfeeding Versus Bottle-Feeding.**   Although breastfeeding has always been considered the natural method to feed babies, bottle-feeding came into vogue during the mid-1950s when AI/AN were told that exposing their breasts was "uncivilized." Now, health care practitioners are being challenged to increase breastfeeding among AI/AN once again. Women with more education tend to prefer breastfeeding, but bottle-feeding may be more convenient for most mothers who work outside the home.

**Infant Protection.**   Infants are perceived to be vulnerable to illness, cold temperatures, the wind, bad dreams, and excess activity. Methods of protecting them include wrapping them tightly in blankets on cradleboards; tying an amulet to their cradleboard, carrier, or clothing; or placing a juniper bracelet around their wrists to provide protection from nightmares. Parents may show off their babies to friends, family, and clan members.

**Primary Caregiver.**   Mothers are the primary caregivers of their infants and children. The traditional lifestyle had separate gender roles in which men had limited childcare responsibility because they did external chores. Now, men are becoming more engaged in childcare. In many settings, the extended family remains strong, and family members may participate in childcare. In nuclear families, however, it may not be practical to have this help.

## Middle Age

### Cultural Attitudes and Expectations

A woman is considered to have reached elder status when she becomes a grand-mother, reaches middle age (which may be in her mid-thirties), or experiences menopause. Middle-aged AI/AN women accept changes that come with the aging process more comfortably than do European-American women. Because AI/AN hold elders in esteem, many of them do not mind graying hair, increased wrinkling, reduced level of activity, or other age-related changes. Indeed, some people frown upon middle-aged women who intentionally "act young," especially when they have grandchildren.

### Psychological Response

The psychological response to the aging process may vary by tribe or individual. The most common difficulty is dealing with pain from arthritis or, if there is no obvious illness, abrupt changes in activity level.

### Menopause

Generally, the onset of menopause is observed quietly without the public recognition that is common at onset of menses. AI/AN do not anticipate menopause negatively or equate it with hot flashes and other adverse physiological changes. Women do, however, enjoy the cessation of monthly periods.

**Onset and Duration.**   Because menopause is seen as a natural occurrence and a new phase of life, it is not viewed as a disruption to the woman's normal life pattern. Most tribes do not celebrate menopause publicly, but menopausal women can now proudly consider themselves elders.

---

**NOTE TO THE HEALTH CARE PROVIDER**
Some AI/AN women may be unaware of their increased need for calcium, estrogen, and the like. Providers should explain such issues as osteoporosis to these women. They should encourage women to report any unfavorable physiological changes to a health care provider so that they do not suffer needlessly. They also should encourage them to see a traditional herbalist if they so desire.

---

**Sexual Activity.**   Sexual activity declines among menopausal AI/AN women although it does not cease completely. It is safer to ask rather than to make assumptions since women's sexuality patterns vary individually and by tribes. Health and disability may also be important factors as to whether a woman remains sexually active.

**Coping.**   AI/AN tend not to dread the onset of menopause or mourn the end of their fertility. They accept menopause quietly—it actually puts most women in an admired status. Those who may have difficulty coping with menopause are the more acculturated and more educated women.

## Old Age

Grandmothers, postmenopausal women, and gray-haired women are valued since they are considered to have attained the highly respected role of elder. Elders are respected for their years of life experience and revered for hardships they have endured throughout their lifetimes. They are also seen as possessing wisdom and are much sought to teach the young about AI/AN traditions. Indeed, elders may be relegated to the role of storyteller as they pass on cultural norms, lessons learned, moral obligations, and observation of taboos.

Although aging people are revered, changing tribal societies may not always protect elders from physical or psychological harm from relatives or the community. Elder abuse has been reported, although statistics are unreliable at this time. Disability, chronic conditions, and inability to perform activities of daily living may require institutionalization of elders. Many elders dread this situation and consider it to be the final sign that their contributions are ending and that their loved ones will abandon them to die alone. Most tribes do not operate their own long-term care facilities. Families who cannot care for elders may be forced to send them off the reservations or into unfamiliar towns.

## Death and Dying

The most frequent causes of death among AI/AN women are heart disease and malignant neoplasms. The rates of these conditions, however, are lower in AI/AN women than in the general U.S. population of women.

### Cultural Attitudes and Beliefs

Death is considered part of the circle of life. Dying alone far from home and in an unfamiliar environment, however, is considered the worst way to leave the earth. Some tribes, such as the Diné, may avoid the deceased or articles belonging to them for a certain time.

---

**NOTE TO THE HEALTH CARE PROVIDER**
Death rituals vary by tribe and level of acculturation. Providers should ask each family or tribe about their rituals. For example, they should always ask the family how to handle clothing and jewelry belonging to the deceased.

---

### Rites and Rituals

Death most frequently occurs in the hospital or a long-term care facility; many American Indians avoid home death. Some tribes believe that the spirit of the dead may linger longer than expected and cause illness or prolong the grief process. Grieving, burial, and behavioral practices vary by tribe, as do burial rituals. Examples of different burial rituals are wrapping the body in a simple white shroud, as practiced by some Pueblo people, or using brand-new and elaborate clothing, as practiced by the Diné and others.

### Mourning

After the death of a family member, some women cut their hair, others wear black paint for four days, and still others may remain home or not bathe for four days following the burial. Mourning is observed differently by region, tribe, and family. It may last one year or longer and is definitely longer than in European-North American populations. A traditional practitioner may be sought if mourning is considered to have gone on too long or begins to interfere with normal life functions.

## Coping

Coping also varies by individual, family, or tribe. Women who lose a child take it very hard, feeling as if they have lost a part of themselves. If death followed a prolonged terminal illness, a woman may cope by feeling that it is better that her loved one is no longer suffering and feeling physical pain. Members of organized religions, like Christianity, may take comfort in the belief that their loved one has gone to heaven. More traditional people may talk about the deceased having gone to the happy hunting grounds or joined other relatives, or that the Creator has reclaimed the person. The deceased's spirit may be thought to exist within an animal or bird or in the wind.

Women have great difficulty accepting the loss of parents. Often, women may have cared for old or ill parents prior to their death. Friends and family may be comforting, but in urban areas some women may feel alone when coping with their loss.

---

**NOTE TO THE HEALTH CARE PROVIDER**

Women may be reluctant to ask questions or offer information about themselves. Thus, providers must be perceptive and ask a woman whether she has mental health concerns, especially if the woman has experienced a recent loss. If the health care facility has access to traditional counselors, providers should offer women that choice.

---

## IMPORTANT POINTS FOR PROVIDERS CARING FOR AMERICAN INDIAN AND ALASKA NATIVE WOMEN

### The Medical Intake

Not all AI/AN women are eligible for health care coverage or insurance. The U.S. IHS covers only those enrolled in federally recognized tribes, those who live in an area with IHS services, or those referred by the IHS for specialized care or contract services. Trained intake personnel are expected to assist women who need it. A referral to a social worker may be necessary.

#### Literacy and English Proficiency

Older AI/AN who live on reservations or in rural communities may speak only their native tongue; even if they speak English, they may not read it. If the health provider does not speak the patient's language, he or she should make every effort to use a trained interpreter. Providers should never use children as interpreters as they may become privy to personal medical information about their elders. Moreover, this is a daunting task for a small child. They should ask if the woman prefers an interview or instructions in her native language.

---

**NOTE TO THE HEALTH CARE PROVIDER**

Practitioners should speak slowly and not use a hurried manner. They should speak *with* women rather than *to* them and encourage active involvement in their own care. Older women may consider direct eye contact aggressive or rude, but younger women may prefer it. Providers should accept and respect periods of silence as times of reflection, not disinterest.

---

### Status of the Provider

As most health care providers are outsiders, AI/AN typically view them with suspicion. Often, IHS health providers average two years tenure before they move on; as a result, many AI/AN describe them as being temporary and there just to "practice on us" before they move. To enhance trust, practitioners should convey acceptance and respect for women, including their physical appearance, beliefs, and practices. If health providers come to be trusted, their advice will ultimately be respected.

### Communicating Illness and Symptoms

When provider and patient differ in cultural background, a cultural translator is very important. The provider may need to use the third person to convey risk factors or a possible course of a condition, which may be interpreted as "wishing them" on people. For instance, rather than stating that "you might develop complications," it is preferable to say, "some people develop diabetes complications." The provider should take the time to learn the local language and engage in community activities to learn more about the clients' worldview. Sharing one's own culture with clients will also help earn their respect and acceptance.

---

**NOTE TO THE HEALTH CARE PROVIDER**
Storytelling may be a useful way to explain illness; it is an effective method for all age groups, but providers must make sure that they allow enough time. When doing health teaching, they should consider the following culturally appropriate methods: a talking circle for family or small group education where all have a chance to speak without interruption; a modified focus group approach; allowing elders to lead the discussion; or use of storytelling. Health providers who emphasize comprehensive and culturally competent care are likely to be more successful than those who do not.

---

## The Physical Examination

Women older than childbearing age believe that female examinations are no longer needed. They tend not to have annual examinations or Papanicolaou tests.

---

**NOTE TO THE HEALTH CARE PROVIDER**
Providers should not assume that all patients understand why certain procedures are performed (e.g., why a patient needs to undress for a podiatry examination). They need to explain what is to be done and why.

---

### Modesty and Touching

Older women prefer to be examined by female practitioners. In general, AI/AN people are modest and may not be comfortable being touched by providers, especially when they are of the opposite gender.

### Expressing Pain

It may be very difficult for some AI/AN to express pain when they believe that pain is part of their life experience. Although these women may have a higher pain tolerance than women in the general population, they are often more expressive than are the men. The provider should ask the patient to describe the pain and to point to the part of the body that hurts. Frequently patients will describe "hurting all over."

## Prescribing Medications

Providers need to explicitly explain medication actions, side effects, dosage, and frequency, particularly to elder patients. Some patients may require the help of a caretaker or calendar or instruction on how to prepare daily doses in a pill container to take medications as prescribed.

### Drug Interactions

Providers should always ask patients if they also take any traditional medicine or tea (e.g., camas, bitter root, juniper, and various berry teas) because of possible detrimental interactions.

### Medication Sharing

Family and relatives may share medications, particularly when patients do not have health insurance coverage and live on fixed incomes. Providers should ask patients about possible challenges, such as transportation or finances, that may encourage medication sharing.

### Compliance

Adherence issues are ever present, particularly when the patients and providers are from different backgrounds. Every effort should be made to use local people to serve as culture brokers to bridge communication problems. Providers cannot admonish or blame patients every time an adherence problem arises. Rather, they must inquire how best to improve communication to avoid such problems in the future.

## Follow-up Appointments

AI/AN keep appointments for the most part, particularly when these patients trust providers. Practitioners should provide positive feedback to patients who keep appointments and ask for their input in appointment-making, setting, and maintenance.

Most AI/AN are present-oriented and past-oriented, which can pose a challenge when, for example, teaching prevention to older women. They are future-oriented, however, with regard to making the present better for their valued children, grandchildren, and future generations. Accordingly, teaching the concept of being healthy now "to take care of and enjoy your grandchildren" often encourages older women to consider their own future health. Indian time is not hurried or oriented to watching the clock. Many believe that the clinic will be there later today or tomorrow and, thus, may not keep appointments. Others may have more pressing priorities at home or lack transportation to keep clinic appointments. It may help to advise clients to try to come at the designated time so that other clients can also be seen.

## Prevalent Diseases

The IHS reports that AI/AN populations, including women, have higher prevalence than national rates for the following conditions: alcoholism (627%), tuberculosis (533%), diabetes mellitus (249%), and accidents (204%). The rates are lower for suicide (72%) and homicide (63%). Risk factors for heart disease and cancer include the highest smoking rates of all ethnic women (31.4%), obesity (at least 22% of native women have a body mass index greater than or equal to 30), and physical inactivity (at least 40% are sedentary).

## Health-Seeking Behaviors

Cultural views of health and illness are holistic, and health is associated with balancing physical, mental, spiritual, and kinship realms. Harmony is associated with appropriate attention to health, growth, gender roles, family, and community dynamics. Disharmony exists when there is illness, disease, violence, stress, or family or community discontent. Illness is believed to relate more to how persons experience or interact with their surroundings than to a specific disease process.

To do health teaching and encourage healthy behaviors, the provider should use traditional health promotion concepts to promote physical activity, observations of taboos, and healthful practices. Culturally specific teaching-learning approaches include (1) the Medicine Wheel, Sacred Directions or local native philosophy, holism, caring, spiritualism, and humor; (2) a talking circle for family or small group education where all have a chance to speak without interruption; (3) allowing elders to lead discussions; and (4) using storytelling. Patients should be told that they have the right to request a traditional practitioner.

## 🌐 BIBLIOGRAPHY

Denny, C. H., & Holtzman, D. (1999). *Health behaviors of American Indians and Alaska Natives: Findings from the Behavioral Risk Factors Surveillance System*, 1993–1996. Centers for Disease Control and Prevention, Behavioral Surveillance Branch. Atlanta, GA.

Indian Health Service, 1998–1999. *Regional differences in Indian health*, 1998–99. U.S. Department of Health and Human Services. Rockville, MD.

Strickland, C. J., Squeoch, M. D., & Chrisman, N. J. (1999). Health promotion in cervical cancer prevention among Yakama Indian women of the Wa-Shat Longhouse. *Journal of Transcultural Nursing*, 19(3), 190–196.

Tom-Orme, L. (2000). Native Americans explaining illness: Storytelling as illness experience. In B. Wholly (Ed.), *Explaining illness: Research, theory, and strategies*. Yahweh, NJ: Lawrence Album Associates, Inc., pp 237–257.

Wilson. U. M. (1983). Nursing care of American Indian patients. In M. S. Orque, B. Bloch, & L. S. Monrroy (Eds.), *Ethnic nursing care*. St. Louis: C.V. Mosby, pp 271–295.

# CHAPTER 4

# Arab Americans

## MARIANNE HATTAR-POLLARA, DNSC, RN, FAAN

### INTRODUCTION

### Who are the Arab-American People?

Arab-Americans originated from any of 21 independent Arab states (Algeria, Bahrain, Egypt, Iraq, Jordan, Kuwait, Lebanon, Libya, Mauritania, Morocco, Oman, Qatar, Saudi Arabia, Somalia, Sudan, Syria, Tunisia, the United Arab Emirates, Yemen, and the Palestinian Authority). Three factors unify the Arab world under a common Arabic identity: (1) Semitic ancestry, (2) a common history, and (3) the Arabic language. English is spoken in most Arab countries, but French is spoken in Algeria, Lebanon, Morocco, and Tunisia.

Past and present political discourse in the Middle East affects ethnic identity. Arabs in North America may identify themselves as Middle Easterners, by their country of origin, or by their town or village. Ethnic minority groups (e.g., Armenians, Chaldeans, Assyrians) maintain their own ethnic identities but also self-identify as immigrants from the Arab Middle East.

Despite the common use of Arabic, different countries and regions have different accents and dialects. Generally, people can communicate if they clarify some words; for example, "how are you" is **Eziak** (Egyptian), **Kief Hallek** (Jordanian), **Kiefik** (Lebanese), or **Shlonick** (Bedouin or Syrian).

### Arabs in North America

Close to 5,000,000 Arab immigrants and their offspring currently live in the United States. Fifty-four percent are foreign-born and entered the United States between 1970 and 1979. Of this group, more than half speak a language other than English at home, but 86% speak English well. More than 50% have some higher education.

Waves of Arab immigrants followed economic or political instability or war in the Middle East. With the first wave, occurring between 1880 and 1938, some 250,000 Arabs immigrated to the United States from Greater Syria, now known as Jordan, Syria, and Lebanon. Of this group, about 47% of those who migrated between 1899 and 1915 were reportedly women. Likewise, in the 1920s, more than half of these immigrants were also women.

The second wave (1947 to 1967) of 154,000 Muslim and Christian families included a sizable number of refugees who came to the United States following the 1948 war and creation of the State of Israel or because of general political instability in the Middle East. The most recent third wave (1968 to 1990) consisted of the more highly educated and professionals, seeking a better qualify of life in the United States, resulting in a "brain drain."

In the United States, large established Arab-American communities are found in New York (Yonkers), New Jersey, Michigan (Detroit), Ohio, Virginia, Texas, Florida, Arizona, and California. Regionally, about 30% of Arabs live in the Northeast, 27% in the North Central States, 21% in the South, and 21% in the West.

In Canada, people of Arab origin number 274,205, of whom 46% are women. They live predominantly in Montreal and Toronto, with a smaller group found in Ottawa. Lebanese Arabs are by far the largest Canadian group.

## 🌐 BEING FEMALE IN THE ARAB CULTURE

Arab cultures socialize women to be wives and mothers. Women should not demonstrate sexual attractiveness in appearance or behavior because Islam, a strong religious influence in the region, views women as *fitna*, a source of temptation from which men should be spared. Thus, women must cover their heads and bodies. Women are also referred to as the weaker sex and in need of male protection and guidance. A good reputation is extremely important for a woman's marriage and her family's good social standing.

## At Birth

### Preference for Sons

Despite social change that has led to valuing both males and females as potentially productive members of society, the Arab patriarchal family structure continues to favor male children. The boy carries on the family name and lineage, and the parents will turn to him in their old age. The boy will also keep most of the family's assets within the family. Girls are considered a liability throughout their parents' lives because they need to be guarded and protected even after marriage. The proverb **"Ham el Banat li ba'd el mammat"** means "the burden of the parents."

### Response to the Birth of a Female

Generally, families greet the birth of a boy with much rejoicing and celebration, while they receive the birth of a girl with more emotional restraint, if not outright sadness. If the family was already "blessed" with one or more boys, it may better welcome the birth of a girl. If the first and subsequent births are girls, however, the parents will keep trying for a male child. A woman who gives birth to only or mostly girls may feel less valued and express herself in those terms. Extended family members may reinforce negative feelings about the birth of a female child and pay less attention to the mother.

Usually, mothers hold and cuddle a boy more and nurse him longer than they would a girl. But families never disregard or neglect girls. After the parents adjust to the birth of a girl, they love and care for her appropriately.

### Birth Rituals

Birth rituals differ by country of origin. Distributing sweets and candies **(hallawan)** is common after a birth, although families give more expensive candies for the birth of a boy. Some families slaughter a lamb and distribute the meat among the poor, a gesture of thanksgiving to God and a means to ward off evil spirits. In some countries, the first week after birth **(sebú),** especially of a boy, is filled with celebration and festivities.

Male circumcision is an Islamic practice followed throughout the Arab world and in Sudan and Egypt. Rural or suburban people of lower socioeconomic class still widely practice female circumcision. Some families seek circumcision for baby girls in North America because of pressure from extended family members.

## Childhood and Youth

### Stages

There are no actual stages of childhood, but families encourage children to become independent as quickly as possible. While women may breastfeed their infants beyond the first (and sometimes after the second or third) year of life, they toilet-train their children within or shortly after the first year. Parents and extended family rear children with love and attention; they also discipline children. A clear definition of "youth" is not established; however, the concept is recognized in the use of **"lisato walad"** or **"listaha bint,"** terms indicating that this boy or girl is still young enough not to know better.

The word for children is **awlad,** from **wiladeh,** meaning to be born. If the children are only girls, however, they are called **Banat.**

### Family Expectations

Children are expected to respect their elders; obey parents; and demonstrate filial piety, devotion, and loyalty to the family. Both nuclear and extended families value interdependence over independence. Because parents put their children's needs ahead of their own when the children are young, parents expect children to put the needs of their parents first when they become adults.

Children are not allowed to participate in adult conversations. Immigrant parents perceive children who talk back or argue with parents or other adults as having assimilated to the American way of life, which is highly distressing.

Girls are traditionally socialized early to fulfill women's roles. Thus, they are expected to help with household chores and work hand-in-hand with the mother. They are also expected to submit their will and desires to the approval of male family members, including their younger brothers.

### Social Expectations

Loss of family honor is the worst calamity that can befall the Arab family. Family honor is the family's stock for social survival. Women are entrusted with protecting family honor by upholding proper cultural conduct at all costs. Chaste, modest public conduct of females is an indicator of socially expected behavior.

### Importance of Education

Education is important for both boys and girls, but higher education is more emphasized for boys. Female illiteracy is a product of role expectations. Girls must work doubly hard to succeed in school because they must also do household chores; and if finances are limited, boys' higher education is the priority.

## Pubescence

Beginning adolescence is called starting **Murahaka,** which refers to being torn between the forces of childhood and adulthood.

### Psychosexual Development

The average age for the onset of puberty is 12.5 years for girls. Physical changes and the onset of menses are considered tangible proof of sexual development and potential fertility. Sex education is rarely provided in an open or neutral way. At the onset of puberty or shortly before menses are expected, a girl's mother or an older female sibling will educate her about the menstrual cycle and the required hygienic practices during and after the menses. However, girls who have not been educated on this topic may wake one morning with menstrual blood and have no notion for its occurrence or meaning.

Delayed onset of menses (beyond age 14 or 15) may be a cause for alarm and to seek professional advice. Irregular menses at the early stage of sexual development is of little concern and attributed to hormonal imbalance.

### Rituals and Rites of Passage

No specific rituals celebrate a girl's transition to puberty. Female circumcision, however, may be done around puberty in regions where this is still practiced. The menstrual cycle is not welcomed openly. Although parents, especially mothers, may be relieved to know that their daughters are developing normally, they will usually handle the subject privately and with some degree of embarrassment.

### Teen Sexuality

**Social Restrictions and Pressures.** Pubescent girls are considered young women **(sabaia)** and should not dress as girls do. They are expected to be conservative in their play and laughter in public and to demonstrate more "lady-like" behavior. Parents and brothers restrict and guard their freedom to socialize and play.

**Teen Pregnancy.** Dating and courtship are not acceptable in the Arab culture. A man may court his fiancée with a chaperone, but only after their official engagement. Sexual relations before marriage are taboo. Parents fear out-of-wedlock pregnancy more than any other occurrence for daughters. They make enormous efforts to socialize their daughters about its grave consequences, and they reinforce moral values and social measures to prevent its occurrence.

### Menstruation

**Relationship to Health.** Regular menstruation with a medium flow of 4 to 5 days' duration is considered ideal. Irregular periods with heavy or scant flow may be considered abnormal and indicate a need for medical consultation and intervention.

**Relationship to Fertility**   Fertility is closely linked with regular and consistent menstrual periods. The motive for seeking treatment for irregular periods or irregular/abnormal flow is concern about ability to conceive.

**Taboos and Restrictions During Menstruation.**   During menstruation, women are considered unclean. They are supposed to abstain from such religious duties as fasting during the Islamic month of Ramadan, holding the Holy Koran, and bathing. These restrictions are more prevalent in some countries than in others and among those of lower socioeconomic classes.

**Dysmenorrhea.**   Menstrual pain and abdominal cramps are common and considered normal. Hot herbal teas or drinks made of mint, rosemary, sage, or any combination of them are used to treat cramps. Women avoid cold (temperature) foods believed to diminish the menstrual flow and cause clots. They typically use anti-inflammatory or pain medications to control excessive pain from cramping.

Women may interpret missed periods as a sign of either pregnancy or illness. Deviation from the usual blood flow (scant or heavy) may also be cause for alarm.

### Female Modesty and Touching

Female modesty is expected in the Arab culture. From an early age, girls learn to guard their behavior at all times and to be especially aware of how they dress, play, and sit. They learn early about the potentially dire consequences of immodesty, and that their modesty is linked to family honor. As girls mature, they are no longer allowed to freely interact with males, and modesty is emphasized in terms of maintaining virginity. Because of concern over the potential loss of virginity, unwed young women do not undergo pelvic examinations; and physical examinations are conducted with extreme respect for modesty. A chaperone (either the girl's mother or another female family member) will generally be present during such examinations.

---

**NOTE TO THE HEALTH CARE PROVIDER**

When a gynecologic examination is considered essential for a young unmarried woman, the practitioner should exert extreme care to maintain an intact hymen.

---

# Adulthood

### Transition Rites and Rituals

Young adult women have little autonomy or freedom of choice until they are married and have at least one child. Unmarried Arab women, regardless of age, are referred to as girls and are often restricted in their choices. In contrast to young men, young women have no rites of passage into adulthood; instead, their entry into adulthood is marked by more restrictions. They are excluded from the carefree play that their male counterparts enjoy and enter exclusively into the women's world, where they are further socialized into domestic roles.

### Social Expectations

A young Arab woman knows that her own family and families into whom she may potentially marry carefully observe her conduct. Whether they choose to pursue their education, become gainfully employed, or remain at home, young women must conduct themselves with social honor, responsibility, and accountability toward themselves and their families. In North America, extended family and Arab-community members similarly observe Arab immigrant women and their daughters.

### Union Formation

Marriage at a young age is desired in more traditional areas, but the marriage age is rising with more female education. Between 20% and 30% of Arab women marry by age 20; 80% marry by age 30. Arranged marriages are the norm, and young women are often pressured to accept a marriage proposal for fear that there will not be another, to prevent gossip and potential slander, or both.

The prospective groom seeks the hand of the prospective bride through her father, brothers, and extended family members. The women in both families unofficially initiate a marriage arrangement, but it is the groom, accompanied by his elder and most distinguished extended male family members, who makes an official announced visit to the bride's family to request marriage from her father.

Polygamy is acceptable in Islam, which permits up to four wives concurrently, as long as the man can be just, fair, and even-handed with all his wives. Polygamy has become less common over the past two decades, however, as a result of higher educational levels, better living standards, and economic constraints.

Unmarried women older than 30 years are considered undesirable for marriage and are quickly labeled "old maids" **(awanes)** with dim futures. Choices for unmarried women are limited despite higher education or other qualities. They may marry an older widower or become a second wife simply to escape domination by their fathers or brothers.

Age of marriage among Arab immigrants and Arab Americans varies by country of origin and generation. For example, Yemeni families tend to protect the chastity of their daughters by arranging marriages at very young ages, while women from urban educated professional families have a choice of mate and time of marriage that resembles the dominant norms.

### Domestic Violence

Abused women typically do not openly discuss domestic violence. Shame and social disgrace prevent an Arab woman from seeking outside help. Women may rationalize their spouses' abusive behavior by attributing it generically to men's volatile tempers and nervous tendencies. Domestic violence is a family affair and usually dealt with within the immediate family.

### Rape

Women who are raped are doubly victimized and punished, first by the rape and second by social reaction to the incident. Thus, victims will not report the rape and may endure the trauma alone. People in some Arab countries consider raped women to be at fault for the incident and may punish them by death to curtail the family's social disgrace.

---

**NOTE TO THE HEALTH CARE PROVIDER**

Practitioners should handle young women seeking treatment or abortion for rape with strict confidentiality and understanding. They should try to understand and respect the woman's refusal to report the crime of rape in light of the grave cultural consequences she is likely to face.

---

### Divorce

**Sociocultural Views.**  In Islam, divorce is permissible but undesirable. A man can divorce his wife by simply saying "you are divorced" three times. The wife has no choice but to return to her parents' house to await settlement. Women, on the other hand, must seek a divorce through the court system, which may take years and sometimes may depend on the husband's consent. Christian Arabs view divorce as an unacceptable solution to marital problems, except in specific or extreme circumstances. In some countries, the divorce rate is nearing 50%. Causes are primarily women's sterility, lower level of education, and bearing only female children.

**Women and Divorce.**  Divorced women are viewed negatively, especially if they are Catholic. Culturally, divorce is considered a source of disgrace and shame. People outside the immediate family may view divorced women as potentially problematic and socially avoid or treat them tentatively. The immediate family, on the other hand, may express open displays of pity and sorrow to ward off blame and project it on the ex-spouse.

**Child Custody Practices.**  According to Islamic law, the male partner may have full custody of the children following a divorce, once the children reach the age of 7. Some countries have modified the law to give the mother the right to keep her children until they reach age 14. The father, meanwhile, has the right to see his children frequently. Since the children ultimately belong to the father, he remains active in their upbringing and provides financial support.

---

**NOTE TO THE HEALTH CARE PROVIDER**

Divorced women or women going through divorce may display an array of psychological symptoms. While these women readily accept emotional support, they may interpret referral to counseling as an indication that they are mentally sick or that the health care provider views them as such.

---

### Fertility and Childbearing

**Family Size.**  With fertility comes higher status for women and proof of virility for men. Women are expected to become pregnant as soon as they get married, and childbearing continues throughout the reproductive span. Families tend to be large in most regions. Families in rural farming areas commonly have 8 to 10 children, because they view children as the future economic and social support of the parents. The average family size among highly educated and employed couples is declining.

**Contraceptive Practices.**  Although knowledge about birth control and contraception is widespread throughout the Arab world, cultural, religious, social, and political factors hinder effective implementation. Family planning in the form of spacing births may be more acceptable than other types of birth control.

Only a small percentage of couples use contraception regularly and efficiently. They usually use oral contraceptives and intrauterine devices (IUDs), but condoms are now more prevalent than a decade ago. Catholics do not believe in contraception but may use the safe-period or "rhythm" method to time or space births.

**Role of the Male Partner in the Couple's Fertility Decision-Making.**  The male partner has the right to allow or deny the woman a choice regarding childbearing. Women can negotiate with their partners but can decide only after ensuring their partners' consent. Health professionals need to understand the cultural context, particularly the couple's role relations, the high value of fertility and conception, and the social forces surrounding the woman's decisions about family planning.

---

**NOTE TO THE HEALTH CARE PROVIDER**
Since the woman cannot solely make decisions about family planning, the health care provider needs to involve the husband. Educating and seeking the cooperation of the husband are essential if compliance with a selected method is to be expected.

---

## Abortion

**Cultural Attitudes.**  Given the high value placed on children and big families, abortion is uncommon in the Arab world. Christian Arabs, especially Catholics, consider abortion a mortal sin. Abortions of undesirable pregnancies (pregnancies in violation of social and cultural norms) may be performed in secrecy.

**Teen Abortion.**  Pregnancy of married teens is encouraged; thus, abortion is uncommon. A common health problem in this society is the result of early teen pregnancy, when the mother has not completed her own physical growth, leading to miscarriage.

Medically justified abortions are done in hospitals under the direct care of an obstetrician-gynecologist. Women are likely to seek abortion in early pregnancy, but late abortions are performed in adverse medical or social situations, such as out-of-wedlock pregnancy. Some women may try to lose the fetus by lifting heavy objects, jumping, and doing strenuous activities. Some women insert a metal object into the vagina in an effort to break the amniotic sac and abort, with the common outcomes of bleeding and infection.

Immigrant women or their offspring are more likely to use abortion for accidental pregnancy, but even for these women it is a difficult choice.

---

**NOTE TO THE HEALTH CARE PROVIDER**
Young, inexperienced women may display emotional reactions in connection with spontaneous abortion of desired pregnancies. Outward displays of grief through crying and losing interest in self, including refusal to eat, may mimic postpartum depression. Such behavior, however, may well be related to the culturally learned manner of expressing grief.

---

## Miscarriage

Given the high prevalence of grand parity and poor spacing of pregnancies, the rates and risks of miscarriage are high. Women tend to view miscarriage as a natural occurrence that most women experience at some point in their reproductive lives. Often, they attribute miscarriage to fatigue, carrying heavy objects, or a weak or weakened body. To avoid future miscarriages, women are encouraged to eat well and to avoid fatigue or carrying heavy objects. Women who habitually miscarry are regarded as having weak bodies that are incapable of carrying a fetus to full term.

After several miscarriages, women may seek traditional treatment, medical treatment, or both. Traditional treatment may involve a suppository made of camel bone marrow mixed with dry herbs and wrapped in lamb's wool. This suppository is supposed to cleanse the uterus, rid it from impurities or coagulated blood from previous miscarriages, and strengthen the wall for successful pregnancy and full-term delivery.

---

**NOTE TO THE HEALTH CARE PROVIDER**

Providers should educate women about the danger of repeated pregnancies without adequate spacing. Young, newly married immigrant women may be at risk because they lack knowledge or women kin, but they also do not know how to take care of themselves or access the health care system. Once they come to the health care facility, they need detailed information about proper health behavior related to pregnancy and beyond.

---

## Infertility

The importance of fertility puts unusual pressure on the newly married woman to get pregnant as soon as possible. Her status depends on her ability to bear children, especially sons. Women who fail to immediately conceive are blamed and expected to seek treatment from medical as well as folk healers or religious or spiritual leaders to help them conceive. Belief in sorcery (**ámal**) as having prevented conception leads women to seek the help of Sheiks or religious people to uncover and rid them of the evil. Infertile women (**áquer**) are stigmatized and feel less whole or without God's blessings. They may be divorced, deserted, or forced to agree to a polygamous marriage.

Arab immigrant women who have difficulty conceiving are likely to seek infertility treatment. In light of the strong value placed on bearing children, husbands are likely to provide support and resources.

---

**NOTE TO THE HEALTH CARE PROVIDER**

Arab men may resist fertility screening and treatment, viewing such measures as denigrating their manhood. Education and counseling during the early period of screening can provide support and understanding for the couple's infertility issues.

---

## Pregnancy

**Activity Restrictions and Taboos.** During the first trimester, pregnant women are not allowed to carry heavy objects or do strenuous physical labor for fear of miscarriage. They are also spared from actively participating in mourning a loved one's death because emotional upset is believed to affect normal fetal growth. Sexual intercourse may diminish during the first and last trimester for fear of causing fetal injury.

Some countries and people from lower socioeconomic groups believe that fetal deformity or handicap results from a pregnant woman viewing a person with the deformity. They may also think that fright can harm the fetus. Some frightened pregnant women are given sacred water in a special copper cup to relieve the fright and its negative consequences. They are also revered and given seats or preferences when standing in line.

Pregnant women are encouraged to eat large portions of protein-rich foods, to "eat for two." Depending on the husband's financial situation, the woman eats meat, chicken, liver, and lentil soup, along with vegetables, rice, milk, and other dairy products. Women are given any foods they crave **(waham)** for fear that the fetus may develop a birthmark in the shape of the craved food.

**Prenatal Care.**   Maternal health clinics in rural areas are now widespread, as are urban maternity clinics and hospitals. Women seek prenatal care earlier than they did some decades ago but not with the regularity that health care providers expect. A pregnant woman may seek pregnancy confirmation during the first trimester, and she may make follow-up visits for emerging problems but rarely for preventive care.

In the weeks or days before delivery, women prepare the infant's clothing and consume herbal drinks to manage their discomfort. In some rural areas, when the full-term woman experiences abdominal pain, she is expected to walk over a metal plate with smoking herbs to discern if the pain is the result of simple colic or actual labor.

---

**NOTE TO THE HEALTH CARE PROVIDER**

Prenatal childbirth classes are foreign to many Arab immigrant women. Thus, providers may need to spend additional time caring for and coaching the laboring woman.

---

## The Birthing Process

**Home Versus Hospital Delivery.**   Hospital delivery is becoming the norm in the Arab Middle East, often in state-of-the-art specialized labor and delivery hospitals. Because of transportation problems, rural women may deliver at home, assisted by certified midwives. A **daia** (woman recognized for her skill and experience in assisting home deliveries), however, may be entrusted with birth. Whether at home or in a hospital, female relatives support the birthing process.

**Cesarean Section Versus Vaginal Delivery.**   Women prefer vaginal delivery, but a recent trend is toward the least painful method. Some upscale urban women prefer scheduling a cesarean section with anesthesia, but poorer rural women view a cesarean section as an interference with a normal process. They also may consider such delivery a disgrace because subsequent deliveries, it is believed, will be cesarean in the hospital.

**Labor Management.**   The husband remains close by but does not participate in the labor and delivery process. Female family members act as coaches, encouraging, supporting, and providing direct care as needed. Usually, they rely on their own birthing experience and provide care accordingly. During contractions, they encourage the woman to push and bear downward. The laboring woman may be given a rug to bite on to help with the pain and to keep her mouth closed. Herbal hot drinks of rosemary or thyme are offered to enhance the contractions and speed delivery. The laboring woman is allowed to express her pain loudly, but she is also encouraged to invoke God's help with prayers. If the presentation of the baby is breech, the woman's abdomen may be manipulated externally to maneuver the fetus toward occipital presentation.

**Placenta.** The placenta is usually examined for intactness or abnormalities. It is typically buried deeply in the ground at the periphery of the woman's household because it is considered part of the human remains of the birth and should be disposed of properly by burial.

---

**NOTE TO THE HEALTH CARE PROVIDER**
Providers should not coerce men into participating in the birthing process. While some Arab men wish to be part of the process, most think it is taboo.

---

## Postpartum

Arab women observe 40 days postpartum, during which they are relieved from household duties and attended by their mothers or female in-laws. Women are considered impure during the postpartum period, and sexual intercourse is not permitted as long as there is vaginal bleeding. Women are not allowed to carry heavy objects or do strenuous work for fear of back injury (after labor, the woman's lower backbone is believed not to be fused back in place [*daher mftuoh*]) or further bleeding. Women avoid drafts or changes in temperature for fear of catching a cold in the womb. When the flow of milk is inadequate, it is encouraged by use of hot compresses or breast massage; putting a hot bottle over the nipple may produce suction.

---

**NOTE TO THE HEALTH CARE PROVIDER**
Postpartum immigrant women may refuse to bathe, sit near air conditioning vents or in drafts, or drink cold drinks because they fear exposure to cold. Providers should support these practices whenever possible.

---

## Newborn and Infant Care

**Breastfeeding Versus Bottle-Feeding.** Women breastfeed their babies for an average of two years, but marketing and distribution of free formula milk have interfered with complete breastfeeding in some countries. During the first 40 days postpartum, women are encouraged to drink fresh goat milk and to eat candied sesame seed butter and chicken soup with large pieces of chicken and *melokhia* (a spinach-like vegetable eaten with soup) to increase the milk flow. Citrus fruits, garlic, and hot pepper are believed to reduce milk flow and cause infant colic.

**Infant Protection.** Newborns are tightly wrapped in cotton blankets to protect them from drafts, provide safe handling, and enhance their sense of security. The umbilical cord is protected by wrapping with a clean cotton belt to prevent umbilical hernia. To strengthen the joints and give the muscles a firm tone, warm olive oil is massaged over the infant's body; in some areas, olive oil and salt massages are thought to strengthen the infant's character. Amulets or written religious verses in a small cotton pouch are attached by safety pin to the infant's outer blanket to ward off the evil eye. Colicky babies are often given herbal drinks of mint or chamomile with sugar.

Many children are now immunized because of the development of maternal child community clinics and increased public awareness of the importance of immunization. Nonetheless, immunizations may not be obtained at suggested intervals. Growth and development may be monitored, but not regularly.

> **NOTE TO THE HEALTH CARE PROVIDER**
> Practitioners should provide the new mother with information about the infant's follow-up care, especially as it pertains to immunization.

**Primary Caregiver.** The primary infant and toddler caregivers are mothers. Older female siblings also care for infants and toddlers and take care of chores associated with younger siblings' care. Other women in the house (e.g., aunts, grandmothers, sisters-in-law) lend a hand whenever needed. Men are not expected to provide direct care of infants; they are shamed and labeled not true men if they are seen changing a diaper or feeding an infant.

# Middle Age

## Cultural Attitudes and Expectations

Middle-aged women are expected to demonstrate seriousness and maturity in their physical appearance and behavior. They are expected to be wise and to mentor younger women.

## Psychological Response

Given the usually large family size and the tendency of adult sons to live in or near their parents' home after marriage, the empty-nest syndrome is unheard of in this culture. Similarly, the Arab culture has no concept of midlife crisis because the lives of middle-aged women still revolve around caring for children. Arab immigrants and Arab Americans, however, may experience midlife crises.

## Menopause

**Onset and Duration.** Menopause, the cessation of menstrual periods, occurs on average at about 49 years. It is believed that early menopause is associated with the early onset of menses or becoming drained by numerous pregnancies. Late onset is attributed to late onset of menses or being active and healthy. Early or late menopause may also be explained by genetic differences, but rarely by differences in diet.

**Sexual Activity.** Menopause means the end of reproduction and the beginning of old age. It is often greeted with relief among women who are expected to produce a child every year. Others may fear that the end of their fertility will push their husbands to marry another young and fertile wife. Menopausal women generally remain sexually active, although sexual activity *may* decrease as they grow older.

**Coping.** Arab women handle the symptoms of menopause with dignity. They do not discuss symptoms openly, but their children often perceive such symptoms and respect them. Women are often relieved of family responsibilities and are provided time for socializing with their peers. They use this time to seek support and understanding and to learn from one another how to handle discomfort, symptoms, and emotional issues. Most women regard menopause as yet another normal phase of life to which they will adjust. They rarely use hormone replacement therapy (HRT), but they do use herbal remedies, cooling drinks, humor, and disregard of physical symptoms.

## Old Age

The average life expectancy varies among Arab countries. For example, it is 55 years in Egypt, but 65 years in Lebanon and Jordan. The Arab population is extremely young, with about 45% of the population younger than age 15. Women's life expectancy is slightly higher than men's.

Women gain recognition and respect as they age, and their experience and wisdom are highly regarded. Older women are worshipped by their children, who give them the attention, time, and money they need. Sons and daughters strive to please, care for, and demonstrate appreciation and respect for their mothers. They ask mothers for advice and help in decision-making. Mothers are usually at the center of their children's lives. An older woman will live in her house with her spouse, and married children may continue to live in the same household. When in need of housing, older women tend to live with their oldest son or daughter.

## Death and Dying

### Cultural Attitudes and Beliefs

Death is perceived as the result of God's will. Death of elderly people is more tolerated than the sudden death of middle-aged or young people. Dying from complications of childbirth produces agony and sympathy for the newborn child, surviving children, and spouse.

Muslims believe that the deceased should be buried immediately after preparation of the corpse, and that the soul of the deceased will face final judgment right after the burial. Any delay in burial will increase the spiritual agony of the deceased.

### Rites and Rituals

Muslims follow strict rites and rituals in preparing the body for burial. With the body facing Mecca, it is washed, and all body orifices are cleaned and sealed with pieces of cotton to keep the deceased soul contained in the body. Then the body is wrapped with white cotton fabric and taken to the Mosque for final special prayers of the dead. The body is buried directly in the ground without the use of a coffin. Christians, who do not practice immediate burial, may keep the body in the morgue until notification and arrangements for a religious funeral are completed. Prior to the funeral, the body is taken home for a brief wake before being taken to the church. Arab immigrants use funeral homes for the wake, and funeral homes are slowly growing more common in the Arab countries.

---

**NOTE TO THE HEALTH CARE PROVIDER**
Practitioners should provide the family members with water so that they can cleanse and prepare the body for burial. Respecting their privacy and need to recite prayers is essential.

---

Mourning

**Cultural Expectations.**   Mourning lasts 40 days. Christians believe that the departed spirit may go to heaven, hell, or purgatory (Catholics); Muslims believe that the departed soul will go to either paradise or hell.

Women and girls in the family express grief by loud wailing and crying. The men and boys are expected to remain in control and mindful of their responsibility to take care of the details related to the death and mourning. All members of the extended family, friends, and social acquaintances who come to share grief or take part in the mourning wear black. Make-up and jewelry are not worn in the home of the mourning family. The extended family is expected to relieve the immediate family of all chores related to cleaning and eating and to help them in expressing their pain and grief. Chanting the good attributes of the deceased encourages crying and allowing grief to run its full course so that family members can move on with their lives after the mourning period. A relative or friend may care for young children to shield them from the open displays of grief and mourning, and children are not allowed to view the deceased.

**Coping.**   Traditional rituals help the bereaved express their grief and receive direct help and support from extended family and friends. Mothers of young children have a hard time with the death of the spouse because of the burden of raising the children alone and lack of financial means. They may have to move in with in-laws to receive the support and protection of the extended family. Young children may be subject to shared custody by their mothers and members of the extended family. If the mother remarries, the extended family may become the sole custodian of the young children.

Following the death of a mother, children generally remain in the father's home, where he maintains sole custody over his children, even if he remarries.

---

**NOTE TO THE HEALTH CARE PROVIDER**
Family members of the dying may cry silently and pray, but women in the family receive death with loud crying and wailing. Providers should respect demonstrative grief and provide a room or private quarters in which the family can grieve.

---

## 🌐 IMPORTANT POINTS FOR PROVIDERS CARING FOR ARAB WOMEN

### The Medical Intake

#### Literacy and English Proficiency

Recent immigrants need an interpreter and help with filling out forms. While some may be proficient in English, they are likely to have difficulty understanding medical terms.

#### Status of the Provider

Arab immigrants highly regard health care providers who demonstrate knowledge and expertise through age or rank (e.g., chief of surgery). They may not take a young-looking or lesser-ranking provider seriously.

## Communicating Illness and Symptoms

Because of modesty, women may appear passive, but they will respond when spoken to. They tend to defer to their spouses to communicate the nature of their illness. Otherwise, they are usually spontaneous and will volunteer information based on their own understanding of their symptoms. Other companions may act as interpreters or historians, giving information and seeking answers to the patient's questions and concerns.

---

**NOTE TO THE HEALTH CARE PROVIDER**

Direct and continuous eye contact between a male provider and a female client may cause discomfort. Glancing rather than continuous eye contact is more culturally tolerated.

---

## Physical Examination

### Modesty and Touching

Modesty and the need to cover the female body are cultural values that seriously influence the physical examination. Embarrassment with revealing the body is readily obvious, especially in relation to gynecologic examinations. Health care providers should be careful not to expose the whole body and should arrange for a female health care provider to conduct the physical examination.

Same-gender touch is the norm and considered appropriate from female health care providers. Indeed, some traditional women expect and relish same-gender touch. They may interpret opposite-gender touch, however, as a sexual advance. Male providers are permitted to touch women within the limits of a physical examination and direct care only; any form of touching beyond direct care is considered inappropriate.

---

**NOTE TO THE HEALTH CARE PROVIDER**

Directly questioning women about sexual activities may create severe embarrassment. If the companion of a women patient is a son or daughter, questions about female disorders can be quite distressing to both patient and companion.

---

### Expressing Pain

Women are permitted to loudly and demonstratively express labor pain. Otherwise, they endure pain without much complaining.

## Prescribing Medications

Practitioners should assess herbal, over-the-counter, or other medications the patient is using to determine potential drug interactions. Asking clients what they did when symptoms first appeared also may elicit the patient's explanation of the illness.

### Drug Interactions

While most herbs traditionally used in the Arab Middle East are mild and generally harmless, herbal and tree bark treatments from other cultures have recently become popular. Controlled medications such as minor antipsychotic and anticonvulsive agents are prescribed freely; practitioners sometimes prescribe antipsychotic medications for hypertension or anticonvulsive medications for neuropathy. If patients are taking such medications without knowing the original intent, they may increase the dose if they experience symptoms of high blood pressure or increased pain.

### Medication Sharing

Generally, Arab and immigrant clients are less informed about health and the exact nature of their illnesses than are European North Americans. Clients suffering from hypertension, diabetes, and sometimes heart disease may share their medications with others who seem to have the same type of disease. Adverse reactions are common and, at times, deadly. Clients may not understand the different types of antihypertensive medications and may use someone else's medication if they forget their own or run out. Other patients double their dose, skip a dose, or stop taking prescribed medications altogether without medical consultation.

---

**NOTE TO THE HEALTH CARE PROVIDER**

Clients may or may not understand the significance of drug interactions, and they are unlikely to talk about concurrent use of other prescribed medications, unless asked. The health care practitioner must inquire about medications prescribed by other health professionals.

---

### Compliance

Compliance may be a major issue with some patients. Older adults, non-English speaking adults, and recent immigrants, in particular, may view medication as simply treating symptoms they can feel; when such symptoms subside, they do not see the relevance of continuing the medications. Cost and fatalism also affect compliance; they tend to view their health as predestined, "in the hands of God."

---

**NOTE TO THE HEALTH CARE PROVIDER**

Providers should elicit the patient's knowledge of the illness, which practitioners she has seen, what medications were prescribed, how long she has been using them, and whether she is currently using them. Arab women may not understand the importance of following prescribed medication regimens, including consequences of failing to comply, without a full explanation.

---

### Follow-up Appointments

Immigrants may not continue with medical treatment when the initial symptoms subside unless they understand the need for follow-up medical visits. Some will simply discontinue treatment without informing the practitioner of their decision.

Arabs are past and present oriented. They believe that time is created for man rather than man being created for time. Tardiness is less important than human relationships; for example, the woman who has an appointment with a health care provider will risk being late or missing her appointment altogether rather than face the social embarrassment of excusing herself from her unexpected guest. Career-oriented Arab Americans, however, are not likely to miss or be late for an appointment.

---

**NOTE TO THE HEALTH CARE PROVIDER**
Questions as to how the client plans to get to the next appointment (e.g., driving or depending on another) may reveal potential problems with tardiness or missing appointments. Usually, when clients understand the ramifications and consequences of their illness, they tend to comply eagerly. Similarly, informing the clients that they need to call to cancel an appointment is important.

---

## Prevalent Diseases

Hypertension, heart disease, cerebrovascular accidents, cancer, diabetes, and renal disease are prevalent. Common nutritional problems include iron-deficiency anemia; anemia of pregnancy; vitamin A deficiency (pellagra); vitamin D deficiency (rickets in children); vitamin $B_1$ deficiency (beri beri); and goiter as a result of iodine deficiency in the water in Sudan, Jordan, Iraq, Lebanon, and Egypt. Parasitic diseases include ancylostomiasis and bilharziasis.

Arab women tend to become overweight as they age, mainly because of a sedentary lifestyle and neglect of their health after menopause. Obesity contributes to diabetes, hypertension, and heart disease. Younger women tend to start smoking after age 30 since, unlike their male counterparts, they were not permitted to smoke when younger.

## Health-Seeking Behaviors

Health is perceived as the ability to carry out one's role functions without pain, and it is maintained by eating fresh food, protecting oneself from the elements, and having adequate rest. Pain is perceived as proof of illness; it requires immediate relief and investigation as to its cause.

### Preventive Health Care

Typically, Arabs and Arab Americans do not practice preventive care or use yearly screening and regular follow-ups. They seek medical attention only when they experience symptoms, especially pain. In lower socioeconomic groups, economic constraints and lack of health knowledge delay seeking medical attention until advanced stages of illness. Depending on the severity of symptoms, they may first consult medical health care providers or jointly seek medical care and the care of folk healers.

### Self-Care of Minor Illnesses

Arabs often use herbal treatments for such minor illnesses as the common cold, intestinal disturbances, and menstrual cramps. They rely on herbal poultices for stiff muscles and abdominal pain. They may use castor oil and Epsom salts for constipation and castor oil for minor burns. They use yogurt with garlic and dried mint flakes for diarrhea. For severe cold symptoms, they depend on cupping and ointment.

### Self-Care of Major Illnesses

In major illness, the sick person is relieved from daily role functions and is cared for by family members, who also oversee the delivery of care and make decisions for the sick person. Family members act as buffers to protect the sick person from emotional upset or concern.

## Culturally Relevant Communication

The most effective approach to potential cultural conflict is identifying the family spokesperson and developing a friendly alliance so that management of care is smooth. A younger family member who is fluent in English may appear to be the spokesperson but may not be the actual decision-maker. Arab Americans expect to be treated with warm regard and respect, and they try to avoid loss of face at all costs. If an alliance is formed early, they will adhere to the expectations of the health care providers and abide by verbal agreements between themselves and the providers.

## BIBLIOGRAPHY

Barakat, H. (1994). The Arab family and the challenge of social transformation. In E. W. Fernea (Ed)., *Women and the family in the Middle East*. Austin, TX: University of Texas Press.

Hattar-Pollara, M., & Meleis, A. I. (1995). The stress of immigration and the daily lived experiences of Jordanian immigrant women in the United States. *Western Journal of Nursing Research*, 17(5), 521–539.

Hattar-Pollara, M., & Meleis, A. I. (1995). Parenting their adolescents: The experience of Jordanian Immigrant women in California. *Health Care of Women International*, 16, 195–211.

Meleis, A. I., & Hattar-Pollara, M. (1995). Arab Middle Eastern American women: Stereotyped, invisible, but powerful. In D. Adams (Ed.), *Health issues for women of color*. Thousand Oaks, CA: Sage Publications, pp133–163.

Zahr, L., & Hattar-Pollara, M. (1999). Nursing care of Arab American children: Consideration of basic cultural factors. *Journal of Pediatric Nursing*, 13(6), 349–355.

# CHAPTER 5

# Brazilians

## DEANNE K. HILFINGER MESSIAS, PhD, RN

### ⊕ INTRODUCTION

### Who are the Brazilian People?

Brazil is the largest country in South America, in both size (8.5 million square kilometers) and population (currently more than 165 million). The Portuguese first colonized Brazil in 1500. The native indigenous population, estimated to be between 2.4 and 6 million in 1500, has faced genocidal attrition dating from the arrival of the first Europeans. Such persecution and rights violations have continued into the 21st century, with the national and international exploitation of the vast resources of the Amazon basin.

The current Brazilian population is a result of widespread racial and ethnic mixing of the native indigenous groups, Portuguese colonizers, and African slaves. Other immigrant groups incorporated into the population during the 20th century include Europeans (Italians and Germans), Middle Easterners (Lebanese and Syrians), and Asians (Japanese and Koreans). Various terms are used to identify and describe the resulting racial blends and skin colors in the Brazilian population. The long tradition of miscegenation between individuals of European and African descent has resulted in a wide range of mixed race blends and shades of black and brown, commonly referred to as *mestico, mulato, moreno,* or *pardo.* In Northern Brazil, *caboclo* is the designation for the combined heritage of Amerindians with Portuguese settlers and later with migrants from the Northeast. People of color make up about 45% of the population. Social class and status are strong components of Brazilian society and are highly correlated with race and color. The strong presence of African elements in Brazilian culture, food, dance, music, language, and spirituality, as well as widespread biological miscegenation, has contributed to the myth of Brazil as a "racial democracy." Recently, however there has been more open and public acknowledgement of racial prejudice and inequalities in Brazil.

Brazil has tremendous social disparities, ranking equal to or above all other countries in measures of socioeconomic inequalities. Once a predominantly rural country, 80% of the population is now urban. The South and Southeast are the most economically and socially developed regions, but urban poverty, unemployment, underemployment, and violence are all major social concerns. Rural poverty, malnutrition, illiteracy, and unemployment are chronic social issues in the North and Northeast regions.

The language is Brazilian Portuguese. Brazilians are Latin Americans, but Brazil is culturally and ethnically distinct from the Hispanic nations and cultures. Although most Brazilians are Catholic, the numbers of Evangelicals and Protestants are growing, in addition to Brazilian Spiritists and followers of Afro-Brazilian religions and voodoo cults **(candomblé). Umbanda** is an indigenous, syncretic Brazilian religion that borrows from Amerindian, African, Catholic, and occultist doctrines and practices.

---

**NOTE TO THE HEALTH CARE PROVIDER**

Brazilians speak Portuguese, so practitioners should not assume that a Brazilian client speaks Spanish. Most Brazilians do not speak Spanish, although some immigrants may have acquired knowledge of Spanish through contact with U.S. Hispanic populations. Brazilians frequently take offense at being classified as Hispanics; although they are South Americans and Latinos/as, they usually prefer to identify as *brasileiras/os*. Similarly, second-generation or third-generation Asian Brazilians are usually monolingual Portuguese speakers.

---

## Brazilians in North America

Very few Brazilians immigrated to North America before 1980. Brazil's chronic economic instability, inconsistent growth, and extremely high inflation fueled the wave of emigration that began in the early 1980s. Many Brazilians came to North America as temporary economic migrants, hoping to obtain employment, earn and save money, and return to Brazil. Others have come as students, professionals, or to join family members. Most recent Brazilian immigrants settled in New York, New Jersey, Massachusetts, Florida, California, and Texas; cities with large concentrations of Brazilians include New York, Newark, Boston, Miami, Fort Lauderdale, San Francisco, Los Angeles, Philadelphia, Washington, D.C., Austin, Houston, and San Antonio.

Brazilians have been undercounted in official U.S. Census data because of the lack of appropriate choices among the ethnic categories and since many undocumented Brazilians have not participated in the census. Unofficial estimates of the Brazilian population in the United States during the 1990s ranged from 330,000 to 600,000 or more. The Canadian Census listed 6520 Brazilians, who live mostly in Toronto and Montreal.

Many recent Brazilian immigrants are young adults in their 20s and 30s. Although they may have some family ties in the United States, relatively few Brazilian Americans have parents or grandparents who also immigrated to the United States. The recent Brazilian immigrants vary along the Brazilian socioeconomic spectrum from lower working class to middle and upper classes. Rarely are immigrants from the poorest of Brazil's social classes, although occasionally very poor women may come as domestic employees of Brazilian officials, diplomats, or multinational business executives.

Although some middle-class Brazilian immigrants are employed in professional positions in the United States, many are employed in low-status service jobs they would not normally hold in their own country, such as domestic or food service employment. Limited English proficiency is one of the barriers for professionals who are required to pass examinations in order to practice in the United States. The number of Brazilians employed in technical and professional fields, however, is increasing. Economic and social transitions related to migration are a source of stress, family discord, or embarrassment for some; others view such experiences as enhancing their personal growth and development.

Family is at the center of Brazilian social life, and it also serves as a resource for mutual aid and social and economic assistance. **Saudades** is a cultural construct that refers to an intense longing and yearning for that which is not present; that is, home, friends, and good times, both past and future. Brazilian immigrants frequently express saudades for their families of origin and the social networks and emotional and material safety nets they provided. Being separated from their traditional family support system may be a source of stress, sadness, and loneliness for immigrants.

---

**NOTE TO THE HEALTH CARE PROVIDER**

A Brazilian immigrant woman's current occupation (e.g., domestic help, baby-sitter, food-service worker) may not reflect her previous educational, occupational, or socioeconomic status in Brazil. A good way to uncover possible sources of stress, identify personal health resources, and evaluate her ability to cope and adjust to life in North American is to explore the client's perceptions of how her immigration and occupational transitions have influenced her health practices.

---

## 🌐 BEING FEMALE IN BRAZILIAN SOCIETY

Traditional Brazilian society is family-based and patriarchal. The male head of household (*chefe de família*) is expected to provide for the family's material and economic necessities. Traditional roles of Brazilian women are housewife (*dona de casa*) and mother (*mãe*).

The number of Brazilian women employed in the formal workforce is increasing, with the proportion of those who are economically active currently more than 35%. On average, women earn only 63% of what men earn. Women are employed in domestic and service sectors, agriculture, and the professions (education, nursing, medicine, pharmacy, law, and information technology). More than 30% of all practicing physicians are women, and 13% of professional health care workers are nurses. In addition to employment in the formal sector, many Brazilian women engage in paid work in the informal sector, producing goods (e.g., birthday party favors, clothes, and jewelry) and services (e.g., manicures and hair styling) in their homes. Across social classes, women entering the paid labor force is often a response to a decline in the purchasing power of family income. Some men may not approve of their wives' employment as a matter of male pride or jealousy.

## At Birth

Although Brazilians highly value male children, they do not disregard or neglect girls. Many families desire children of both sexes. Male circumcision is not routinely performed at birth, but it may be performed later for phimosis. Baby girls often have their ears pierced soon after birth. The baby's parents choose godparents, whose role in current society is primarily symbolic. Among lower-class families, however, the choice of godparents may reflect the expectation of future assistance with clothing, education, or guardianship in the case of the parents' death.

Infants are referred to as **nenê** or **bebê.** Poor, rural families often do not give their babies a proper name until they have reached the first birthday. The first birthday is a significant social event, usually marked by a large celebration **(festa de aniversário)** for extended family, friends, and neighbors.

# Childhood and Youth

## Family and Social Expectations

From ages 2 to 12, children are referred to as **crianças.** Girls are expected to be more docile, submissive, calm, and interested in school and family than are boys. Boys are considered more competitive, given more freedom, and not held to same standards of discipline as are girls. Parental and societal treatment and expectations differ for sons and daughters, and they are class- based. In poor and working-class families, girls are expected to participate actively in domestic responsibilities such as helping with the care of siblings, housecleaning, laundry, and meal preparation; boys may be expected to find employment, often in the informal sector. Rising rates of child labor and abandonment are indications of the deteriorating social and economic situation of poor Brazilian families. Middle-class Brazilian girls and boys are often exempt from any type of domestic or outside work or employment expectations.

## Importance of Education

Education is valued by society, but it is class-based. In Brazil, poor and working-class children usually attend public schools, whereas middle-class and upper-class children attend private schools. In the United States, public school enrollment is more frequently the norm for Brazilian families.

# Pubescence

## Psychosexual Development

Menarche commonly occurs between ages 11 and 14 years, the average age being between 12 and 13 years. Female family members are the usual source of information about menarche. No particular social or cultural rituals or celebrations are related to menarche itself.

## Rituals and Rites of Passage

The 15th birthday marks a girl's transition into adulthood. Middle-class and upper-class families usually fete girls with a debutante party **(baile)** or a trip abroad. In working-class families, girls may seek employment, which may result in dropping out of school.

College entrance examinations **(vestibular)** are highly competitive and constitute a major rite of passage among middle-class Brazilians. In addition to their regular high school studies, many students attend commercial preparatory courses before attempting the vestibular examinations.

Family gatherings are the mainstay of Brazilian social life. In addition, adolescent social activities often include group outings to clubs, bars, and beaches. Many families no longer require teens to follow the strict traditional dating (***namoro***) etiquette in which the young man is required to formally ask for parental permission to date a girl.

### Teen Sexuality

Although not formally sanctioned, teenage sexual activity is widely acknowledged. Despite recent decreases in overall fertility rates, pregnancies among adolescents have been increasing. Recent studies show that among girls age 15 to 19 years, 50% report an active sex life, 33% have been pregnant, and 14% have given birth. In cases of adolescent pregnancy, families generally provide material and emotional support; mother and child often continue to reside at home, and the father of the child may also move into the maternal household. Brazilians tend to view teen pregnancy as a family issue rather than a societal issue. Because no school-based programs for pregnant teens are available, girls must interrupt their studies, at least temporarily, during pregnancy.

Drug use is a major health concern, with Brazilian adolescents most frequently using alcohol, tobacco, solvents, tranquilizers, amphetamines, and marijuana.

### Menstruation

Menstrual regularity is viewed as a sign of health.

**Taboos and Restrictions During Menstruation.**   Most women rarely adhere to such traditional taboos as abstaining from bathing, exercising, or eating certain foods during menstruation; some abstain from sexual activity. Cleanliness is emphasized, for example, using a soap and water periwash during menstruation (***higiene íntima***) and vaginal douching (***lavagem, ducha vaginal***) for hygienic as well as contraceptive practices. It is customary to hand wash one's intimate apparel daily.

**Dysmenorrhea.**   Self-medication for menstrual cramps and discomfort is common. In Brazil, women and girls may request injections of pain medication at local pharmacies. Limited access to prescription and injectable drugs in the United States is one of the principal reasons given by Brazilian immigrants for bringing their own stock of medications into the United States.

### Female Modesty

Certain attire and dress practices (e.g., revealing bathing suits, tight pants or skirts) of Brazilian girls and women may be considered immodest by North American standards. The design of Brazilian clothes, particularly bathing suits, is a reflection of the traditional cultural tendency of Brazilian men to pay more attention to women's buttocks than to their breasts. In Brazil, where young people do not have access to private automobiles (in particular, those not of the upper-middle and upper classes), intimate behaviors such as kissing often take place in public (e.g., in parks, on buses, at the beach).

Personal hygiene, including daily baths and changes of clothes, is integral to Brazilian women's daily life. (Attention to personal hygiene is traced to the native Amerindian women, who bathed several times a day and applied coconut oil to their hair.) Females bathe before meals because it is commonly believed that bathing after a meal can interfere with digestion.

# Adulthood

Weddings and graduation ceremonies (from both high school and university) mark the significant social transitions to adulthood, regardless of age. Large parties or extended family gatherings often accompany these ceremonies.

## Social Expectations

Social expectations for women include marriage and motherhood. Single women may live alone or with parents and often take their role as aunt (*titia*) very seriously.

Men have traditionally been expected to have premarital heterosexual experiences, often with prostitutes. Social acceptance of premarital sexual activities for women has increased. Although this represents some degree of change, gender inequality persists.

Career and employment expectations vary according to class. The women's liberation movement among upper- and middle-class Brazilians has encouraged them to pursue employment and professional careers. Other, lower-class women provide the labor to maintain their households, doing the cooking, cleaning, laundry, and child care. Many social, cultural, and gender norms related to women's work may be challenged as the result of immigration to the United States. Middle-class Brazilian immigrants who were accustomed to having paid domestic help frequently identify the fact that they must assume the entire domestic workload in addition to outside employment as a significant source of stress and frustration. Another result of migration may be that these middle-class immigrants, particularly recent arrivals, may themselves engage in paid domestic employment, a social and cultural experience they would not have in their home country. In some cases Brazilian men may even join their wives or partners in paid domestic employment.

## Union Formation

Many Brazilians have both civil and religious weddings, although only civil marriages are binding. Brazilian law also recognizes common-law marriages or domestic partnerships of more than five years. The number of female-headed households is higher among poor women but on the rise across all social classes.

The Brazilian Civil Code considers a married woman to be her husband's companion, consort, and collaborator. Married women have joint legal custody over children, but fathers are considered to have authority over "jointly held property." Illegitimate children not recognized by their fathers remain under the authority of their mothers. Marriage serves to legitimize children conceived or born prior to a couple's wedding.

## Domestic Violence

Despite the centrality of the family in Brazilian culture and society, the structure and function of families in Brazil have not been based on principles of gender equality or human rights. The use of force or control to dominate or subjugate women is related to the traditional cultural values and norms of **machismo**. Until recently there was little social recourse for women who were victims of domestic violence (**maus tratos**). Domestic violence, however, is now recognized as a women's health concern, and much progress has been made in the past decade. Although services tend to be concentrated in urban areas, shelters and special "Police Posts for Women" (**Delegacía da Mulher**) are available to provide legal, social, psychological, and health assistance to battered women and their families. Federal laws protecting rights of victims and witnesses have been recently enacted.

---

**NOTE TO THE HEALTH CARE PROVIDER**
In cases of suspected domestic violence, providers should work first toward developing a trusting relationship with the woman before bringing up the issue. A woman is likely to interpret a practitioner's reporting directly to authorities as evidence of a lack of respect and trust.

---

## Rape

Like other forms of violence against women, only recently have sexual assault and rape been recognized as societal and women's health issues in Brazil. Laws that offered men special protection at the expense of violence against women (such as allowing a rapist to avoid punishment if he marries the victim) are evidence of the legal and social barriers Brazilian women have had to overcome. Various Brazilian cities have now instituted assistance programs for victims of sexual violence. Where such programs exist, they encourage women to report a rape immediately to a Police Post for Women to receive assistance and health care, including a legal abortion, if desired.

Immigrant women may be reluctant to share with providers their personal histories of sexual violence. They may, however, seek assistance from health care providers in the case of rape.

## Divorce

**Sociocultural Views.**   Separation, divorce, remarriage, and blended families are common in contemporary urban Brazilian society. Societal views and practices related to divorce have changed significantly over the past several decades. Despite the official position of the Catholic Church, divorce is now legal in Brazil, and women can remarry in civil ceremonies. Previously, Brazilian women could obtain a legal separation but could not remarry.

**Child Custody Practices.**   Women who remarry do not lose parental rights to children by a previous marriage. In the absence of either parent, the remaining parent has sole responsibility for children.

## Fertility and Childbearing

Brazilians highly value fertility and childbearing. Voluntary childlessness is uncommon. Large families were previously the norm, but fertility rates have been rapidly decreasing over the past several decades, to the current level of approximately 2.5 children per woman. Maternal mortality rates have declined to a current average of 124 deaths per 100,000 live births, but regional disparities exist as to rate, largely because of high-risk pregnancies and lack of access to health services.

Married or partnered women tend to use some form of contraception despite Brazil being a predominantly Catholic country. Female sterilization and oral contraceptives are the most frequently used methods. Less popular methods include condoms, abstinence, withdrawal, male sterilization, injectable contraceptives, intrauterine devices (IUDs), and lactational amenorrhea. Strong resistance to barrier methods is a factor that compromises HIV/AIDS prevention efforts.

Tubal ligation is often performed in conjunction with a cesarean section and is sometimes the primary indication for that procedure. Nearly one-fourth of the sterilized women in Brazil have opted for this contraceptive method before age 25. Sterilization was legalized in 1997 for married women older than age 25 who have at least two living children, with the consent of the husband. Formal consent by the male partner is not required for dispensing other forms of contraception, and men rarely participate in women's decisions about the type of contraceptive method used.

---

**NOTE TO THE HEALTH CARE PROVIDER**
Providers should carefully review use of oral contraceptives with patients. Brazilian women may have obtained oral contraceptives in Brazil without prescription; incorrect use is also common.

---

## Abortion

Abortion is illegal, characterized by the Brazilian Penal Code as a "crime against life," and punishable by a jail sentence for the woman who induces or consents to an abortion as well as for the person who performs it. Legal abortions are extremely rare and are allowed only as a last resort to save a pregnant woman's life or in rape cases. Postabortion curettage, however, accounts for about 8% of obstetric hospitalizations, an indirect indication of the extent of illegal abortions. Clandestine abortion clinics of varying quality exist for those who can pay; poor women frequently risk their lives and their health, often depending on friends, neighbors, or a drugstore clerk for access to means to induce abortion. Women use various herbal teas and drugs (estrogens, progestagens, and misoprostol) to "induce menstrual flow" in cases of suspected pregnancy.

### Miscarriage

Miscarriage **(aborto espontâneo)** may be attributed to "God's will" **(vontade de Deus)**, falls, blows to the stomach, other accidents, or defective sperm. Miscarriage may be directly attributed to domestic violence, as in the case of physical assault, or indirectly, as in the case of defective sperm, attributed to the partner's use of alcohol.

When identified, high-risk pregnancies are followed medically, which may include extended hospitalization or bed rest at home.

### Infertility

Because voluntary childlessness is uncommon, others usually assume a childless couple to be infertile. The male partner may view infertility as a threat to his manhood, leading to a source of marital discord. Despite familial pressure to have children, it is not a social norm for a husband to leave his wife solely on the basis of infertility. Fertility treatments are available to upper-class women who have access to private pay health care services.

### Pregnancy

Pregnant women are given special attention. Family members feel obligated to satisfy a pregnant woman's specific desires or cravings **(desejos)** and to provide larger quantities of food because of the need to "feed two." It is common to seek prenatal care early in pregnancy. Women may request a sonogram to determine the baby's sex. Friends or family members may discourage some pregnant women from heavy work, sexual relations, and eating specific foods, although such restrictions vary widely by region of origin and social class.

Women generally continue to work throughout pregnancy. Maternity is valued by family and society and is afforded special protection by Brazilian law. Mandatory maternity leave is 120 days for employed women, and a special maternity salary of 120 days is given to women who are not employed in the formal sector, such as rural and domestic workers. Brazilian immigrants may not be aware of the differences in labor policies, particularly the lack of standard maternity leave in the United States.

## Birthing Process

**Home Versus Hospital Delivery.**    Most births (96%) occur in hospitals and are attended by physicians. Trained obstetric nurses perform some hospital deliveries; traditional birth attendants (*parteiras*) practice in poor, rural areas of the North and Northeast. Presence of the father in the labor and delivery room is often actively discouraged because of the belief that he may become faint or "not be able to take it."

**Cesarean Section Versus Vaginal Delivery.**    The rate of cesarean sections is very high in Brazil, ranging from 50% to 85% in some private hospitals. A high cesarean section rate has also been reported among some Brazilian immigrant populations. A woman's preference or choice of a cesarean section may be related to fear of a difficult delivery, desire for a tubal ligation, or belief that vaginal birth following a cesarean delivery is not possible or advisable. Physician convenience and pressure have also been documented as factors related to the high rate of cesarean sections.

**Labor Management.**    Women often become passive, reacting to pain with fear, crying, or screaming, as well as requests for pain medication or anesthesia. Episiotomy is thought to restore a tight vaginal opening and to afford the male partner sexual pleasure.

## Postpartum

The social norm is for the new mother to rest at home, assisted by her mother, sister, or other family member. She is to avoid strenuous physical activity and outside social engagements for 40 days following birth (*resguardo*). Extended visits to the home by family and friends, however, are expected. The prevalence of postpartum depression is comparable to that reported in other countries.

## Newborn and Infant Care

**Breastfeeding Versus Bottle-Feeding.**    Breastfeeding is socially desired, and its average duration is eight months. Brazilian labor law gives employed mothers the right to two special half-hour rest periods during working hours for the purpose of breastfeeding an infant during the first four months of life. Common deterrents to successful breastfeeding include beliefs that breast milk is "weak" (*fraco*) or insufficient in quantity, fear that milk has dried up (*o leite secou*), and employment and work obligations.

**Infant Protection.**    During the first 40 days, the newborn is usually not taken out in public except for doctor's appointments. In public, newborns are often completely covered because of the common belief that infants and young children can become ill if exposed to gusts of fresh air or wind **(pegar vento).** Childhood immunization rates are generally high, and free vaccinations are provided at all public health services. Routine infant vaccination series includes BCG (bacille Calmette-Guérin).

Childhood illnesses may be attributed to spiritual origin, such as the evil eye **(mau-olhado),** spells **(feitiço, quebrante),** or jealousy **(inveja).** In conjunction with or as alternatives to folk remedies or allopathic medical treatments, mothers may seek spiritual healing through prayer, blessings by folk healers **(benzedeiras, rezadeiras),** or laying on of hands **(passes)** by spiritist practitioners.

---

**NOTE TO THE HEALTH CARE PROVIDER**

When taking a health history of a Brazilian woman or her child, the practitioner should inquire about history of BCG vaccination and carefully explain the possible implications of a positive tuberculin skin test (PPD test) following BCG vaccination.

---

**Primary Caregiver.**   Mothers have primary responsibility for child health, including both preventive and medical and sick care. They often share or delegate childcare responsibilities to others. Among the poor and working classes, other female family members (e.g., older siblings, grandmothers, aunts, and cousins) often participate in childcare activities. Middle-class and upper-class families hire live-in or daytime nannies or maids who take on childcare and household duties, regardless of whether the mother is employed outside the home. Childcare and household responsibilities may overwhelm Brazilian immigrants who do not have access to the support of extended family, paid domestic help, or both.

## Middle Age

### Cultural Attitudes and Expectations

Women are the principal family caregivers, and middle-aged women have an important role in kin-based social networks. Most Brazilians welcome the role of grandmother, which affords them a certain positive social status. Unmarried adult children frequently continue to live with their parents. Visitation by married children and grandchildren is a common practice, particularly on weekends. The concepts of "empty nest syndrome" and "midlife crisis" are not relevant in this population.

### Menopause

The age at menopause varies, but the average is between 49 and 50 years. Women generally regard menopause as a natural function of aging. It is of little concern to many women; some view it as a welcome reprieve from the worry of unwanted pregnancy. Women may express concerns related to menstrual irregularity, increased menstrual flow, nervousness, headaches, and hot flashes. The first choice of treatment may be herbal or homeopathic remedies. Brazilian physicians do prescribe hormone replacement therapy (HRT), although long-term use by women is not widespread. Sexual practices vary among postmenopausal women.

# Old Age

In 1999, the life expectancy at birth for Brazilian females was 71.2, compared with 64.8 for males. Older women usually remain at home, and their social contacts revolve around family. They are respected and may be seen as a source of wisdom or counseling. Adult children are expected to provide both economic security and social companionship for parents in old age. It is rare for an older woman to live alone; widowed or single older women usually have live-in domestic help or live with family. Most Brazilian immigrants retain the cultural preference for home care rather than institutionalization or nursing home care.

# Death and Dying

## Cultural Attitudes and Beliefs

If a loved one is dying from a chronic disease, families may prefer to have the patient remain at home. The family may not accept hospice care if it requires denial of aggressive therapeutic measures, however, because of not wanting to "give up hope."

Grief is often accompanied by the belief that an unexpected death, such as that of a child, was "God's will."

## Rites and Rituals

In Brazil, bodies are not embalmed, and burial takes place within 24 hours. Wakes are held in funeral chapels at the hospital or cemetery. Open expressions of grief, such as crying, are common. Family and friends maintain a constant vigil by the open casket until the time of burial. Final good-byes may involve kissing and caressing the body and perhaps taking a photograph. Organ donation and autopsy are not common practices.

---

**NOTE TO THE HEALTH CARE PROVIDER**
When dealing with the death of a relative or friend, Brazilian immigrants may not be familiar with U.S. hospital and mortuary procedures. They require a careful explanation of the available options as well as expected practices. Providers should offer support and the opportunity to ask questions and explore alternative options.

---

## Mourning

In modern Brazilian society, the traditional mourning practices **(luto)** are rarely practiced. Catholics celebrate mass in honor of the deceased on the 7th day, one month, and yearly anniversaries of death. Family members may make regular visits to the cemetery; annual visits occur on November 1, the Day of the Dead **(Dia dos Mortos).** The bereaved may wear black, but it depends on age and relationship to the deceased. Some families hang a photograph of the deceased near a household altar. On the anniversary of the death, the deceased may be honored at home and church.

Extended family is the primary source of support for women in mourning. It is generally expected that women will need time to put their lives together following the death of a child or spouse. Women who are employed may want to take an extended leave.

## The Medical Intake

### Literacy and English Proficiency

The level of English fluency in immigrants varies widely; recent immigrants, particularly those of lower socioeconomic class, may have very limited comprehension and speaking ability. Family members or friends may accompany a woman to provide support and assistance with English. Spanish-speaking interpreters are of limited use.

### Status of the Provider

Among Brazilian women, interpersonal contact is generally easy and warm, personal space is quite close, and women often touch each other's clothing while conversing. Kissing on the cheek is part of greetings and farewells. Contacts with professionals, however, are usually more formal. Handshakes between provider and patient are appropriate, both in greeting and saying goodbye. In addressing a person of higher status, a lower-class woman may use the title "doctor" **(doutor/doutora)** as an expression of social deference and respect. She may also avoid direct eye contact with health professionals.

---

**NOTE TO THE HEALTH CARE PROVIDER**

Providers need to be careful about nonverbal communication that Brazilians might misinterpret. For example, they need to avoid making the American sign for "OK" (making an "O" with thumb and forefinger), which is an obscene gesture for Brazilians. An appropriate nonverbal sign for "all is well" is "thumbs up."

---

### Communicating Illness and Symptoms

Clients may associate the onset of acute physical illnesses with physical activity, temperature changes, food ingestion, or strong emotions. Brazilian women are generally considered to be more tolerant of pain **(dor)** than are men. They usually describe pain in terms of location and intensity; providers must not assume that patients will be familiar with or understand a numerical pain scale.

Including an assessment of emotional status is important. Folk syndromes known as **nervos** (nerves), **ataque de nervos** (nerve attacks), **mal olhado** (evil-eye), **peito aberto** (open chest) and **susto** (shock sickness) are associated with suppression of strong negative emotions such as anger **(raiva)**, fear **(medo)**, envy **(enveja)**, worry **(preocupação)**, sadness **(tristeza)**, or grief **(pena, luto)**. Physical symptoms, such as bruises, headaches, trembling, or limping, may be perceived as evidence of women's suppression of these strong emotions, colloquially referred to as "swallowing frogs" **(engolir sapos)**.

Providers should inquire about liver function and self-medication for liver problems, because Brazilians tend to attribute gastrointestinal symptoms to liver dysfunction **(doença de fígado).**

## The Physical Examination

Young girls and older women tend to be modest and may prefer female practitioners. No cultural restrictions are placed on male providers, although some women (or their husbands) may prefer that they see female providers. There are no particular restrictions or taboos related to the physical examination, although the provider should make sure to appropriately cover the woman at all times.

## Prescribing Medications

### Drug Interactions

Health providers should realize that professional health care is rarely the first line of care and many Brazilians self-medicate. Most medications, including antibiotics, contraceptives, antidepressants, and analgesics, are sold at Brazilian pharmacies without prescriptions. Immigrants often bring these medications with them or obtain them through Brazilian social networks. Homeopathic remedies, medicinal herbs, acupuncture, aromatherapy, and spiritual healing are also widely used, often in conjunction with allopathic medicine. Herbal teas are regularly used for common ailments such as colds, influenza, or gastroenteritis, and they can interact with allopathic medicines.

### Medication Sharing

Brazilians may seek advice from family and friends first; women freely share their knowledge, experiences, and prescription drugs and folk remedies with others, particularly when they have found the treatments to have helped. Regardless of whether a woman has used home remedies or treatments, she expects prescribed medications when she consults a medical doctor.

---

**NOTE TO THE HEALTH CARE PROVIDER**
Providers should ask, in a polite and nonjudgmental manner, what home remedies, Brazilian medications, or alternative therapies the woman is using. They should explain the potential dangers of drug interactions and the importance of completing a course of antibiotics or other treatment regimen.

---

Many Brazilians do not consider over-the-counter analgesics (e.g., aspirin, acetaminophen) to be effective pain medications. The belief by some Brazilian immigrants that U.S. providers "only prescribe Tylenol" for pain is one reason why they often will rely on medications from home.

### Compliance

Brazilians have a strong respect for "doctors' orders," which contributes to adherence to medical advice. Explicit instructions may also improve adherence.

## Follow-up Appointments

Clients may not understand the necessity or advisability of coming to follow-up appointments; they also may miss appointments because of economic or time constraints. They often receive phone reminders well, perceiving them as a positive "personal" touch.

Time is subordinate to personal and social relationships. Brazilians do not follow clock time in social situations and expect guests to arrive after the appointed hour. Social events are usually open-ended, without a predetermined time for guests to leave. Punctuality is an expectation for employment, however. Most immigrants arrive on time for health care appointments.

## Prevalent Diseases

Cardiovascular disease is the major cause of mortality among Brazilians. Breast and cervical cancer are the major causes of cancer death in Brazil. North and Northeast Brazil have the highest incidence of cervical cancer in the world, yet 40% of Brazilian women between ages 35 and 49 years have reportedly never had a Papanicolaou (Pap) test. The high incidence of breast cancer in some regions of Brazil is comparable to other regions of high incidence such as the United States and some European countries.

Infectious diseases, including malaria, tuberculosis, viral hepatitis, HIV/AIDS, Chagas' disease, and dengue fever, are significant sources of morbidity. Sickle-cell anemia is prevalent among blacks. Neurotic disorders, especially anxiety and phobias, are the most prevalent mental illnesses.

## Health-Seeking Behaviors

Brazilian women utilize health care facilities more than men, especially during the reproductive period, with use decreasing sharply after age 60 years. They consult medical professionals primarily for treatment of existing illness rather than for health promotion or prevention. They may be reluctant to seek screening when no symptoms are present because of fear of uncovering disease or not wanting to face "bad news." In illnesses that require hospitalization, family members may want to have someone stay with the patient in the hospital.

Brazilian women may be unaware of nurses in health education and advanced practice. Professional nurses comprise only a minority of the Brazilian nursing workforce, and people of that country often consider nursing a "second-class" health care profession. However, within the Brazilian public health force, nurses and midwives perform vaginal examinations and Pap smears and provide comprehensive prenatal care. Many, if not most, middle-class Brazilians as a rule use the private health sector rather than the public health sector for their personal health care.

Women are often comfortable combining medical treatment with folk traditions in health, healing, and religion. Herbal and medicinal teas are one of the mainstays of Brazilian folk medicine, particularly for gastric symptoms such as indigestion, heartburn, or diarrhea. Traditionally, medicinal teas were made at home from ingredients such as lemon grass (*cidreira, capim santo*), orange rind (*casca de laranja*), guava flowers (*a guía da goiaba*), cinnamon leaves (*canela*), nutmeg (*noz moscado*), garlic (*alho*), and ginger (*gingibre*). Because many urban Brazilians lack access to a home herb garden, the use of commercially available herbal teas, such as chamomile **(camomila)**, boldo, and anise **(erva doce)** is increasingly common. Among those from the Amazon region, folk medicines include various indigenous plant oils, such as *copaíba* and *andiroba*, used for inflammations and wound healing.

Belief in miracles, miracle cures, and faith healings is prevalent. Parapsychology, spirit mediumship and spiritual or faith healings are part of popular Catholic and spiritist religions. Pentacostal believers may include exorcism as part of their healing strategies. Spiritists practice laying on of hands **(passes)**; blessings and prayers by folk healers **(benzedeiras, curandeiras)** are often given in conjunction with herbal remedies. Catholic faith healers **(rezadeiras** or **rezadores)** use prayers, rituals, advice, herbs, and pharmaceuticals in their treatment of common ailments. Antisorcery rituals and consultations with spirit guides are part of **Umbandista** healing practices.

Lack of information, assumptions, and misinformation about North American health care systems, in addition to economic and time constraints, contribute to Brazilian immigrants' putting their health "on hold." As a result of an "I'll take care of this when I return home" attitude, immigrants may delay seeking care from health care professionals or may seek it only in emergencies. Women frequently first seek the advice of family members or friends regarding health or illness issues or they talk informally with a family member, friend, landlord, acquaintance, or employer who is a health care professional prior to taking action to seek formal health care. Thus, seeking formal health care signifies acknowledgment of a significant or urgent health or illness concern that warrants attention by a professional.

## ⊕ BIBLIOGRAPHY

Barbosa, R. M., do Lago, T. G., Kalckman, S., & Villela, W. V. (1996). Sexuality and reproductive health care in São Paulo, Brazil. *Health Care of Women International*, 17(5), 413–421.

Giffin, K. (1994). Women's health and the privatization of fertility control in Brazil. *Social Science and Medicine*, 39(3), 355–360.

Hopkins, K. (2000). Are Brazilian women really choosing to deliver by cesarean? *Social Science and Medicine*, 51(5), 725–40.

Margolis, M. L. (1994). *Little Brazil: An ethnography of Brazilian immigrants in New York City*. Princeton, NJ: Princeton University Press.

Messias, D. K. H. (in review). Transnational health perspectives, practices and resources: Brazilian immigrant women's narratives.

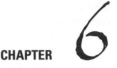

# Cambodians

## JUDITH C. KULIG, DNSc, RN

### 🌐 INTRODUCTION

#### Who are the Cambodian People?

The Cambodian, or Khmer, people are from what is now known as the State of Cambodia (SOC). During the civil war, the country was referred to as Kampuchea; nationalist Cambodians do not prefer this name. Historically, the SOC was more influenced by India than by other Asian countries; for example, Khmer, the Cambodian language, is based on Sanskrit.

At one time the SOC was a protectorate of France. Intermarriages occurred between upper-class Cambodians and French individuals affiliated with the government. Thus, some Cambodians speak French. A small number of minority tribal groups maintain their own languages.

#### Cambodians in North America

The arrival of Cambodians in North America began in the middle to late 1970s. The Vietnamese conflict spilled over into Cambodia at the same time the country was in the midst of a civil war. The educated were often killed outright, while the more agrarian Cambodians were forced into becoming laborers for rebuilding the country. Common estimates are that up to one million Cambodians were tortured and died. Others escaped into Thailand or Malaysia and lived in refugee camps during the period from 1978 to 1988.

As of 1998, the number of Cambodians living in the United States was estimated to be 168,863, most of whom live on the West Coast, particularly Stockton and Oakland, California. Cambodian communities also are found in New York, Texas, and Minnesota. According to the 1996 census, about 21,435 Cambodians live in Canada, of whom 55% are women. Most live in Montreal, followed by Toronto, Vancouver, and Edmonton.

Well-educated professionals arrived first (as early as 1977), followed by individuals and families who had spent up to 10 years in refugee camps in Thailand or Malaysia. Many Cambodian refugees in North America have suffered greatly from loss and the brutality of life around them throughout the war years and as a result have both physical and mental health problems. For example, headaches are caused from injuries related to shovel blows in the labor camps. Many Cambodians suffer from posttraumatic stress syndrome as a result of the loss of numerous family members and having witnessed torture and killings. When Cambodian refugees who were familiar only with village or camp life relocated to North America, they lacked the life skills and knowledge necessary for living in technologically, fast-paced countries. Resettlement workers invested considerable time and effort in helping Cambodians to learn the basics of purchasing groceries, understanding modern transportation systems, and securing employment.

Since the return of a more stable government to the SOC, Cambodians have been able to return and visit their homeland and family members. Younger Cambodians are fluent in spoken and written English and will act as interpreters for their elders.

## 🌏 BEING FEMALE IN CAMBODIAN SOCIETY

This culture regards women positively. The social class structure within Cambodian society influences the number and type of roles that women hold. Women are wives and mothers, and wives are expected to maintain household budgets. They also routinely contribute to family income through farming or gardening and have businesses in which they sell such articles as silk and jewelry. Women continue to be obligated to care for and maintain immediate and extended families. Thus, the women hold multiple roles and are expected to simultaneously assist elderly parents and their children and grandchildren. Stress from such role overload is not uncommon.

Since arrival in North America, some Cambodian women have added other roles, such as taking advantage of educational opportunities and employment in specific fields. Most Cambodian women, however, work for minimal wages in factories or similar establishments.

Being female is also influenced by Buddhism, which includes an elaborate series of celebrations and events throughout the year. Women mainly prepare food and appropriate clothing, but they also organize the events, accept prayer money, and are **yiey chii** (Buddhist nuns). In North America, however, a number of Cambodians have accepted Christianity, so Buddhism is not the only religious influence.

## At Birth

### Preference for Sons

There is no outright preference for sons. Women who do not bear sons are still treated with respect by their husbands and the community. All children are welcomed and cherished, which may also be related to Cambodians' loss of so many family members during the war years.

### Birth Rituals

No specific birth rituals are observed for either gender, but baby showers are routinely held to celebrate a new baby's arrival. The shower is family-based and includes both men and women. Food is cooked and shared, and gifts are presented to the couple for their new child.

# Childhood and Youth

### Stages

In the Khmer language, children are referred to generally as **kone**. There are five loosely set developmental stages for girls: baby, child, premenstrual, menstrual, and young adulthood. Boys have but one child stage. Young women and men are expected to be ready to marry and have families of their own by their late teens or early 20s.

### Family Expectations

Girls as young as 7 years are expected to watch over their younger siblings or cousins. Girls also learn from an early age (8 to 10 years) about such domestic activities as cooking and cleaning. These expectations do not apply to boys. It is not uncommon, however, for young men to help their wives with domestic tasks.

### Social Expectations

Overall, girls are expected to become good wives and mothers. In adolescence, a girl is expected to demonstrate such desirable behaviors as speaking in a soft and low tone, walking with minimal noise, and respecting elders.

### Importance of Education

Education in Cambodia was restricted to the upper classes, and boys and men received more education than women. Consequently, some older Cambodian women cannot read and write in Khmer. In North America, despite opportunities for Cambodian girls and women to attend postsecondary schools, the number taking advantage of these opportunities remains low compared with other Asian groups.

## Pubescence

### Psychosexual Development

Historically, most girls reached puberty at 15 or 16 years of age. In North America, this age has decreased to about 14 years. Boys and girls reach puberty at about the same time. Menstruation and sexuality are not discussed among Cambodians, although older women will make jokes about sex and menstruation.

### Rituals and Rites of Passage

Historically, an elaborate ceremony called **coul mlop** was held to signify a girl's transition to womanhood. The ceremony includes such activities as the girl stepping on three steps to her parents' home to ensure that her menstrual period lasts only three days and sharing of food.

This ceremony is not practiced in North America. As recently as the late 1980s, however, young girls were still taught how to prevent "love magic" (the power of a young man to influence a girl's or woman's emotions) to ensure that their virginity is not lost before marriage. To guard against love magic, the young woman takes a dried piece of her used menstrual cloth, sews it into a small bag, attaches it to a string, and wears it around her waist. The power of the menstrual blood combined with the circular string (which symbolizes keeping the emotions safe from men) protects her from love magic. All women who adhere to this practice continue to wear the bag even if they are menopausal.

### Teen Sexuality

**Social Restrictions and Pressures.** When girls begin to mature, their families become concerned about the girls' potential to act inappropriately, that is, to become sexually active. Sexual activity causes family shame; accordingly, girls' activities are increasingly restricted. If a girl and her family are shamed, it will be difficult to ensure that she will marry well.

**Teen Pregnancy.** Dating is often done secretly, and teen sexual activity is not acceptable. Teen pregnancy is considered shameful for both the girl and her family. Some families prefer their daughter to marry young, without completing school, rather than take the risk that she may become pregnant before marriage. There is less criticism of boys' premarital sexual behavior.

### Menstruation

**Relationship to Health.** Cambodian women believe that a good menstrual flow is important for their health, and they expect to have monthly periods. They are concerned about passing blood clots, however, and may take traditional medicines to ensure that they have a "clean flow." Menstrual blood is considered powerful. For example, if a husband commits adultery, the wife may secretly give him a glass of water containing a few drops of her menstrual blood in an effort to stop such behavior.

**Relationship to Fertility.** Not all Cambodian women understand the association of menstruation with fertility. Hence, they will not consider some types of contraception because their effectiveness is unclear.

**Taboos and Restrictions During Menstruation.** No restrictions are placed on a menstruating woman except that she should not participate in activities that may lead to an embarrassing situation, such as swimming. She is also expected to exercise care when sitting in the traditional way (squatting) so that "nothing" (e.g., pad or menstrual blood) shows. Sexual activity is avoided during menstruation.

**Dysmenorrhea.** Cambodians use the term "stuck blood" to refer to difficulties with menstruation such as missed periods, passing clots, and light periods. This condition is seen as being undesirable and possibly leading to the woman's overall poor health. These women take traditional medicines to alleviate stuck blood. Painful menstruation is not a great concern among Cambodian women.

### Female Modesty and Touching

Female modesty is very important to Cambodian women, and women should not expose their bodies. Modesty is intertwined with sexuality. A woman should not overtly display sexuality, but she should be feminine (very ladylike). Adolescent boys cannot touch girls. Married couples touch each other, but it is less apparent than in mainstream American or Canadian cultures.

**Relationship to Health Care.** Cambodian women visit male practitioners; but their comfort level varies, depending on their age and acculturation to North American society. Pelvic examinations will likely be a concern to both older and younger women.

## Adulthood

### Transition Rites and Rituals

Traditionally, a young woman was considered an adult when she got married. Now, however, with the age of marriage at times delayed, some young women are considered adults when they can be responsible for themselves in terms of completing their education or holding a job. There are no specific rituals for either young women or men to mark the transition to adulthood.

### Social Expectations

It is more acceptable for upper-class women to delay marriage and pursue education and employment than it is for people of the lower classes. Ultimately, all women are expected to marry and have children.

### Union Formation

**Union Types.**   Historically, marriages were arranged in Cambodian society. Although such arrangements are now less common, it is still expected that a representative from the man's family will discuss a potential marriage with someone from the woman's family. There are some common-law arrangements, but they are not viewed positively. Interracial marriages with Caucasian or Hispanic individuals also occur; family and community members view them with mixed feelings.

**Social Sanctions for Failing to Enter into Union.**   There are pressures to marry because of concern about pregnancy before wedlock. Most women expect to be married by their mid-20s. Although an unmarried woman is not looked down on, she is viewed with concern related to who will look after her and whether she will be lonely.

### Domestic Violence

Domestic violence is not acceptable in Cambodian society since women are to be treated with respect. When abuse does occur, however, the woman is justified in divorcing her husband. It is unlikely that an abused Cambodian woman will seek assistance from the authorities. Instead, she will seek the advice and help of her mother, sisters, and female friends. There are no safe houses (shelters) specifically for Cambodian women. Although they can use other safe houses, where available, it is unlikely that Cambodian women will do so because domestic violence is the type of family problem that should be kept within the family unit.

### Rape

The incidence of rape is unknown among this culture, but historical documents suggest that it was not common. The protection of a woman's sexuality is paramount among Cambodians; hence, rape is considered a horrendous crime. Depending on the circumstances, there may be questions about the woman's role in a rape, but she usually is not considered directly responsible for it. Women do not openly share their experience of rape with people outside the family because of the shame and concern it causes. Recent Cambodian immigrant and refugee women living in the United States are also unlikely to report this sexual crime.

### Divorce

**Sociocultural Views.**   The social view of a divorce depends on the reasons for it. A woman can legitimately divorce a man who interferes with the household budget. Another legitimate reason for divorce is the husband's taking a "second wife" (e.g., he has an affair with another woman or literally takes a second wife). Otherwise, divorce is disfavored in Cambodian society.

**Women and Divorce.**   Until the community determines the reason for the divorce, it will treat a divorced woman with caution. If there is any question that she was sexually unfaithful during her marriage, the community will treat her with disrespect.

**Child Custody Practices.**   In the context of trauma and flight in Cambodia and the harsh conditions in refugee camps, some young Cambodian men have not taken responsibility for their children and, hence, have abandoned them. This behavior may be attributable to their experiences in the war years and the loss of parents and adults to guide them. An ex-husband is nonetheless expected to assist financially with his children.

### Fertility and Childbearing

**Family Size.**   Historically, upper-class families had two or three children. In other families, the number of children ranged from five to nine. The war, however, influenced family size, as all families lost members to starvation, hard work, or torture. Women also ceased having normal menses because of poor nutrition. When families moved to refugee camps in Thailand and their nutritional status improved, women could conceive again, and there was a baby boom that was perceived as a replacement of the children lost in Cambodia.

After resettlement in North America, families realized that they could not afford so many children, and family size decreased. Today, young couples in North America may commit to having only two or three children.

**Contraceptive Practices.** Since resettlement, women have more options for contraception than they did previously. In Cambodia, village women neither had access to family planning nor did they understand their body's fertility cycle or that they could conceive on a monthly basis. Even upper-class women did not usually use contraception.

Some types of contraception are less acceptable than others because of the manner in which they are used. For example, diaphragms require being familiar and comfortable with one's body, which is not always true of Cambodian women. If a woman is concerned about "stuck blood," methods that exacerbate it will also be unacceptable. Condoms are often associated with men's use of prostitutes. There have also been rumors that tubal ligations release passion in women, after which they cannot control their passion and have sexual intercourse with multiple men.

---

**NOTE TO THE HEALTH CARE PROVIDER**
Prescribing contraception for teenage girls is a potential source of cultural conflict. When educating about contraceptive methods, simple, jargon-free language is best. Drawings can be helpful as long as they are simple. Practitioners should be aware of the meanings attributed to different types of contraception. They should explain different methods using the traditional beliefs of the Cambodian people (e.g., Cambodian women believe that to become pregnant, they need to be in a cool state). They can use this basic premise to explain the birth control pill as increasing the heat in the body to prevent conception.

---

**Role of the Male in the Couple's Fertility Decision-Making.** The male has less say than the woman in deciding the type of contraception to be used. In many marriages, it is also the wife's decision when to have children.

Abortion

**Cultural Attitudes.** Historically, women did not view a missed period as the early stages of pregnancy but instead conceptualized it as a late period. Hence, actions could be taken to "help the period come." Village women sought an abortion from a *kru khmer* (Cambodian healer), who prepared a mixture that would cause an abortion. Since resettlement in North America, women have relied on abortion as another form of birth control. They were overwhelmed by the horrors of war and the loss of family members, lacked understanding of their bodies and fertility cycles, found few contraception methods acceptable, and could not financially or emotionally deal with many children. Abortion was seen as a reasonable option. However, some families consider abortion unacceptable because of their Buddhist beliefs. Such beliefs are that abortion negatively affects one's karma and thus negatively influences one's future lives.

**Sources of Abortions.**    In Cambodia, abortions per se were not performed, although women were given hormone injections to "help the period come" and abort a fetus in a socially acceptable manner. Village women sought help from a kru khmer; but these healers are hard to find in North America, and now there is less use of traditional medicines and treatments. Most abortions in North America are obtained in the same settings that other women use. Cambodian born-again Christians do not accept abortion as an alternative.

**Complications.**    Abortions are sought early in pregnancy. Thus, there are fewer complications. There is no available information on complications related to abortions in the SOC.

---

**NOTE TO THE HEALTH CARE PROVIDER**

Asking about the woman's religious beliefs is important. If she is Buddhist or a born-again Christian, she may find the suggestion of an abortion unacceptable and upsetting.

---

### Miscarriage

There are no particular beliefs regarding miscarriages. In any event, they seem to be relatively rare among Cambodian women.

### Infertility

Although there is little information about infertility, generally speaking it is relatively uncommon in Cambodian women. When it does occur, however, the woman is not blamed.

---

**NOTE TO THE HEALTH CARE PROVIDER**

There is no known cultural conflict with fertility treatments, but the cost may be prohibitive for Cambodian women.

---

### Pregnancy

**Activity Restrictions and Taboos.**    During pregnancy, women use preventive behaviors to avoid miscarriage, particularly activity restrictions. They include avoiding walking fast, carrying heavy objects, working too hard, and eating or drinking hot substances. It is believed that if the mother reaches too high, the umbilical cord can break and the fetus will lose its supply of nourishment. Women may avoid showering or bathing late at night because they believe that these activities can lead to having a large infant. Sitting in a doorway can result in the infant becoming stuck in the vagina during delivery. Sexual activity in the last months of pregnancy is believed to thicken the amniotic fluid, leading to respiratory distress in the fetus. Similarly, vernix is believed to be sperm; women ingest a liquid to avoid a baby with vernix.

If a woman falls during pregnancy, it is believed that the fetus can be born with malformations. Other problems with the fetus are attributed to beliefs in reincarnation. For example, one who acted improperly in his or her past life can be born with a defect, such as a missing finger or hand. Birthmarks are believed to be from soot or red coloring that had been placed on the body at death, thereby allowing relatives to recognize the individual during a subsequent life.

**Dietary Practices and Observances.**   Women avoid foods (such as red peppers) that can cause excess heat in the body to prevent miscarriage. Maternal nutrition is seen as being vital to the birth of a healthy infant. Some women believe that the fetus sucks on the placenta for nourishment. Medicines such as coconut milk or a drink prepared from a tree root or bark is ingested to ensure a short and easy labor.

**Prenatal Care.**   Historically, midwives and the woman's own female family members provided prenatal care. Today, Cambodian women access mainstream health resources for their care during pregnancy at much the same time that other women do.

---

**NOTE TO THE HEALTH CARE PROVIDER**
Women may ingest herbal or traditional medicines during pregnancy. These medicines may interact with medicines prescribed by health practitioners.

---

## Birthing Process

In Cambodia, most deliveries occurred at home; few women had access to a hospital. In North America, women deliver in hospitals. They generally do not have their male partners present. There is a preference for vaginal deliveries, but cesarean sections are also accepted. If female relatives are present, they are expected to support and encourage the birthing woman. Women are quiet and sedate during labor and delivery. There are no specific practices for the placenta.

---

**NOTE TO THE HEALTH CARE PROVIDER**
Women may refuse pain medication even when they actually need it. Providers should encourage it when needed.

---

## Postpartum

A new mother is supposed to rest for several weeks after the birth. Her mother and mother-in-law prepare meals, help care for the baby, and provide advice. The new mother is advised to wear warm clothing and ingest foods and drinks to regain her body's balance. During delivery, she loses "heat" and is in a cool state during the postpartum period. The drinks are prepared during the last six weeks of pregnancy and include herbal mixtures or pieces of porcupine stomach placed in about 960 mL of white wine to soak. After the baby is born, 15 to 30 mL of this mixture are ingested up to four times each day. If the heat is not regained, the mother is believed to expect such health problems as arthritis during menopause.

---

**NOTE TO THE HEALTH CARE PROVIDER**
A new mother may be required to take the advice of her mother and mother-in-law during this phase even though it conflicts with her own knowledge or advice from the health provider. If her mother died during or after the war, she may find it difficult to learn such practices and potentially requires more attention and intervention in collaboration with the practitioner. Do not be overly concerned about her ingestion of wine since the amount is rarely excessive.

---

### Newborn and Infant Care

**Breastfeeding Versus Bottle-Feeding.** Bottle-feeding became the preferred method after Cambodians immigrated to North America. Many women believed that Western women do not breastfeed; consequently, some imitate them to be "modern" and may not be aware of the positive health effects of breastfeeding. It is not uncommon to feed infants "rice soup" (rice overcooked with water; it has a sticky consistency) as early as 3 to 4 months of age.

**Infant Protection.** Some families use such traditional practices as herbal drinks and coining (rubbing the infant on the upper back and chest with a warmed coin to release excess heat in the body). Families immunize their infants. An infant may wear an amulet, a small container holding a blessing in Pali script, on a chain around the neck to keep it from harm and ensure good health.

The mother is the primary caregiver, although some fathers are also involved in childcare. Extended family members also assist in the care and upbringing of children. Cambodian infants are held down and away from the mother's body. Cambodians show affection to their infants by sniffing them in an affectionate manner.

---

**NOTE TO THE HEALTH CARE PROVIDER**
Practitioners should not assume that maternal-infant bonding is not occurring because of the way the mother holds her infant.

---

## Middle Age

### Cultural Attitudes and Expectations

Women are considered middle-aged in their 40s. They are expected to dress more conservatively and be less concerned about their physical appearance than when they were younger.

### Psychological Response

Cambodian children are not expected to leave their parents' home as early as mainstream North American children do; hence, dealing with the "empty nest" syndrome is less important in this population. The notion of a midlife crisis is not a part of Cambodian culture.

### Menopause

Menopause normally occurs in the late 40s to early 50s. Women still have sexual relations with their husbands. Some women welcome menopause because it allows them to become **yiey chii** (Buddhist nuns) and live in the **wat** (temple) on a routine basis. In Buddhism, it is not uncommon for women to follow this practice because it is an opportunity to enhance their religious beliefs. Postmenopausal women are considered to have less power because they no longer have menstrual blood, a powerful substance.

In Cambodia, postmenopausal women were relieved of domestic and child-care duties, and their children and grandchildren cared for them. In North America, opportunities for older women to relax in this way are fewer. For financial reasons, many women must work outside the home or take care of grandchildren while their children work. Thus, they cannot realize the status and roles that should come with middle life.

---

**NOTE TO THE HEALTH CARE PROVIDER**

A postmenopausal Cambodian woman may experience depression or other psychological symptoms, because she cannot fulfill the traditional role of an older Cambodian woman and there are few opportunities for her to become a nun and live in the temple.

---

# Old Age

Women older than age 60 are considered old. Elderly women are respected and addressed with specific titles to display that respect. They are thought to be sources of wisdom, although their experiences may not be considered useful or relevant to young Cambodians who have lived predominantly in North America. Elderly women live with relatives who care for them until they die or can no longer be managed in the relatives' home.

# Death and Dying

## Cultural Attitudes and Beliefs

Cambodians are primarily Theravada Buddhists, but they also practice a combination of animism and Christianity. Their beliefs and practices regarding death and dying vary depending on their adherence to these different beliefs. Cambodians who practice Theravada Buddhism and believe in reincarnation perceive that dying relatives will have additional lives in the future.

## Rites and Rituals

Buddhist monks and the **accha** (Cambodian layperson) may be present at a dying person's bed. Incense may be burned. Prayers may be recited after the person has died. The family is expected to wait quietly for the death of their relative. There are no gender-based differences in practices regarding death.

## Mourning

Community prayer rituals are held at different periods following an individual's death (e.g., 30 or 365 days). The formal mourning period lasts for several months after the death. Family members are expected to accept the death with stoicism. If a mother dies, the husband is expected to continue to care for the children with the help of extended family members.

---

**NOTE TO THE HEALTH CARE PROVIDER**

Practitioners should inquire whether a woman has family support during this time of mourning and ensure that the woman is caring for herself.

---

 IMPORTANT POINTS FOR PROVIDERS CARING FOR CAMBODIAN WOMEN

## The Medical Intake

### Literacy and English Proficiency

Older Cambodian women are likely to be illiterate in both English and the written version of Khmer. Family members commonly assist with interpretation and completing medical forms.

### Status of the Provider

Health providers are automatically given respect because of their perceived higher status. Direct eye contact is not generally acceptable and, hence, is not acceptable with health providers. Women tend to be passive and quiet when interacting with health providers. Cambodians often use indirect communication, such as asking questions or making requests in vague terms. It is not "polite" to say "no" directly, so these women may indicate "no" by failing to respond, changing the subject, or even saying "no problem."

### Communicating Illness and Symptoms

Cambodians are not always comfortable discussing traditional treatments or medicines because of lack of their acceptance by mainstream society. The provider should routinely ask whether the client is using any home remedies or drinks that elders have suggested. In general, patients will answer questions in short, abbreviated form rather than providing lengthy explanations. Some illnesses may be attributed to hexes or love magic, but the treatment of these illnesses depends entirely on traditional means and is therefore unlikely to be discussed with health practitioners. Family members, such as the husband or a sister, tend to be involved in the care of female clients and can provide assistance to the practitioner in understanding the situation.

---

**NOTE TO THE HEALTH CARE PROVIDER**

Practitioners need to remember to ask all questions about sexuality sensitively. Forthright questions about sexual behavior and activities are likely to be considered offensive.

---

## The Physical Examination

### Modesty and Touching

Cambodian women are modest and shy and expect to have their bodies covered during physical examinations. Talking to the woman during the examination is important, as is explaining what is being done and why. It is more appropriate for a woman to see a female health practitioner, but she will see a male health provider if necessary. Touching the head is not appropriate at any time for either gender because it is believed that a person's soul is found there. Touching elsewhere is acceptable but not commonly done.

### Expressing Pain

All Cambodians, female or male, are expected to withhold their reaction to pain and be stoic and quiet. Complaining about physical symptoms is not acceptable in this group.

## Prescribing Medications

### Drug Interaction

The health care practitioner should ask the client whether she takes traditional medicines and advise her that there may be an undesirable interaction with prescribed drugs. Use of a translator is apt to be necessary, since elderly clients are more inclined to use such medicines.

### Medication Sharing

Medication sharing is common. It is important to talk with the client about the importance of finishing the full course of prescribed medication and not giving any of it to others.

### Compliance

Education about the importance of the medication and the manner in which it works is essential if compliance is expected. It is helpful to relate how the medication works in the context of how traditional medicines work. For example, because "coining" (rubbing an infant on the upper back and chest with a warmed coin to release excess heat in the body) is believed to release heat, acetaminophen can be described as also releasing heat.

## Follow-up Appointments

Reminders about follow-up appointments are helpful. Missing appointments may be related to a lack of transportation or assistance in getting to the health facility. Otherwise, Cambodians tend to be compliant and anxious to please such authority figures as health practitioners.

Elderly Cambodians in particular tend to be past-oriented. Cambodians generally subscribe to social time and are not especially concerned with punctuality. They are becoming more westernized and, hence, are more likely to be on time for appointments, but they still tend not to differentiate time between social time and appointment or business time. People can be up to one hour late, even for a party.

## Prevalent Diseases

A number of Cambodians suffer from mental health symptoms and illnesses (e.g., posttraumatic stress disorder) because of their experiences during the war years. They may not be inclined to seek assistance for these problems, however, and Western psychiatric approaches are often ineffective. Diabetes and cardiac problems are also becoming much more prevalent in North American Cambodians because of dietary changes; hepatitis B is common.

## Health-Seeking Behaviors

Many Cambodian families try traditional treatments before seeking professional health advice. Cambodian healers (kru khmer) are not common in North America, but some of them are still practicing. Seeing these healers provides psychological comfort to the ill individual and family. Husbands and wives may decide together to seek care. Once they have sought professional advice, Cambodians trust their health practitioners and usually adhere to their suggestions.

As Cambodian women have become more accustomed to health care in North America, they have been more amenable to accepting health prevention activities such as breast self-examination, blood pressure screening, and annual check-ups.

## BIBLIOGRAPHY

Becker, E. (1986). *When the war was over: Cambodian's revolution and the voices of its people.* New York: Simon & Shuster.

Kulig, J. (1995). Cambodian refugees' family planning knowledge & use. *Journal of Advanced Nursing,* 22, 150–157.

Kulig, J. (1994). "Those with Unheard Voices:" the plight of a Cambodian refugee woman. *Journal of Community Health Nursing,* 11(2), 99–107.

Kulig, J. (1994). Sexuality beliefs among Cambodians: implications to health care professionals (1994). *Health Care for Women International,* 15, 69–76.

Ngor, H. (1987). A *Cambodian odyssey.* New York: Warner Books.

# Chinese

## BETTY L. CHANG, DNSc, RN, FNP-C, FAAN, and LIN ZHAN, PhD, RN

### 🌐 INTRODUCTION

## Who are the Chinese People?

The Chinese culture is one of the oldest recorded, from around 2200 B.C. to the present People's Republic of China. The Chinese consider the country and its people to be the center of the world (China, or **Zhong Guo,** translates literally to "center of the world"). The values and beliefs of the Chinese people are based on the teachings of Confucius, who promoted the importance of education, the family, and a harmonious community. Religion plays a less important role in the Chinese culture than in other cultures, although people of older generations believe in Buddhism. Christianity, however, has made significant inroads in the cities during several periods of Chinese history.

China is more than 3.7 million square miles, roughly the same size as the United States. The majority of Chinese people are Han; about 10% are minorities, such as the Miao, Dai, Tu, and Yi ethnic groups. Most minorities are located in the poorer Western areas of China and do not immigrate. Although the national language is **pu tong hua** ("the common language"), the main dialect spoken in the southeastern part of China is Cantonese **(Guangdong hua)**. Each city and county has its own dialect and local idioms, which can make comprehension difficult for outsiders. The written language is the same for most of the country. Some minority ethnic groups also have their own written language.

Some useful Chinese phrases in Mandarin are "how are you" **(ni hao),** "please" **(please),** "thank you" **(xie sie),** "very good" **(hen hao),** "where" **(na lee),** and "not available" **(may yo).**

## Chinese in North America

The Chinese are the largest Asian subpopulation in the United States. Chinese immigration dates back to the California Gold Rush in the middle 1800s. Between 1840 and 1882, men were brought in without their spouses or families as cheap laborers to work in mines and railroads and later in agriculture and service trades. Their transition in America was very difficult because of the political and xenophobic climate and the lack of family support. The Chinese Exclusion Act of 1882 drastically limited Chinese immigration. It prohibited immigration of spouses and families, as well as any new laborers to the United States. This ban remained in effect until 1943.

Prior to the 1960s, Chinese immigrants came mainly from the southeastern part of China, where Cantonese is spoken. After 1965, with the easement of immigration laws, more educated professionals and families from Taiwan, Hong Kong, and China came to the United States and Canada. Since the 1970s, immigrants have been predominantly from mainland China, and most speak Mandarin (**Guoyue** or **pu tong hua**). These Chinese immigrants came mainly seeking political freedom, professional advancement, economic opportunities, and to rejoin families.

Chinese migration to Canada has also increased substantially in recent years. The 1996 Canadian Census found that between 1991 and 1996, the number of people who reported Chinese as their mother tongue increased by 42% to 736,000, representing 2.6% of Canada's population, up from 0.4% of the population in 1971. According to the 1996 Canadian Census, Chinese is now the third most-spoken language after English and French.

There are wide variations in health beliefs and health practices among Chinese-Americans. In traditional Chinese culture, good health means to have a "balance of two forces": **yin** and **yang**. The yin represents the female and negative force: darkness, cold, and emptiness. The yang represents the male and positive force: light, warmth, and fullness. All things or beings in the universe consist of yin and yang. An imbalance is thought to cause catastrophe and illness. One of the major premises of traditional Chinese health care is the holistic view of the person. The belief is rooted in the idea that all body systems interact with one another and with the environment to result in a balanced state that maintains wellness. Fundamental concepts include **qi** (vital energy force), and "yin" and "yang." Names of organs are used to represent systems in the body and elements to represent phases (e.g., wood, fire). Channels of communications in the body are conceptualized as "meridians."*

Differences in cultural beliefs and practices are based on birthplace, degree of assimilation, education, occupation, and socioeconomic status. Such differences also depend on whether the immigrants are urban or suburban residents; early or new immigrants or born in the United States; northerners or southerners; or Catholics, Protestants, or Buddhists. Since it is difficult to encompass all groups of Chinese, this chapter focuses on Chinese immigrants from 1970 to present.

In 2000, more than 2.4 million persons of Chinese descent resided in the United States. Approximately 63% of Chinese-Americans were not born in the United States. California has the largest population of Chinese-Americans, and New York has the second largest, followed by Hawaii, Illinois, and Texas. Most Chinese-Americans reside in New York City, San Francisco, Los Angeles, and Boston. Each of these cities has a "Chinatown" in which recent immigrants settle. Immigrants who speak English, however, tend to settle in the suburbs.

In Canada, most ethnic Chinese flock to Vancouver or Toronto, attracted by the availability of economic opportunities and established ethnic communities. The Chinese community across Canada is said to be prosperous. Many arrive from Hong Kong with sizable financial assets; others work hard and save, later investing in business ventures.

---

* Brief chapters on complementary health care including acupuncture and herb use can be found in Freemen LW, Lawlis GF. Mosby's Complementary & Alternative Medicine. St. Louis: Mosby, 2001.

Being a woman meant a lesser social status in the traditional Chinese society. The traditional Chinese view was that a woman should be passive and genteel and subject to her husband. She was not expected to work outside the home or pursue a career. The women's movement and economic reform, however, have changed this way of thinking among many Chinese, both men and women. This is especially true in the younger generations, who may not hold traditional views. In North America, many young women are expected to achieve a good education and career and to be independent.

## At Birth

### Preference for Sons

Many families adhere to the strong traditional view of preferring sons **(er ze).** This preference has much to do with the group practice of passing family inheritance to the son and the son's obligations to take care of his elderly parents. Also, sons are expected to continue the family name from one generation to the next. This view is strongest among the working class, peasants, and rural residents, who need the additional labor that a child provides. In educated families, this preference may not be as strong or may even have been eliminated.

### Response to Birth of a Female

For new immigrants, the "one-child policy" in China may enhance the desire for sons. The Chinese government subsidizes only the first child by providing living expenses and education. Conversely, parents experience negative societal pressure for having a second child. For this reason, some parents attempt to determine the gender of the fetus before birth so that they can make the decision to abort a female fetus. The one-child policy applies to the Hans but not to ethnic minority groups in China. However, if a child is born with a birth defect, the family is allowed to have another child regardless of ethnic origin.

Today the one-child policy is less strictly enforced than in the recent past. The desire for a boy is less compelling among urban families. In rural areas, however, sons are the major laborers on the farm. A farmer who is economically well off can afford to have additional children, although he may have to pay a fine to the local government. If he is poor, however, he may abandon a female child. As a result, orphanages are full of girls, and China is now the country of choice if one wants to adopt a girl. Nevertheless, it is rare for city residents to abandon a girl, since they more readily accept the one-child policy.

As a consequence of the one-child policy, the pressure on an only child to excel can be detrimental to the child's mental health. Obesity and problems with interpersonal relationships may also occur. Although there is no one-child policy in North America and the preference for sons may be weaker, the history of this policy in China may still influence some families.

### Birth Rituals

Traditional families celebrate when a son is born. They give dyed red eggs to the guests. There is no traditional ritual when a girl is born, although some families also hold a celebration. These practices are slowly changing in some Chinese families in North America.

# Childhood and Youth

## Stages

The stages between childhood and adult status are infancy, to 2 years *(yin)*; child, 3 to 10 years *(haize)*; teens, 11 to 17 years *(shaonian)*; youth, 18 to 25 years *(qingnian)*; and adult, 25 years and older *(chenren)*.

## Family Expectations

Family expectations for boys and girls differ. Traditionally, boys are expected to be strong; girls are expected to be gentle and soft. Children are expected to obey their parents' wishes, be good students, and demonstrate proper behavior. This view is changing as the expectations of Chinese society change.

## Social Expectations

Children are taught to respect their elders and those in authority. Proper behavior is always expected of the youngster in public. They are expected not to question the decision of their parents. Grandparents play a strong role in decision-making about family welfare and health care. Boys are expected to excel and advance the family status; girls are trained to fulfill the roles of housewife and mother. Young girls today, however, are also expected to be educated and to pursue a career.

## Importance of Education

The literacy rate is very high in China, and education is compulsory. There is an expectation, however, that parents will pay the teachers. Most children receive the equivalent of a ninth-grade education. The quality of the schools varies in China, and the emphasis is on conformity and rote learning. Nonetheless, education is one of the most important values in Chinese culture, and parents sacrifice for their children's education. In the United States, Chinese-American graduation rates from high schools and colleges for both men and women are higher than the national average. Children are highly encouraged to excel in school, but expectations are higher for boys than girls in terms of pursuing a formal education. The family's social and economic background may influence this expectation. Educated and economically well-to-do families in the United States are more likely to hold the same expectations for both boys and girls.

# Pubescence

## Psychosexual Development

The first menses defines puberty. The Chinese term for menstruation is *"yue jing."* The average age of onset is around 12 or 13 years, but poor nutrition or ailments may delay it. A boy reaches puberty when his voice changes, usually between 15 and 18 years of age.

## Teen Sexuality

**Social Restrictions.**  Chinese culture disapproves of sexual relationships prior to marriage. Engaging in a premarital sexual relationship will bring "shame" on the family. A woman would not talk about her sexual experiences that occurred prior to marriage. In the younger generation of Chinese Americans, however, some teens may date and engage in sexual behavior in the same manner as their Caucasian counterparts. Traditional parents generally do not discuss sexual topics with their children. As a result, teenagers may not seek contraceptive advice. There is also a great reluctance in Chinese society to acknowledge sexually transmitted diseases (STD), human immunodeficiency virus (HIV), or acquired immunodeficiency syndrome (AIDS).

**Teen Pregnancy.**  Dating for Chinese Americans starts at a much later age than for the majority of the U.S. population. Young people tend to go out in groups rather than as couples. Teenage pregnancy is uncommon, since sexual relationships prior to marriage are disapproved. A teenage girl who is sexually active may take precautions to prevent pregnancy, because she will disgrace her family if she gets pregnant. There is always the fear that she might be expelled from the house.

## Menstruation

**Relationship to Fertility.**  Menstruation indicates that a woman is "normal," healthy, and fertile. Women who are not menstruating may be advised to get treatment with traditional Chinese medicine such as **Xiao Yao San,** which contains bupleurum **(chai hua),** tang kuei **(dong gui),** and other herbs. If the traditional medicine fails to work, however, many Chinese women will accept that failure and not seek help from Western medicine.

**Taboos and Restrictions during Menstruation.**  During their menstrual period, some women avoid drinking cold water or cold beverages, swimming, taking a bath, or performing heavy physical work. They believe that a menstruating woman is less healthy since she is losing blood and that water may contaminate her vagina. Intercourse is not permitted, based on the belief that the woman is unclean during menses.

**Dysmenorrhea.**  Menstrual cramping is considered normal. Traditional Chinese medicine (pills) such as **Wu Ji Bai Fong Wan** are commonly used to treat dysmenorrhea.

## Female Modesty and Touching

This culture emphasizes modesty according to Confucian beliefs about female privacy and modesty. It is especially apparent in older women, who are reluctant to do monthly breast self-examinations. This inhibition is decreasing in the younger generation.

## Relationship to Health Care

Ninety percent of obstetricians and gynecologists in China are women, and most Chinese women prefer a female practitioner, especially for breast and pelvic examinations. Chinese women who are very modest may avoid having a male practitioner perform such examinations altogether. Chinese are reluctant to discuss any problems related to sex, such as vaginal infections, STDs, or HIV.

## Adulthood

### Transition Rites and Rituals

A woman is considered to have entered young adulthood (*chennian ren*) between 20 and 30 years of age. There are no special rites of passage or ceremonies to mark this transition.

### Social Expectations

Young educated women are expected to marry at about age 23 to 24 years or after obtaining a college degree and to begin a family before age 30. Young women who do not go to college or live in rural areas are likely to marry much earlier. A woman who has never married is often treated as if something were wrong with her, because no man has asked her to be his wife. A single woman who has a career and is well educated, however, may be viewed with respect.

### Union Formation

**Union Types.** Most couples in China formalize their marriages by registering at a local government office and celebrating with families and friends in a wedding banquet. In North America, Chinese observe monogamy as required by law. Prior to the 1930s, it was not unusual for a wealthy man to have several wives, but this custom is no longer practiced. A woman is free to find her mate, although it is not uncommon to be matched with a husband whom family members recommend. After marriage, women in China, as well as frequently in North America, retain their own family names, although the children take the father's family name.

**Social Sanctions for Failing to Enter into Union.** If a woman becomes pregnant, she is expected to marry the father of the baby.

### Domestic Violence

The extent of domestic violence is not well reported. If domestic violence occurs, it may not be mentioned by the woman. Instead, she is likely to accept her situation and feel that it was her fault. With the rise of unemployment, domestic violence may also be on the increase. Health care providers need to be alert for signs and symptoms of such abuse. As Chinese women in North America become more westernized and informed about their legal rights, they are more likely to seek legal actions for domestic violence.

## Rape

The incidence of rape is unknown. Many women view rape and sexual molestation as shameful **(xiu chi)**, and a victim, called a "lost person" **(dui ren),** is apt to feel decreased self-worth. Victims are often blamed for having behaved provocatively and somehow causing the rape. Therefore, they tend not to report or talk about it and merely accept the situation in a conspiracy of silence. As Chinese rape victims become more aware of their legal rights and available support services in North America, however, they are more likely to seek help.

## Divorce

**Women and Divorce.**   Divorce was traditionally viewed as being shameful **(xiu chi),** a loss of face **(dui lian),** or a failure; however, this view is changing in the younger generation. Today, divorce is more acceptable in the Chinese culture. Remarriage may occur, although a traditional Chinese man may not value a divorced woman as highly as a woman who has never been married. It is typically much easier for a man than a woman to enter into a new relationship following a divorce.

**Child Custody Practices.**   In China, the legal system traditionally was biased toward the father, who would usually be granted custody of the children after a divorce since children belong to the father's family. Often, the father's parents opt to care for the children. Because of recent reforms in the Chinese legal system, more and more divorced women in China are being granted custody of their children. In this event, the father is expected to maintain ties and provide support, although this obligation is not enforced.

---

**NOTE TO THE HEALTH CARE PROVIDER**

Divorced women appear to accept their fate. More traditional women may not see the need for psychological counseling, and the family will probably not be responsive to accepting it because of their reluctance to seek psychological counseling and mental health care. They believe that the problems of rape, domestic violence, and divorce are private affairs that individuals or family can work out. Practitioners can expect difficulty in obtaining information from the client, especially since Chinese do not openly display their emotions. In the case of rape, for example, asking the "right" questions is important. It may be helpful to use a phrase such as "it has helped others in a similar situation," and to acknowledge possible feelings of shame and guilt. For an immigrant with English difficulties, a medical interpreter may be more appropriate than a family member.

---

## Fertility and Childbearing

**Family Size.**   In China, the "recommended" family size is one child per family, as dictated by the government. In rural areas and minority regions, however, many families are likely to have more than one child. In North America, family size is typically two or three. Family size also differs depending on age cohort and working status of the parents in the United States and Canada. At present, many families with two working parents have one or two children.

**Contraceptive Practices.**   Contraceptive choices are governed by the individuals' religious beliefs and society's attitude. In China, the government mandates that all sexually active women use some form of birth control, such as birth control pills, the rhythm method, intrauterine devices, home remedies, folk medicines, condoms, abortion, or tubal ligation. However, certain groups (e.g., Catholics) may not practice contraception because of their religious beliefs.

---

**NOTE TO THE HEALTH CARE PROVIDER**

Chinese women are usually shy and modest about sexuality. When recommending contraception, practitioners should keep in mind that some terminology applicable to reproduction may be unknown to a recent immigrant. If there is no language barrier and no accent, however, one might assume that the client was raised in North America and knows the terminology.

---

**Role of the Male in the Couple's Fertility Decision-Making.** In traditional Chinese culture, the individual (male or female) does not usually make important decisions. Typically, decisions are made by a group of family members consisting of the senior one, the most educated one, and the most respected one. This practice is called "collective decision-making." Chinese social relations are buttressed by the Confucian model, which espouses the primary importance of the father-son relationship. It is important to have the family's approval for decisions.

Abortion

**Cultural Attitudes.** To enforce the one-child policy in China, abortion (**da tai,** meaning "getting rid of the fetus") is commonly performed when birth control fails. It is neither perceived as a sin nor hidden. Religion does not play a role in this decision-making process. Chinese Americans, on the other hand, influenced by religious, societal, and cultural views are likely to view abortion as others in the United States and Canada do. Chinese women in North America seek abortions through the same sources as other women; however some may consult a Chinese herbalist for alternative home remedies.

**Teen Abortion.** Teen abortion is not commonly practiced, although parents may force an unmarried teen to have an abortion to save the family from shame.

---

**NOTE TO THE HEALTH CARE PROVIDER**

When talking about the possibility of an abortion or miscarriage, practitioners should be especially considerate if the woman is unmarried. The first practical step in communicating is to tone down the interchange and soften the voice, keeping in mind that Chinese people often appear agreeable. They will generally avoid offending others by responding "yes" to all questions or remaining silent rather than saying "no." Thus, providers should attempt to verify answers with restatements or interpretations that will avoid giving the woman a sense of being disagreeable.

---

Miscarriage

Miscarriage or **liu chan** ("loss of birth") is often seen as a divine intervention and viewed as an ill omen. Rest and good nutrition (such as chicken, soups, eggs, green vegetables) are encouraged following a miscarriage. A woman with repeated miscarriages may be perceived as being less of a woman, because of her inability to carry a pregnancy to term. Sometimes a miscarriage may be viewed as the woman's own fault (working too hard, being too physically active, or not being careful), as well as "bad luck." To avoid miscarriage women will generally take such precautions as avoiding heavy work or stress, eating nourishing foods, and thinking only "good thoughts."

---

**NOTE TO THE HEALTH CARE PROVIDER**
If repeated miscarriages occur, the woman needs emotional support and health care appropriate to her condition as determined through a careful health evaluation.

---

## Infertility

It is generally believed that infertility is the woman's fault, as well as bad luck. She may be perceived as having had "bad" thoughts or perhaps not really wanting to be pregnant. It is socially and culturally acceptable in China for a husband to divorce his wife because of infertility. This custom is diminishing in North America, and it is not evident in the younger generation.

---

**NOTE TO THE HEALTH CARE PROVIDER**
Fertility treatment is generally acceptable to the younger generation of Chinese. More traditional Chinese, however, may seek fertility treatments through herbalists and other traditional Chinese medicines; they are apt to be reluctant to seek Western methods involving modern reproductive technology.

---

## Pregnancy

**Activity Restriction and Taboos.**   Many traditional families observe some aspects of folk medicine, although these practices vary. Expectant mothers should have good nutrition (eggs, soup, chicken, fish, vegetables) and good thoughts (such as imagining beautiful places, listening to lyrical music, picturing a beautiful and healthy baby, and thinking about good deeds) to ensure a healthy and happy baby. Some folk beliefs include avoiding "frightful" situations, seeing anything ugly, attending funerals, and touching animals, out of fear of catching diseases. Pregnant women are encouraged to restrict physical activities because many believe that such activities may cause a miscarriage.

**Dietary Foods.**   Nutritious foods such as eggs and soups with chicken, fish, or meat are promoted. Shellfish is prohibited during the first trimester since it is believed to cause allergies in the baby. Taking iron supplements is believed to harden the bones and make delivery difficult. During the seventh and eighth months, some expectant women take ginseng as a general strengthening tonic.

**Prenatal Care.**   Although the Chinese government mandates and provides prenatal care, in actual practice there is a rising expectation that people will pay for health care. Women receive prenatal care after the confirmation of pregnancy. If the woman is older than 30 years, she will receive closer monitoring since a pregnancy at an older age may be at risk for more complications.

## Birthing Process

**Home Versus Hospital Delivery.**  Most Chinese women prefer hospital deliveries to home deliveries. Home deliveries are more common in rural areas when hospitals are not available.

**Cesarean Section Versus Vaginal Delivery.**  Most deliveries are vaginal, which is preferred and considered normal. A cesarean section is performed only when medically necessary.

**Labor Management.**  It is uncommon for the father to actively participate in the birthing process, although this custom is changing with the younger generation. Family members, especially grandmothers, may wait outside the delivery room for the birth.

**Placenta.**  In China, the placenta holds no particular significance and is usually disposed of after delivery. Sometimes the hospital may give it to a pharmaceutical company for use in manufacturing traditional Chinese medicines.

## Postpartum

Traditionally, there is a one-month postpartum period, during which the new mother's dietary and health practices are directed toward decreasing the yin energy forces or cold air in her body. The mother, during this period, is encouraged to eat nutritious foods, especially chicken and fish soups. New mothers avoid fruits and cold beverages, which are considered "cold foods." The typical postpartum diet is high in "hot foods," such as ginger, chicken, eggs, fish, and pork. The basic mainstay diet consists of rice, eggs, and a chicken soup containing pig knuckles, vinegar, ginger, rice wine, and sometimes peanuts and walnuts. Vinegar is believed to help transfer tricalcium phosphate from the knuckle bones into the soup and may supply the essential calcium requirements. The alcohol in traditional rice wine may stimulate bleeding, so women postpone drinking it for at least two weeks postpartum.

The "pores" are believed to remain open for 30 days postpartum, during which time cold air can enter the body. The new mother is forbidden to go outdoors during this period, and windows are typically kept closed to avoid the cold air. In China, the woman does not take showers or tub baths; most Chinese Americans are unlikely to observe this restriction. Sexual intercourse is also discouraged to avoid infection and prevent interruption of vaginal healing, at this time.

### Newborn and Infant Care

**Breastfeeding Versus Bottle-Feeding.** Breastfeeding is promoted in China and likely to be the method of choice. Many Chinese are not accustomed to drinking cow's milk and are lactose intolerant.

**Infant Protection.** Chinese are very conscientious about complying with directions as to infants' health care. Infants and toddlers generally receive their immunizations, and growth and development are monitored regularly.

**Primary Caregiver.** The mother is generally the primary caretaker of her new infant. In traditional Chinese culture it is customary for the grandmother to assist during the first few months. Chinese grandmothers play an important role in the care of newborn babies. Grandmothers provide support to new mothers, but they may also cause stress based on their "old-fashioned" restrictions during the baby's first month. Such restrictions include limiting visitors and preventing new mothers from going outside the house. A new mother is likely to receive conflicting information from the health practitioner and her mother.

---

**NOTE TO THE HEALTH CARE PROVIDER**
A new mother may seem negative when, after being complemented about her baby, she responds that "he is ugly." She is merely being humble.

---

## Middle Age

### Cultural Attitudes and Expectations

Women are considered middle-aged at about 40 years of age. There are no specially sanctioned behaviors or clothing other than the usual expectations of North American societies. The "empty nest" syndrome does not receive much emphasis in the Chinese culture since adult children are expected to maintain close ties with their parents. In North America, however, parents may feel a sense of loss when their youngest child leaves home, because the younger generation may resemble their non-Chinese counterparts in maintaining less contact with their parents.

### Menopause

Little attention is given to menopause. The age of onset is between ages 42 and 55.

**Sexual Activity.** Chinese do not usually talk about sexuality after the onset of menopause. A woman's husband will generally still consider her attractive and valued, since being "sexy" is not considered important in this culture. Most couples are faithful to each other. Divorce rates are low; but if one is divorced, dating and marriage at middle age is culturally acceptable.

**Coping.** Chinese women seem to exhibit fewer menopausal symptoms than do Caucasians. This may be partly attributable to the reluctance to discuss sex-related symptoms and their self-treatment of symptoms, using Chinese herbs such as **tang kuei (dong gui),** and exercises such as **Tai Chi Tuan,** or meditation.

> **NOTE TO THE HEALTH CARE PROVIDER**
> Hormone replacement therapy is not commonly prescribed in China; however, these women may be receptive to hormone replacement therapy, if offered. Chinese women drink and eat foods that are high in phytoestrogens. But assessment for osteoporosis should be routinely performed since the Chinese diet is low in calcium. These women are reluctant to talk about sexual relationships, intercourse, or private body parts. Asking the sensitive questions toward the end of the clinical session will be helpful.

## Old Age

Women consider themselves to be old at age 60 or 65. Chinese women from China may consider 55 years as "old age" since it is an age identifier for retirement from work. Unlike American culture, the status of elderly women increases with age in Chinese culture.

According to tradition, filial piety ensures that children will take care of their elderly parents in their later years. This custom, however, is changing. Most elderly and widowed women live alone in North America. Family members may care for those who cannot care for themselves, or may place them in assisted living or nursing home facilities. Cultural conflicts may arise when a woman expects to live in an extended household as she would have done in her homeland.

## Death and Dying

### Cultural Attitudes and Beliefs

According to cultural beliefs rooted in Taoism, Buddhism, and Confucianism, death has a natural time. Both the moral framework of Buddhist ethics and the philosophy of Confucius require a holistic, humanistic, organic view of life and death. Those who hold a strong Buddhist view believe in other lives following death.

### Rites and Rituals

Rituals depend on the family's religious beliefs. Some traditional Buddhist families bury or burn fake paper money with departed ones so that they may spend it in the afterlife. Food offerings such as steamed chicken or rice cakes may be made at the gravesite. Men generally play a more important role than women in burial ceremonies and rituals.

### Mourning

In China, the appropriate mourning period is about one month, during which time family members may wear a black armband. Family members are expected to wear black or white clothing at the funeral ceremony. There are no rules for others who attend the funeral.

### Coping

Following the death of her husband, the surviving wife may feel lonely and lack direction in her life. Coping strategies include seeking emotional support from family members and friends, sharing feelings with these people, cherishing good memories of the deceased person, and moving on with life.

Chinese are reluctant to have autopsies performed following death. They believe that bodies need to be buried intact, and they have great reverence for the dead, particularly their own ancestors. If an elderly Chinese patient dies in the hospital, family members may be reluctant to accept his or her clothing if they consider it to contain evil spirits. The family may return later, however, and request all or part of the deceased person's clothing. Sometimes elderly people will have large amounts of money hidden in the linings of their clothing. Therefore, providers should itemize all clothing and keep them in a safe place.

## IMPORTANT POINTS FOR PROVIDERS CARING FOR CHINESE WOMEN

### The Medical Intake

A lack of proficiency in English is the greatest barrier to health care for most Chinese immigrants, especially the elderly. If the immigrant was accustomed to traditional methods of diagnosis, she may have expectations about the initial examination derived from traditional Chinese medicine, for example, expect elaborate assessment of the radial pulse, examination of the tongue, and minimal undressing/exposure. Communication may be impeded by the various dialects within Cantonese (e.g., **Toisan),** spoken by most Chinese who emigrated from the southern part of China prior to the 1960s. Most Chinese who emigrated after 1970 speak Mandarin. Older persons should always be addressed by their last name, preceded by "Mrs." A client with a Chinese name such as Li Lai Mun should be asked whether she is Mrs. Li (with first name Lai Mun) or Mrs. Mun.

For reasons of confidentiality it is better to use a Chinese-speaking health care provider or medical interpreter than a young family member who has accompanied an older woman, especially if the health condition is of a sensitive nature. Printed materials provided should be in the Chinese language.

## Status of the Provider

Since nursing is not a high-status profession in China, Chinese elders may not be amenable to seeing a nurse practitioner (NP), especially if she is a woman. Although respectful of it, many recent immigrants and elders who have not fully acculturated into North America may be skeptical about the effectiveness of Western medicine and its premises. They may perceive Western physicians as being less skilled because of their strong reliance on "machine-based diagnosis" rather than on their clinical experiences. Also, those born in China are accustomed to physicians dispensing medication and charging a nominal fee for their services, whereas in the United States, the major cost of the visit may be the medication.

For those who came to the United States to escape political persecution, obeying authority was common for the sake of survival. As a result, these immigrants may be less likely to question practitioners' decisions and be reluctant to say "no." Nodding the head does not necessarily mean, "I agree with you"; rather, it may simply mean, "I heard you." Chinese clients may sign a consent form to conform, but not to consent, to a proposed treatment. Therefore, it is essential that practitioners thoroughly discuss involved risks and benefits of treatment to ensure clients' understanding.

## Communicating Illness and Symptoms

Many older women will present physical symptoms when the underlying problem may be emotional. Women generally give elaborate explanations or tell lengthy stories about their illnesses. Practitioners need to pay attention to the client's medical history to yield a valid assessment of the given symptom. Family members typically accompany clients to their medical appointments and actively participate in providing information.

---

**NOTE TO THE HEALTH CARE PROVIDER**

Practitioners should avoid discussing such issues as durable powers of attorney, "do-not-resuscitate" directives, and emergency measures, if possible. Women are apt to find these topics delicate and offensive, and the elderly may refuse to discuss them at all.

---

## The Physical Examination

### Modesty and Touching

During a physical examination, the woman's body should be covered to expose only those parts that need to be examined. Women typically prefer to be seen by female providers.

### Expressing Pain

Stoicism is common in China. A client may not complain about her pain so as not to disturb social harmony. Complaining is perceived as a sign of weakness or disturbing others. Therefore, clients try to smile and be as agreeable as possible despite their pain. It is essential to perform specific pain assessments and provide the appropriate intervention.

## Prescribing Medications

### Drug Interactions

Very traditional Chinese (usually first-generation) tend to buy specific herbal treatments for their own use from herbal shops in Chinatown. Health care providers should assess clients' medication patterns, including their use of herbal roots, teas, and the like, and assess for possible drug interactions with prescription medications. Research suggests that Chinese people poorly metabolize mephenytoin and are more sensitive to beta-blockers and the effects of alcohol than many other groups. They also experience increased gastrointestinal disturbances with analgesics. Commonly, Chinese clients use an all-purpose topical ointment called Tiger Balm for headaches or aching muscles.

### Medication Sharing

Many Chinese clients tend to keep all medications ever prescribed and take them at their own discretion for varying ailments. They also tend to borrow and loan medications to friends and family members. It is not unusual to self-medicate when they think they know what is wrong or when past use of a given medication was successful.

Traditional patients may switch doctors and herbalists and may consult two or three specialists at the same time. Therefore, it is particularly important for the health care provider to find out what medications the woman is receiving from each doctor. The patient is apt to be reluctant to tell one doctor that she is seeing others for fear of offending that doctor.

### Compliance

It has been observed that non-English speaking Chinese exhibit poor compliance with Western prescriptions compared with English-speaking Chinese. This problem may be partly attributable to the language barrier and lack of understanding of the purpose for the medications.

Typically Chinese clients tend to take medications based on symptoms; if the symptoms are relieved (or if there are side effects), they will stop using the medication.

---

**NOTE TO THE HEALTH CARE PROVIDER**
Practitioners should carefully question clients about their use of such herbs as St. John's wort, ma huang, and ginseng. Some herbal preparations are contraindicated with use of antihypertensive medications and may also affect blood clotting.

---

## Follow-Up Appointments

Some clients may not attend follow-up appointments because of the need to make follow-up appointments several weeks in advance (long waits discourage elderly Chinese) and the belief that a woman is healthy if she is asymptomatic. Practitioners should be sure to remind clients about their next appointment with a phone call or card, using an appropriate language. Also, an effort should be made to minimize the waiting time necessary to see a doctor.

## Prevalent Diseases

Health statistics show that Asian-American women, including Chinese, born in the United States have a 60% higher risk for breast cancer than those born in the Far East. Heart disease is the second most common cause of death for Asian females. Tuberculosis in Asian Americans is the highest among all groups and nearly four times that of the general population. Suicide is also identified as a major cause of death for Asian women. Depression results largely from tremendous cultural conflict experienced by the more recent Chinese immigrants. Mental health services are underutilized even though some Asian groups are increasingly experiencing psychotic disorders.

## Health-Seeking Behaviors

Disease represents disharmony or imbalance in the body, and clients may use therapies such as herbal medicines and acupuncture to restore the balance. Typically, many Chinese Americans modify their diet as their first approach to treating an illness if they consider it a minor problem *(xiao mao bin).* They also may take herbal or over-the-counter medications. If these measures do not work, they may visit their medical doctor. Only when they have a major condition *(dao mao bin)* are they likely to immediately visit their doctor for prescription medication. In some instances, effective treatment begins late in the disease process, resulting in poor outcomes.

Typically health-seeking behaviors vary by education, socioeconomic status, and level of fluency in English.

---

**NOTE TO THE HEALTH CARE PROVIDER**

Providers need to be cognizant of the numerous variations found within the Chinese population and use their assessment skills in the area of cultural variations. They must always exercise caution to assess the client's level of acculturation, beliefs, and preferences.

---

## 🌐 BIBLIOGRAPHY

Campbell, T, & Chang, B.L. (1981). Health care of the Chinese in America. In BW Spradley (Ed.), Contempary Community Nursing. Boston, Little Brown and Co., pp. 189–197.

Chang, B. L. (1981). Asian American patient care. In G. Henderson & M. Mrimeaux (Eds.), *Transcultural health care.* Menlo Park, CA: Addison-Wesley, pp. 255–277.

Freemen, L. W., & Lawlis, F. G. (2001). *Mosby's complementary & alternative medicine.* St. Louis: Mosby.

Morbidity and Mortality Weekly Review. Behavioral Risk Factor Survey of Chinese-California, 1989. April 24, 1992/41(16):266–270. Accessed 9/19/2000 from **http://www.cdc.gov/mmwr/preview/mmwr.**

Zhan, L. (1999). Xi Young Hong: Health practices in Chinese older women. In L. Zhan (Ed.), *Asian voices: Asian and Asian American health educators speak out.* Sudbury: Jones and Bartlett.

# CHAPTER 8

# Colombians

## PILAR BERNAL DE PHEILS, MS, RN, and DIVA JARAMILLO, MPH, RN

## 🌐 INTRODUCTION

### Who are the Colombian People?

Most Colombians are of mixed origin. Their ancestors were primarily white Europeans (most of whom were from Spain), indigenous people (Indians), or blacks whose ancestors were brought from Africa as slaves. On the Atlantic coast, **mulattos** (black and white) predominate; on the Pacific coast, Afro-Colombians predominate; and in the Andean region, the **mestizos** (white and indigenous) predominate, although some rural indigenous groups have less mixing. Spanish is the national language, yet many indigenous groups continue to speak their native languages and teach these languages in their schools. Natives from the San Andres and Providencia Islands speak a mixed dialect (English, French, and Spanish).

### Colombians in North America

Most emigration from Colombia has been for economic reasons; although in the past 15 years, and especially during the past 5 years, sociopolitical reasons have also been a driving force. Many Colombians are now fleeing their country because of fear of political persecution, kidnapping, and death as the result of increased tension and fighting between guerrilla factions, paramilitaries, drug lords, and the national army.

The approximately 2 million Colombians in the United States live mainly in Florida (800,000) and New York City (1 million). There are also 50,000 to 100,000 Colombians in Los Angeles, Chicago, Atlanta, and Houston. As of the 1996 census, some 8500 Colombians were in Canada, 54% of whom were women. Most Colombians in Canada reside in Toronto and Montreal.

## 🌐 BEING FEMALE IN COLOMBIAN SOCIETY

Women are expected to provide physical and emotional care and support to the family and to maintain the unity of the family group. Culturally, women are expected to be feminine, tender, and affectionate.

## At Birth

### Preference for Sons and Response to the Birth of a Female

Traditional families desire a son, mainly to carry on the family's name. However, the birth of a daughter is also well received, since in most cases the daughter will ultimately take care of the elderly parents. The family, on the other hand, is likely to be disappointed if all children are of one gender, either boys or girls. All children (if wanted) are received as a gift from God, and there is no outright disregard for or neglect of the female child in this culture.

### Birth Rituals

About 95% of Colombians are Catholic. An important ritual a few weeks after birth is baptism and a celebration, with a party after the religious ceremony. Before leaving the hospital, girls commonly have their ears pierced; boys may be circumcised.

## Childhood and Youth

### Stages

The seventh birthday is an important transition for children in this culture because it is thought to be the beginning of the **uso de razon,** meaning that the children can now reason and take more responsibility for their actions. Children also commonly celebrate their first communion at this age, an important religious event that is followed by a celebration with friends and family. For this occasion, girls wear short or long white dresses; boys wear dark suits.

An important female milestone is the **quinciañera** at age 15 years. It is celebrated with a big party with family, family friends, and the young woman's friends. Usually there is dancing, and the young woman dances the first waltz with her father. She then dances with brothers or close male relatives and, finally, with her male friends. This celebration symbolizes her transition from girl **(niña)** to adolescent **(señorita),** the age at which having friendships and relationships with males becomes more acceptable. Boys' transitions are not associated with a specific age but rather with voice change and first sexual experience, the latter being unacceptable for girls outside marriage.

Although there are some regional differences, parents commonly call their children **mijo** (from **mi hijo,** my son) and **mija** (from **mi hija,** my daughter). A boy is called **niño,** and a girl is called **niña**. A youth is most commonly referred to as a **muchacho** (boy) or **muchacha** (girl).

### Family Expectations

Children are expected to stay at home until they begin school. As more women enter the work force, however, children may be cared for at home by other relatives (usually the grandmother) and, to a lesser extent, in child care centers. If the family can afford a maid, the child will stay at home with the maid. As girls approach the teen years, they are frequently asked to help with household chores (cleaning, cooking, and taking care of younger siblings). Boys, on the other hand, are seldom asked or expected to help with household chores.

### Social Expectations

Traditionally, staying home to take care of the husband and children was expected. People from rural and less developed areas of Colombia may not view secondary education as a necessity for young women. Rather, they may expect women to prepare for marriage in their late adolescence or early 20s, and soon thereafter to become mothers.

Although teen dating is acceptable, sexual activity before marriage is discouraged for girls. Norms have changed in the past 10 to 20 years, however, and there is now less condemnation of sexual intercourse before marriage and more acceptance of children born out of wedlock. This is not true in more rural or isolated regions of the country.

### Importance of Education

The literacy rate in Colombia began increasing in the 1960s among both women and men. The average level of schooling for both women and men is about six years. No data are available about the effects of current sociopolitical problems on education.

## Pubescence

### Psychosexual Development

The word for adolescence is **adolecente** or **señorita** for girls; **joven** refers to both genders. Mothers often say **"ya eres una señorita,"** meaning "You are now a young woman," and implying that the girl should no longer behave like a child.

Menarche commonly begins between 10 to 13 years of age, with 11 years the average. The onset of menses symbolizes the onset of puberty. Better nutrition is thought to have reduced the age of menarche since the beginning of the century.

### Rituals and Rites of Passage

The most important rituals or rites of passage have to do with the young girl. An example of this is the important female milestone at age 15 (quinciañera), which symbolizes her transition into womanhood. For the young boy, there is no equivalent celebration to mark this developmental milestone. In the past, the father might take the boy to a prostitute to initiate him, symbolizing his transition to "manhood," but this practice is now a rare occurrence. More often, the adolescent boy has his first sexual experience with a friend, which is implicitly considered the passage to "manhood."

### Teen Sexuality

**Social Restrictions and Pressures.** The only restriction placed on the pubescent girl is on sexual activity. There are no restrictions on clothing, and young women wear whatever they choose. As educational opportunities have increased, young women are less inclined to marry early. In rural areas, however, a young woman may be pressured to marry in her early 20s.

Older sisters are expected to take care of younger siblings, and a teen brother may be expected to accompany his sister at all times when she starts dating to avoid the possibility of a sexual encounter. This restriction has been loosening in recent years. Teen sisters, however, are never expected to accompany teen brothers on dates.

**Teen Pregnancy.** Teen pregnancy is still common in Colombia, and most pregnant teens are unmarried. If the teen mother comes from middle or high social classes, her educational opportunities may not suffer, because in most cases, her family assumes responsibility for childrearing. Disadvantaged teens or teens from lower social classes, however, may have to drop out of school to take care of their babies, starting another cycle of poverty.

### Menstruation

**Relationship to Health.** During the menses, women used to be discouraged from bathing or eating certain types of food (e.g., lemons, other acidic or spicy foods) fearing adverse effects, but these restrictions have lessened in recent years. Some women do not swim during their menses. There are no restrictions as to attending religious services or being in the company of others, including males, during the menstrual cycle.

**Relationship to Fertility.** Many Colombian women have very little knowledge of their bodies' functioning and, therefore, do not usually associate menstrual irregularities with infertility. The ability to bear children is, nonetheless, highly valued and a hysterectomy before motherhood can be devastating to the woman. Although this society does not devalue a woman who has had a hysterectomy, it may be harder for her to find a partner.

**Dysmenorrhea.** Changes in menstrual patterns may be attributed to eating certain foods, particularly acidic foods, or to getting cold, such as by taking a cold shower or getting into a swimming pool. Herbal teas are generally recommended for cramps; the type of tea varies by region.

### Female Modesty and Touching

Colombians are physically very expressive, and touching is common and acceptable between women unless it has a sexual connotation (e.g., touching of buttocks or breast in public). Women friends and relatives greet each other (or greet male friends and relatives) with a kiss on the cheek; they use a handshake when people are first introduced or with mere acquaintances. Women will dance with each other, but a man dancing with a man is not culturally accepted.

**Relationship to Health Care.** Women may see male health providers, but if they have a choice, most women prefer female practitioners. Modesty may prevent many women from obtaining an annual pelvic examination and Papanicolaou's test **(Citología Vaginal)**. It is not unusual for women to avoid Papanicolaou's tests because they are embarrassed to show their genitals to a health care provider, especially a male.

It is customary for a mother to be present during the physical examination of a young girl; in her absence, a female relative or a friend will be present. This is more important if the practitioner is male.

---

**NOTE TO THE HEALTH CARE PROVIDER**

Colombians see physicians and nurses as authority figures and treat them with a great deal of respect. Therefore, a young woman who has never had a pelvic examination may feel reluctant to refuse an examination of her breasts or pelvic area. The practitioner should clearly describe, in advance, how the examination will be performed and the reason for it to gain the young woman's trust and increase her comfort. Also, since these women are quite modest and embarrassed about having their bodies exposed, even to other women, it is important to offer a gown prior to examinations that may cause the breast and/or genitalia to be exposed.

---

# Adulthood

### Transition Rites and Rituals

In general, women are considered adults when they enter their 20s. Another symbol or indicator of adult status is the right to vote, which has for many years been at age 21 but is now 18.

### Social Expectations

Adolescents, especially females, are expected to live at home until they marry. Those who move away usually do so to obtain higher education that is unavailable where they live. Parents are expected to assume all expenses for living and higher education in either case.

Expectations regarding engagement and marriage vary with social class. Formal marriage is expected in middle and upper socioeconomic classes, but common-law marriage is more prevalent in the lower classes. In the past 50 years, young women have been increasingly expected to obtain higher education, and most universities now have equal numbers of men and women undergraduates. Thus, more women have established careers before marrying. In Colombia and in North America more women are also delaying marriage and children beyond the early 20s, although this is still uncommon in families of lower socioeconomic status. Lack of access to higher education is related to lack of economic resources, the need to contribute to family income, and limited space in universities.

Women are expected to provide physical care of elderly parents, but they share the provision of any needed economic support with brothers. It is common for an unmarried woman to continue to live with her parents and to be their primary caregiver; this is not an expectation for male siblings, however.

### Union Formation

**Union Types.**  Common-law union is very common in Colombia. In 1995, 45% of women reportedly lived in such unions. Arranged marriages are uncommon, and polygamy is not acceptable.

**Social Sanctions for Failing to Enter into Union.**  There are social pressures on both women and men to enter into a marriage or common-law union, earlier in life for women than for men. If a woman is not married or in a union by her early 30s, she may be considered a **solterona** (single woman who has been unable to get married). A single man entering his 40s may be called a **solterón,** but most people view him as not wanting to get married rather than being unable to find a partner.

### Domestic Violence

Domestic violence in Colombia is reportedly experienced by 41% of women who have lived with a partner (married or not) at any time. This high rate can be explained in part by Colombian men seeing women as their possessions. Another explanation relates to women's perception of violence in a partner relationship as normal. Reports show that only 54% of women perceived being hit by a partner as domestic violence, and only 20% of battered women reported the violence to the police or welfare system.

In 1995, the government of Colombia enacted legislation intended to prevent and punish violence against women. There have been obstacles in implementing this law, however, and many women are generally not aware either of the law or where to report domestic violence. In Colombia, there are no shelters and no screening for this type of abuse in health care facilities because domestic violence is still not considered a health care problem in this society.

---

**NOTE TO THE HEALTH CARE PROVIDER**

Colombian women may not be aware of North American laws about and services for domestic violence, particularly if they have language limitations. Bringing up the topic of domestic violence in a nonjudgmental way is essential, as is explaining the kinds of support systems that are available for battered women (e.g., legal aid, social services, shelters).

---

### Rape

Eleven percent of women in Colombia have reportedly been raped by their partners and 7% by other persons, according to the 1995 National Demographic Survey and PROFAMILIA (2000), a private family planning institution that provides services across the country. In 29% of the rape cases, the rapist was unknown to the woman, in 32% of the cases he was a friend, and in 24% he was a relative. Other women were raped by their ex-husbands or were reluctant or unable to identify the assailant.

In Colombia, women are frequently blamed for rapes and there are few if any support systems in place to assist rape victims. A few nongovernmental agencies provide companionship when women request it, but these agencies serve only a minimal number of women. As may be expected, few women report this crime. Reasons for this non-reporting included: (1) lack of knowledge about where to report this crime and about police or health care provider orientation; (2) fear of death threats from the aggressor and not trusting the justice system to offer her adequate protection; (3) fear of mistreatment, humiliating interrogations, or examinations by unsympathetic authorities; (4) shame in talking about the rape and bringing disgrace to her family; and (5) fear of losing the love of their boyfriends or husbands.

Beginning in 1995, however, laws enacted to punish rape in Colombia have resulted in a slightly increased reporting and documentation of rape by medical and legal offices. Despite these efforts, the Office for Women's Equity believes that the incidence of rape is still a highly underreported crime, and that victims of rape still have very little access to counseling and other support services. Likewise, women believe that it is likely that perpetrators of these crimes will still go unpunished.

### Divorce

**Sociocultural Views.**   Divorce (*divorcio*) has become culturally acceptable in Colombia even though the Catholic Church does not sanction it. If one partner in a Catholic marriage wants to remarry, he or she must go to great lengths for the church to annul the marriage. Many couples now choose a civil marriage rather than a Catholic one, perhaps because of a 1992 law that sanctions divorce for civil marriages and does not restrict remarriage.

**Women and Divorce.**   As women have become more educated and economically independent, marriage breakdown has become more prevalent and openly accepted. Also, remarriage is more accepted; however, women (and men for that matter) may be looked down on if they remarry in the "near future," conventionally thought to be less than one year.

**Child Custody Practices.**   By law and social expectations, men have economic responsibility for children. In the case of divorce or separation, many men continue their involvement with the children. Nevertheless, a significant number of men do not pay child support, preferring to quit their jobs after the woman files a complaint in the appropriate government office. In such cases, the women end up having full responsibility for childrearing, and they may need and accept financial support from family members.

### Fertility and Childbearing

**Family Size.**   Family size in Colombia has decreased over the last 50 years. In the mid-1950s it was common to have 5 to 10 children, but in 2000, two children per family is the average. Family size, however, varies by region (higher in rural areas) and socioeconomic class. Also, the higher the woman's educational level, the lower is the birth rate.

**Contraceptive Practices.**   Despite the strong influence of Catholicism in Colombia, contraceptive use is now widely accepted. This practice may not hold true for women living in rural areas, where religion still strongly influences many decisions, including family planning. Oral contraceptives are widely available. Most medicines, including oral contraceptives, can be bought in Colombia without a prescription. Other contraceptive devices can be obtained easily in health centers at a reasonable cost.

Indigenous methods that include placing Alka-Seltzer or aspirin tablets, a mixture of lemon with bicarbonate of soda, or a half of a lemon deep in the vagina are still used by women who have little education and lack access to health care.

Of the women who use family planning, 59% reportedly use biomedical methods, 13% use oral contraceptives, 11% use intrauterine devices (IUDs), 26% use sterilization, and 9% use other modern methods. Only 11% of men have vasectomies because of the prevailing belief that vasectomies can cause erectile dysfunction.

Although an IUD is often requested for birth control, fears and myths surround this method. Rural or poorly educated women may believe that if they get pregnant with the IUD in place and it is not removed, the device may become attached to the fetus.

**Role of the Male in the Couple's Fertility Decision-Making.**   Male partners may or may not influence women's decisions about controlling fertility. Today it is more common for women to make fertility decisions unilaterally. This is particularly true if the chosen methods are reversible. Some men, on the other hand, do not accept women's use of contraception, believing that it will free them to have sex with other men. Despite male resistance, however, many women try to use contraceptive methods to avoid unwanted pregnancies. Conversely, most men are not particularly receptive to condom use because of the widely held belief that condoms reduce sexual pleasure.

---

**NOTE TO THE HEALTH CARE PROVIDER**

Education on human sexuality and reproduction will be very beneficial to Colombian clients. Basic education on female genital anatomy and reproductive physiology will help these clients better understand the mechanics of birth control. It is best to educate women and their partners together about reproductive issues. Group education on birth control methods may be most effective if taught to a class consisting only of women. Classes with both men and women may be uncomfortable and intimidating. Open discussion about contraception is not likely to be a problem on a one-to-one basis.

---

## Abortion

**Cultural Attitudes.**   Abortion is illegal in Colombia, although it is often performed by lay persons and, in the past decade, increasingly by health care professionals with little legal prosecution. Based on the teachings of Catholicism, abortion is unacceptable and considered a sin; nonetheless, the prevalence of abortions is on the increase.

Although abortion is not generally used as a method of birth control, it has been suggested that economic considerations, partner's attitude against pregnancy, loss of employment or schooling, family problems, concern for the well-being of other children, health problems, consideration of health risks because of age and, finally, undesired pregnancy are some of the reasons that push these women toward abortion.

**Teen Abortion.**   Teens of all social classes may seek abortions if the pregnancy is not wanted. However, those with little money must use nonprofessional sources for their abortion. Teens are not generally forced to have abortions, although those with family, financial, and other resources have help in childrearing and do not have to interrupt their education. This is not true for teens in lower socioeconomic groups.

**Sources of Abortions.**   Abortions performed by physicians under safe conditions are available only to women who can pay high fees, and the unsafe nature of many abortions is still an important consideration. Because of its illegality, abortions in Colombia are performed privately rather than in clinics.

Local or indigenous abortifacients used by many women include fig leaves, made into a tea to drink or put into the bath, or *ruda* (plant native to Colombia) leaves. There are no data on the efficacy of these methods or whether Colombian women use these plants in North America, but it is unlikely since abortion is legal and relatively accessible.

**Complications.**   Incidence of complications resulting from abortion is believed to be high in Colombia because of its illegality. The potential for a woman to be incarcerated leads to non-reporting of complications, although very few women are prosecuted. Likely complications include perforations, hemorrhage, infections, and toxic shock from unsanitary conditions.

---

**NOTE TO THE HEALTH CARE PROVIDER**

Because of religious influences, use caution when offering abortion to a woman of Colombian origin. Abortion should be presented to the woman merely as a legal and available option if she chooses to avail herself of those services.

---

## Miscarriage

The rate of miscarriage in Colombia, according to a 1993 Ministry of Health report, was 10% to 15% or all pregnancies. Although the cause of most individual miscarriages is unknown, published reports suggest maternal infections, endocrine problems, immunology problems, problems of infertility, and uterine anomalies, most Colombian women attribute miscarriage to "God's will." Occasionally, these women blame a specific vigorous activity, such as riding a horse, for the miscarriage. Some women, especially the lesser educated, may think that the miscarriage was caused by a spell cast by another woman suspected of having an affair with her partner. After a miscarriage, women are cared for physically and emotionally, this culture does not stigmatize the woman who miscarries.

## Infertility

In most cases, infertility is seen as a medical problem with no cultural meaning. An infertile woman is not looked down on or publicly ostracized, although she is likely to be blamed for her inability to conceive.

If a woman is infertile, how she is treated by her male partner or husband depends primarily on the couple's educational level. Among poorly educated couples, the male partner or husband may abandon the woman because of her inability "to give him a child."

---

**NOTE TO THE HEALTH CARE PROVIDER**

Generally Colombian women are receptive to infertility treatment and, in most cases, their families and partners support such treatment, particularly if financial resources are available. Practitioners should meet with the couple and explain all procedures involved, including the importance of partner collaboration to improve chances of success.

---

## Pregnancy

**Activity Restrictions and Taboos.** During pregnancy, women continue working or doing their usual activities until near or at term, unless there are medical restrictions. Some women adhere to the belief that their labor starts because of **susto** (a fright causing physical harm). Others believe that pregnant women should not attend a funeral because their bodies may get cold and they are likely to get sick.

Pregnant women in this culture are treated with respect and given special considerations, such as being given a seat on the bus or being helped to cross a street. In most respects, however, the pregnant woman maintains her pre-pregnancy activities.

**Dietary Practices and Observances.** No special diets are required during pregnancy. Less educated people believe that if a woman's strong desire to eat something, called **antojo** (craving) is not satisfied, the baby can be born with moles or some other marking. Pica (eating non-food items) exists but is uncommon.

**Prenatal Care.** The point at which the woman typically seeks prenatal care depends on her access to it. If access is not an issue, she usually seeks care no later than the end of the first trimester. On average, however, Colombian women have their first prenatal appointment around the 20th week of gestation.

Other than preparing the needed items for the baby, there are no specific rituals to prepare for birth. In upper middle class families, it is customary to have a "baby shower" (adopted from U.S. culture), in which friends and family members give articles of clothing as gifts for the baby.

## Birthing Process

**Home Versus Hospital Delivery.** Most deliveries occur in a hospital or clinic, except in rural areas, where home birth may take place. Deliveries in the hospital or clinic are most frequently attended by a physician and occasionally by a nurse or licensed vocational nurse. Lay midwives assist with home births.

**Cesarean Section Versus Vaginal Delivery.** Most deliveries are vaginal. Cesarean sections (**cesareas**) are reserved for obstetric complications. If given a choice, most women prefer to have the baby under regional anesthesia. Anesthesia is more common if the woman delivers by a private physician.

**Involvement of the Male Partner.**   Families want to be very involved in the birth of the baby, but very few hospitals in Colombia allow significant others in the labor or delivery rooms. The baby's father and the woman's mother, older siblings, grandmothers, and aunts generally stay in the waiting room for news of the baby's birth.

**Labor Management.**   In most cases, the laboring woman admitted to the hospital is kept in bed. Walking is rarely encouraged, and it is not allowed at all after her membrane ruptures.

**Placenta.**   In rural areas, the placenta is typically buried near the house where the family lives in the belief that this will keep the children from abandoning the paternal house. There are no specific cultural beliefs with regard to the placenta in urban areas.

## Postpartum

Early discharge from the hospital (6 to 18 hours postpartum) is now common. Six weeks is considered to be the postpartum period; however, a 1990 law allows all working mothers 12 weeks of maternity leave with pay. In the past, **quarentena,** meaning quarantine or 40 days, delineated the postpartum period.

Women are cared for during the first six weeks postpartum. They are given high-protein foods like meat and chicken soup. Women are no longer confined; rather, they are allowed to resume their normal activities beginning in the postpartum period. In rural areas it is not uncommon to see postpartum women putting dry cotton swabs in their ears and covering their heads if they go outside to avoid exposure to cold wind.

## Newborn and Infant Care

**Breastfeeding Versus Bottle-Feeding.**   Breastfeeding is making a resurgance among Colombian mothers. The child is burped carefully **(sacarle los gases)** to decrease colic, a condition for which apple tea or a stomach massage may be used. For hiccups, it is a common practice for mothers to put a wet cotton swab on the forehead, to give the child a little bit of sugar, or to blow on the fontanels.

**Infant Protection.**   Well-child programs are well-established in Colombia, and it is customary to take the children for all scheduled immunizations. The belief in **mal de ojo** (evil eye) is more common among lesser educated mothers. Dehydration and sunken fontanels from diarrhea is often attributed to mal de ojo. A bracelet made of garlic heads or plastic beads is used to frighten off evil spirits.

**Primary Caregiver.**   The mother provides most, if not all, child care. Fathers may contribute to care, particularly if they are asked to do so. The mother's mother or other female relatives (e.g., aunts or mother-in-law) are frequently closely involved in assisting the mother with child care. If the new mother lives far from the extended family, her own mother is expected to move to her daughter's home for a period that ranges from days to months.

---

**NOTE TO THE HEALTH CARE PROVIDER**

Female members of the extended family play an important role in caring for the newborn, and some may express strong opinions on how to care for the baby. Including these family members in educational activities provided to the parents is important and may bring up disagreements that can be openly discussed and clarified.

---

# Middle Age

## Cultural Attitudes and Expectations

Women are considered middle-aged when approaching menopause, usually late in the fifth decade. Middle-aged women are more discrete in their clothing and may not feel comfortable wearing shorts or skirts above the knees. There are no stated cultural restrictions as to clothing or behavior for women of this age.

## Psychological Response

The "empty nest syndrome" is not widely experienced in Colombia. Only occasionally do children leave home, usually for postsecondary education in another city, and adult children do not move away as often as they do in North America. Also, parents may compensate for their "empty nest" through frequent family gatherings.

Likewise, Colombian women rarely recognize a "midlife crisis," although some men may exhibit this phenomenon when they leave their wives for younger women.

## Menopause

**Onset and Duration.**   Menopause, also called *menopausia* or *cerrar edad,* means "to close the age." The average age of menopause onset is between 48 and 52 years. An early or late onset is typically attributed to genetic or nutritional factors. There are no known lay explanations for this occurrence.

**Sexual Activity.**   Most Colombian women remain sexually active post-menopausally. Vaginal dryness and its accompanying pain and discomfort may eventually temper sexual intercourse.

**Coping.**   Most women respond to the discomforts of menopause by ignoring the symptoms unless they become so intense that they interfere with the woman's activities of daily living. Although hormone replacement therapy (HRT) is available, it is unclear precisely how many choose this form of therapy.

HRT is used mostly by urban and middle- to upper-class women. In the past decade, there has been an increase in the number of health stores, *tiendas naturistas* (or nature stores), that sell health-related medicaments, some for menopausal symptoms. Such alternative therapies are mostly used by middle or upper class urban people. Few if any specific herbal remedies are commonly used for perimenopausal symptoms. But some women treat symptoms with food extracts (e.g., from beets or figs).

# Old Age

In Colombia, the current mean life expectancy for women is 73.7 years. There is no specific age at which a woman is considered old; instead, it is her appearance (gray hair, wrinkled skin, curved posture, and broken speech) that denotes old age. Elderly women are respected, but they are not necessarily seen as a source of wisdom in the community.

If the elderly woman lived with her husband and her children have left home, she is likely to live alone after being widowed, move in with one of her children, or have an extended family member move in with her.

In most cases, when an elderly woman becomes unable to care for herself, family members take care of her in their own home. On rare occasions, the elderly woman is placed in a nursing home. Elderly people who have no money or family members to care for them are generally cared for in charity nursing homes for the poor.

# Death and Dying

## Cultural Attitudes and Beliefs

In most cases, death is seen as God's will, regardless of age, and there is no difference in perceptions or rituals by age or gender. Most Colombians are Catholics who believe that, following death, the soul or spirit goes to heaven, purgatory, or hell, depending on how one lived his or her life. It is up to God, and the type of death determines where one's soul will go (e.g., suicide may be considered sinful).

## Rites and Rituals

When an individual dies, the corpse is prepared and placed in a coffin. Close family members stay with the corpse at all times until burial, which occurs between 24 to 36 hours after the death. Before burial, other relatives and friends visit the deceased and pray frequently. Until 20 years ago, the coffin remained in the home of the deceased until burial, but today the coffin usually stays in a funeral home. People who attend the funeral traditionally wear black or black and white clothes, although this expectation has become more relaxed in recent years.

Catholics hold three masses for the dead person, one each day, which is replacing an old tradition of nine nights in which friends and relatives gathered in the home of the deceased to pray for his or her departed soul.

### Mourning

**Cultural Expectations.**   Close relatives (siblings, the widow or widower, children) typically mourn for one year, although the time for mourning is becoming more flexible in urban areas, and children, teens, and young adults tend to mourn for a shorter period. During the mourning period, close relatives are expected to keep a low profile, avoiding parties, dancing, displaying merriment. Women use little or no makeup. Widows wear black or black and white clothing initially, and it is preferable to continue wearing dark colors for at least one year.

If the deceased is the mother of young children and the father is alive and part of the family unit, he cares for the children. If he is not present, one of the grandmothers or another close relative (e.g., aunt or uncle) most frequently takes custody of the children.

**Coping.**   Most women are supported by their children and their faith to help them cope with the death of a spouse. Support is also offered by extended family and, in particular, by parents, if they are still alive.

## 🌐 IMPORTANT POINTS FOR PROVIDERS CARING FOR COLOMBIAN WOMEN

# The Medical Intake

## Literacy and English Proficiency

If the woman immigrated to North America as an adult and lives with her relatives from Colombia, it is likely that she does not speak English well, if at all. Ideally, medical forms should be printed in Spanish, and the language kept simple. Family members are likely to accompany the woman to the clinic, but it cannot be assumed that the family members are literate in English. Also, for issues of confidentiality, it is best if a medical translator rather than a family member assist with translation.

### Status of the Provider

Health care providers in general are seen as authority figures and treated with great respect. The older the woman, the more likely she is to be modest about her body, nonverbal, and to refrain from asking questions, particularly if the provider is male.

### Communicating Illness and Symptoms

In most cases, women will disclose significant medical information, unless the history includes what is considered a private matter (i.e., sexual history, history of mental illness). It may take more than one appointment to gain the patient's trust. It is important to talk openly with the woman, explaining why the information being sought is necessary for her care, and to emphasize the confidentiality of the history.

Colombian women tend to give elaborate explanations or tell lengthy stories to explain their illness. The provider should let them talk for a few minutes and listen attentively before asking more specific or direct questions. Regarding the cause of illness, some women may explain it, especially mental illness, as having been caused by something evil that has befallen the affected individual, such as being possessed by an evil spirit.

Family members frequently accompany the patient to visit a health provider, particularly if the patient is young (early adolescence or younger) or elderly. Frequently, the companion actively participates in providing information.

---

**NOTE TO THE HEALTH CARE PROVIDER**

As long as the provider asks questions pertaining to personal family or social history with respect, Colombian patients will answer them or at least not be offended by them. Since confidentiality is not observed in Colombia to the extent that it is in the United States, the provider should always review the standard of confidentiality relevant to the specific setting and problem.

---

## The Physical Examination

### Modesty and Touching

Modesty is especially important to women, so the practitioner should cover the woman's body as a sign of respect. Being assigned a female health provider may ease embarrassment during a physical examination, particularly if a pelvic examination is needed. If a relative accompanies the woman, the practitioner should ask whether the relative should stay or leave the office. Some women prefer even female relatives to leave; others prefer their relatives to stay with them, particularly if that relative is the daughter of an elderly woman or the mother of a younger daughter.

Touching the body during an examination is accepted in the context of a health-related visit. Women may feel embarrassed and avoid visiting a health care provider during their menses, particularly if the visit involves an examination of the genitalia.

### Expressing Pain

There are gender differences in expressing pain: men are expected to be stoic and to not complain or demonstrate pain, but women openly demonstrate their suffering by crying or moaning loudly.

## Prescribing Medications

### Drug Interactions

Colombians use traditional remedies, such as herbal teas or roots, and vitamins, particularly vitamin B complex, on a regular basis. A client will usually tell the health care provider what she is taking when asked, but she may not volunteer this information despite its importance.

### Medication Sharing

With the exception of sedatives, medications are sold in Colombia without a prescription. People commonly describe their symptoms to a pharmacist or person working in a pharmacy and ask what medicine to take to "treat this illness." This is particularly true for minor conditions such as headache, skin rash, or diarrhea. Antibiotics are also sold over the counter and may be taken for severe cold symptoms. Likewise, some people will buy and take a medicine recommended by a friend who had similar symptoms. Recent immigrants may continue to share medications or to obtain those requiring a prescription from friends or relatives living in Colombia.

### Compliance

It is common to discontinue a medication when symptoms disappear, particularly if the client has not been educated on the necessity of completing the full course of the medication. It is, therefore, very important to explain in simple terms how the medicine works and how to take it. Involving family members in explaining the importance of adherence may facilitate it, as may a follow-up call from the provider to demonstrate his or her interest and the importance of adherence.

## Follow-up Appointments

Missing follow-up appointments is common and not considered rude, particularly if the patient feels better. Calling the day before to remind the patient about the appointment will be helpful, particularly when the appointment is needed for care of a chronic illness. It is also helpful to involve other family members as "team members" in the care by asking them to remind the client to keep appointments.

### Orientation to Time

Colombians generally do not adhere to "clock" time; being a few minutes late for an appointment is not perceived as being late. In contrast, in "social time," people are expected to be an hour or more late for social gatherings, and arriving on time is unexpected and may cause difficulties.

## Prevalent Diseases

In 1998, the prevalence of cervical cancer among Colombian women was 7 per 100,000—the second highest cause of mortality among women older than 15 years. Other prevalent health conditions reported for women are heart disease (14.8 per 1000), stroke (7.6 per 1000), and hypertension (4.7 per 1000). Because of the current serious sociopolitical problems in Colombia, homicide is now listed as the highest cause of mortality in women 15 to 45 years (5.31 per 1000).

## Health-Seeking Behaviors

Seeking care for illness varies, depending on such factors as access to care, perceived severity of the illness, and educational level.

It is not unusual for lesser educated, poor, or rural women to visit a **curandero** for mental illness (**nervios** or **nerviosidad**) or **sobanderos** to manage musculoskeletal pain. These practitioners typically use special massage to the affected part of the body to alleviate pain or disease.

For minor illness, women first try home remedies, such as teas, or buy vitamins, over-the-counter medications, or medications from Colombia that would require a prescription in the United States.

If the illness is perceived to be major, fatalism may be displayed, for example, by saying **"lo que Dios quiera"** (it is God's will) or telling the health care provider **"lo que usted diga"** (whatever you say). Few risk-reduction or proactive self-care activities are used to prevent major illnesses other than attempting to eat a healthy diet and remaining physically active.

### 🌐 BIBLIOGRAPHY

De la Cuesta, C. (1995). Mujeres y salud. Un estudio cualitativo. *Dirección Seccional de Salud de Antioquia*. Medellín (Women and health: A qualitative study).

De Pheils, P. B. (1996). Colombians. In J. Lipson, S. Dibble, & P. Minarik (Eds.), *Culture and nursing care: A pocket guide*. San Francisco: UCSF Nursing Press, pp. 82–90.

Jaramillo, D. E., y Uribe, T. M. (2000). Violencia Doméstica en Medellín (Colombia). Un problema que afecta la salud de las mujeres. INDEX *de Enfermería*: 30:17–21 (Domestic Violence in Medellín [Colombia]. A problem affecting women's health).

Mora, M, et al. (1995). El aborto. Factores involucrados y consecuencias. *Orientame. Bogotá* (Abortion: Factors and Consequences).

PROFAMILIA. Salud Sexual y Reproductiva en Colombia (2000). Encuesta Nacional de Demografía y Salud. Bogotá, Colombia. (Reproductive and Sexual Health in Colombia: National Demographic and Health Survey).

# Egyptians

## AFAF MELEIS, PhD, RN, FAAN

###  INTRODUCTION

### Who are the Egyptian People?

Egypt had one of the world's most ancient civilizations. A series of colonizations influenced Egypt's culture and people, with every invading people helping to shape the values and normative structure of contemporary Egypt. The most influential cultures, however, have been the ancient pharaonic and the more recent Arabic/Islamic cultures. Egyptians strongly identify with their own country and demonstrate pride in their heritage.

There is great diversity among Egyptians, among whom 50% live in rural areas and 50% in urban areas such as Cairo, Alexandria, Assuit, and Luxor, among other Egyptian cities. Most people live on 5% of Egypt's land, with most of the population concentrated in large cities. About 85% are Muslims; the remainder are Christians, although a small number of Jews reside in Cairo and Alexandria.

Egyptians speak Arabic. Although it is the same language spoken in all Arab countries, Egyptian Arabic is the most popular dialect in the Arab world. This is largely because of the popularity of performing arts and music that originate in Egypt and are enjoyed in all other Arab countries.

### Egyptians in North America

Egyptians came to the United States and Canada in three major waves. In the 1950s, they came to pursue educational goals; in the 1960s, they were escaping an oppressive political regime; and in the 1970s, they came to seek better lives because the country had lost wars, depriving citizens of life's amenities. Among the immigrants were Muslims, Christians, and Jews. Most Egyptian Jews emigrated around the late 1950s and early 1960s. Egyptian Christians emigrated shortly after the Jews. The major reason was the undermining of the acceptance of their minority status by the changing political regime of the 1960s. These groups felt that they were driven out of their homes, losing many of their possessions in the process, and many left reluctantly. The Muslims, who are the majority culture in their home country, left to pursue a better lifestyle, education, or occupational opportunities.

Estimates are that more than 1 million Egyptians are living in the United States as immigrants and about one-half million are in the United States temporarily to work or study with the intent of returning to Egypt. Most Egyptians in the United States reside in New York, New Jersey, Pennsylvania, Illinois, California, and Michigan. Egyptian communities are found in all of these states.

Canada has an estimated 35,570 people of Egyptian heritage living within its borders, 47% of whom are women. Egyptians in Canada mainly live in Montreal and Toronto.

Among Arabs, Egyptian women have been considered the most liberated; however, there is as much diversity among Egyptian women as there is among their North American counterparts. Several variables influence the patterns of responses of Egyptian women. The following factors are integral to assessing women: reasons for immigration, length of residence in North America, age at immigration, religious affiliation, adherence to religious rituals, educational background, and how often they visit their home country.

For Egyptian-American women, as with other Arab women, family comes first. Egyptians are more oriented to their nuclear families than their extended families, and the nuclear family is their primary responsibility and commitment, after which comes the extended family, with parents and parents of spouses taking a primary role. Other Arab families are more extended-family-centered than are Egyptians. This is particularly apparent in processes involving consent to health care and decision-making, which involve nuclear families among Egyptians and extended families among other Arab Americans.

Women are expected to be caregivers to their children, parents, and in-laws even when they have careers. Women continue to predominantly take care of household responsibilities, while men are considered the "head of the household."

## BEING FEMALE IN EGYPTIAN SOCIETY

### At Birth

#### Preference for Sons

While there is always a subtle preference for sons, when girls are born they are treated equally as "God's gift." The preference for sons is slightly more profound in North America because of the fear of raising a daughter within Western values and norms that allow and expect women to date, go to proms, and experiment with premarital sex. The biggest challenge for Egyptian-American women and their families is raising a daughter in North America—simultaneously instilling Egyptian values of chastity, modesty, and compliance, while expecting her to excel in school and be oriented toward a career. Hence, the birth of sons is met with fewer worries, and sons may be more welcome. Egyptian Americans may choose to return to their home country because they are raising daughters.

#### Response to the Birth of a Female

Daughters are celebrated as much as sons. Both parents take a stand of "let's try again for a son." They will usually abandon this idea, however, after a second or third daughter arrives.

## Birth Rituals

Egyptian-American women prefer to avoid the pain of birthing at all costs. Having Lamaze or prenatal classes are new experiences; they attend classes and adopt "natural childbirth" methods only if prompted and repeatedly encouraged to do so. Although husbands usually prefer other female companions to be present at the birth, many husbands will reluctantly support their wives during labor and delivery when the significance of their presence is explained. In retrospect fathers become the best advocates for attending the birth of babies.

Circumcision is expected for boys. While some Egyptian women support female circumcision and expect their daughters to be circumcised, Egyptian families in the United States rarely expect or practice circumcision.

## Childhood and Youth

### Family Expectations

Children are expected to behave as children and comply with their parents' wishes as long as they are students (through college education). This expectation of deferring to parents continues through major decisions in the lives of young adults, including marriage. These expectations create family tension when children follow Western norms of moving out at college age. At this point, there is gender disjuncture in expectations and behavior. Deferring to parents and complying with Egyptian values, while expected for all children, are emphasized more for daughters than for sons. Children are expected to show **ihteram** (respect) and **adab** (politeness) to their elders and those in authority.

### Social Expectations

Girls have the responsibility not to bring "shame" **(aar)** to their families by dating, having male friends, or practicing premarital sex. Girls' **somaa** (reputation) is to be protected at all costs, including deporting the daughter temporarily to Egypt if there are any indications that she is inclined to adopt Western norms of dating, has romantic inclinations, or rejects the value of chastity.

### Importance of Education

Urban families in Egypt consider girls' education to be almost as important as that of boys. Egyptian-American families value education, serious studying, and degree attainment; and they expect their daughters to complete their education. Parents with tangible resources clearly communicate and support the primacy of these values. Some families immigrated to North America specifically so that their children would have better opportunities for higher education.

## Pubescence

### Psychosexual Development

Egyptian girls today achieve menarche between ages 11 and 14 years. Boys achieve pubescence at a slightly older age. The word used for achieving pubescence for girls is **balaget.** Once girls show signs of pubescence, their families may place more restrictions on them because they fear that the girls may want to date. Most importantly, families fear that their daughters may lose their virginity. Parents carefully monitor relationships, restrict absences from the house, and strongly enforce curfews. Most Egyptian families frown upon sleepovers and slumber parties, and many forbid them.

### Rituals and Rites of Passage

No particular rituals serve as rites of passage into pubescence for Egyptian girls. The start of menstruation, however, symbolizes the achievement of a new stage in young women's lives. North American school-based sex education provides girls with enough knowledge to make the event merely one stage in their development, and families welcome the event as a symbol of the family's normal progress. Onset of menstruation also signals the need to impose more vigilant observations on a girl's behavior, lest she stray and develop relationships with boys that go beyond occasional conversations. The fear of loss of virginity, which characterizes the parent/daughter relationship, takes on a different meaning at this milestone.

### Teen Sexuality

Teenage girls are expected to guard their virginity, protect their bodies, and maintain their modesty. Touching the opposite sex is not permitted. Providing information about birth control to teenage Egyptian girls is frowned upon: "Only American girls need this information because they are loose and could have sex." Girls who stray from these norms are punished. Families do not pressure young women to marry until they have achieved their educational goals.

It is the daughter's duty to protect the intactness of the hymen at all costs. For this reason, girls are not expected to have vaginal examinations until after marriage, and they are also discouraged or prohibited from using tampons.

Teen pregnancy is rare among Egyptian girls. Egyptian-American girls, however, experience the pressure to conform to mainstream North American sexual experimentation, and some girls experiment behind their parents' backs and maintain secrets.

---

**NOTE TO THE HEALTH CARE PROVIDER**
Providers should handle the subjects of a young woman's sexuality and potential pregnancy, or protection from it, delicately and in private. They should not involve the family except at the young woman's expressed request.

---

### Menstruation

**Relationship to Health.**   Regular periods are a symbol of health. There is a pervasive fear of missed periods because of the focus on virginity and an intact hymen. This fear is more acute if the family has experienced any concerns about their daughter's connection or intimacy with boys or men. If the daughter is perceived to be following the family's rules of no contact with boys, the family may associate amenorrhea with lack of fertility and seek medical care.

**Relationship to Fertility.**   Egyptians view the regularity of menstruation during adolescence as good preparation for a fertile adulthood. Mothers of adolescent Egyptian-American girls may seek medical care for their daughters if the girls experience any deviation from what is perceived as normal flow. They require assurance of their daughters' future as fertile women. There are no treatments for amenorrhea other than decreasing physical activity and exercise.

**Taboos and Restrictions During Menstruation.** Some Egyptian-American women avoid baths or showers during the menstrual flow, based on such beliefs as fear of infection, an inability to control the flow, or fear of seeing one's blood flowing in the shower.

For Muslim Egyptian girls who observe the ritual of fasting during the month of Ramadan, the onset of menstruation also signals the inability to fast during a menstrual cycle. They have to make up the fasting days later when they are more "pure." For adult women, sexual intercourse during menstruation ranges from being strictly forbidden to merely being avoided, depending on whether the couple holds traditional views or has adopted a more experimental approach to sexual relationships.

**Dysmenorrhea.** Some young Egyptian women experience menstrual cramping that follows them into adulthood. Absences from school during menstrual cycles are common among some young women, and they cannot undergo gynecological examinations to determine reasons for any problems they are having until after a marriage is consummated for fear of rupturing the hymen. These women value medications to control cramps and use them frequently.

## Female Modesty and Touching

One of the most important tasks of Egyptian-American families is to make sure that their daughters develop a sense of modesty. Modesty means wearing clothes that are not revealing, avoiding touching unrelated boys or men, and saving oneself physically for a future husband. These social mandates are cultural and transcend religions, although Muslim girls and women wear the most modest clothing, ranging from wearing generally nonrevealing clothes to covering their hair with scarves, their wrists with long sleeves, and ankles with long skirts. With increasing observance of Islamic rules and various interpretations of Islam, many young girls are adopting more traditional covering of their heads and bodies.

Touching and hugging are typical and acceptable within the same gender but are prohibited across genders. In addition, women do not usually touch their own bodies and must be coached to do breast self-examinations. Helping women become comfortable with their bodies should be a goal of health care providers.

---

**NOTE TO THE HEALTH CARE PROVIDER**
Providers need to be extremely careful to avoid pelvic examinations of unmarried Egyptian women, which are forbidden. Married women usually accept annual pelvic examinations but with reluctance. If an examination is needed, the practitioner should discuss whether the woman is a virgin and if her hymen is intact before suggesting such an examination. If the provider is a man, he should ask whether the patient prefers a female practitioner. The provider should always drape the girl's body as much as possible. Providers should ask the girl in private if she prefers to have a female member of the family present during the examination. It is essential to approach any discussions of sexual activity with a great deal of delicacy if the girl or woman is unmarried. If the family suspects any sexual activity for an unmarried woman (regardless of age), consequences for her may be unpleasant.

---

# Adulthood

## Transition Rites and Rituals

Egyptians call unmarried women "girls"; therefore, marriage is a transition point for girls at any age. Girls and boys leave their parents' homes only when they get married. These traditions are not uniform, however, among Egyptian-American families. Reluctantly, they allow their daughters to leave home to go to college, though they would prefer keeping them home until they are "settled through marriage" in their own homes. Girls' families are involved in all decisions, large and small, and daughters are expected to consult with their families in all their decisions, whether educational or health related. More liberties are permitted once the daughter holds a job.

## Social Expectations

Girls are pressured in two ways: they are expected to continue to focus strongly on their higher education goals and, at the same time, to comply with the equal imperative to marry during their early 20s. The Egyptian-American family's goal is for the daughter to marry an Egyptian Muslim, if the family is Muslim, or an Egyptian Christian, if the family is Christian. If an Egyptian husband is not possible, the next priority is to marry within the faith. Families expect their sons-in-law to convert to the family religion. A Muslim woman is considered to be living in sin if she does not marry within the Islamic faith. While marriage is highly valued for both sons and daughters, it is more imperative for daughters. Arranged marriages by families are also highly valued, and many families follow this practice. The suitor should be acceptable to the daughter, however, even when the families arrange the marriage. Premarital sex or living together is forbidden among Egyptian-American families.

---

**NOTE TO THE HEALTH CARE PROVIDER**
Unmarried women who are more sexually liberal take great precautions to keep their families from knowing about their activities. Thus, providers should always counsel about preventive measures in privacy.

---

## Union Formation

The only acceptable union is marriage. Both partners expect monogamy. Premarital and extramarital relations are totally forbidden for women; they are merely frowned upon for men.

## Domestic Violence

Men are expected to be the breadwinners and the final authority in the family, and as such, the disciplinarians and rule keepers. Based on this authority and their own expectations, battering and abuse of wives and children are prevalent. Battering in families includes verbal and psychological abuse as well as physical assault. Women and children take it so much for granted as part of the male role that they rarely report it. When reporting occurs, men are shocked and consider it an Americanization process that undermines family members' loyalty and commitment to family functioning. A sense of passiveness among women, as well as the practice of male social control, justify the male battering and abuse of women and children.

Men expect to monitor and control some activities of women (e.g., business appointments with men and outings with male work colleagues), and minor deviations prompt verbal or physical abuse.

Stigma associated with domestic violence keeps the violence a family secret. As women become more empowered by a network or career and gain more financial independence in North America, they are better able to put limits on violence and eliminate it from their families. A similar process occurs with children.

---

**NOTE TO THE HEALTH CARE PROVIDER**

Women are reluctant to admit that they are victims of violence and are not willing to leave a violent situation because of their commitment to the nuclear and extended family. They are also reluctant to share their family secrets with non-Middle Easterners for fear of stereotyping. In a case of suspected domestic violence, providers need to be tactful and approach the woman tentatively and with caution. They should not suggest at the outset a move to a shelter. First, they should try to build a trusting relationship and encourage the woman to contact the provider during future episodes.

---

## Rape

Egyptians handle any sexual activity outside marriage with secrecy. Rape in particular is stigmatizing, with blame often placed on the woman. Therefore, women are ashamed of reporting rape and feel guilty about the experience. Rape brings shame to women and their families. Therefore, when mentioned in the family, girls and women tend to be punished and it remains a secret unless revealed through pregnancy or a husband's suspicion. Besides the shame, guilt, and punishment, the woman may be ostracized in her community and restricted in her daily life.

## Divorce

**Sociocultural Views.** Divorce is rare among Egyptian immigrants; when it occurs, it is either kept a secret or one of the two partners leaves North America and re-establishes residency in his or her home country. In this group, divorce is stigmatizing and shameful and is often considered the fault of the wife and the Americanization of the family. The frequency of divorce among young adults is increasing, however; and families are more forgiving of this generation's decision to divorce. Remarriage is common but frowned upon in women.

Living alone for women is discouraged. Therefore, divorced women frequently move in with other family members or their children. Women live with a threat of divorce, which Islamic laws make easier. Men often use divorce as a weapon to keep their authority and control; they easily suggest it in the heat of anger and just as easily withdraw it.

**Child Custody Practices.** Egyptian-American families often experience disputes about custody of children. Customs and religion give custody of young children to mothers and of adolescents to fathers. Unfriendly divorces and hostile custody fights are much more common than is friendly shared custody of children; joint custody and shared responsibilities rarely work well in these families. Many parents use the children as pawns in fights, pressuring the children to take sides. They often drag children through disputes, and there is loss of protective parenting at the children's expense. In-laws, local or international, are often party to these disputes and play major roles in exacerbating them. Many ex-husbands enter into new relationships as soon as divorce is final, which also tends to decrease any potential for amicable solutions to disputes. The major fear of divorced partners is losing children through repatriation to the home country. There are many stories of children being "stolen" and unable to be reunited with the partner in North America because of the protection of Egyptian law. Extended families then are expected to take full responsibility for children of divorced parents.

---

**NOTE TO THE HEALTH CARE PROVIDER**
If the father is given custody, he will need coaching to follow up on immunizations. It is important to carefully monitor the trauma of separation of parents on the children. Providers should watch for signs of stress in families undergoing divorce. They rarely seek professional support during this transition.

---

### Fertility and Childbearing

**Family Size.**    Historically, large families were a goal of Egyptians, and this pattern continues in rural Egypt. Having children is the *raison d'être* for Egyptian Americans to form marital unions. The pace of life in the United States, the nuclear family responsibilities, and the cost of raising children, however, have encouraged reduction of family size to two to three children per family. Producing children continues to be regarded as the cement for families, however; it is the force to help parents mature, and what extended families far and near expect from a couple. Pregnancy allows some women to decrease their responsibilities and affords them the power to enhance their status.

**Contraceptive Practices.**    Birth control and family planning are practiced in urban Egypt and by most couples who immigrate to North America. Women use oral contraceptives and intrauterine devices (IUDs) and may also require their husbands to use condoms. Tubal ligations are acceptable, but vasectomies are not. All contraceptive use is contingent on first having the number of children the family wants. Most Egyptian-American couples do not use contraceptive methods before they are married or before they give birth to at least two or three babies. Religious teachings give mixed messages about the use of contraception based on different interpretations of the religious books (Koran or Bible). Information on birth control should always be provided, but it is usually not welcomed before the birth of the first baby.

**Role of the Male Partner in the Couple's Fertility Decision-Making.**    The use of contraception and the processes used for family planning are considered for the most part the "woman's responsibility." Men, however, reserve the right to veto the use of contraception. It is best to include both partners in discussion of family planning and birth control, so that both can answer questions that are usually directed to the wife, to empower women's negotiation abilities, to defuse resistance, and to emphasize the significance of mutual planning.

---

**NOTE TO THE HEALTH CARE PROVIDER**
Egyptian-American men respect Western health care professionals; introducing and supporting the use of condoms or vasectomy may encourage men's involvement in the process and their active use of male-focused birth control methods.

---

## Abortion

**Cultural Attitudes.**   Abortion is one of the most frequently used methods of birth control in Egypt for accidental or unwanted pregnancies, even though it is legal only for therapeutic purposes. A great deal of secrecy but no stigma, shame, or guilt surrounds its use. Egyptian couples in the United States, however, rarely practice abortion; and when it does occur, it happens in total secrecy. No data support its use in the United States for birth control purposes by Egyptian couples. In Egypt, mothers wanting to abort their babies may resort to heavy lifting, herbal remedies, or seek licensed or unlicensed practitioners. Egyptian Americans have not reported such practices.

**Sources of Abortion.**   If they have medical or health care insurance, women seek abortion services in the United States. The only reasons for Egyptian-American women to seek abortions elsewhere may be the lack of insurance or if abortion is illegal or subject to criminal prosecution. Women are likely to seek abortions very early in the pregnancy, not beyond the first trimester.

**Teen Abortion.**   If the teen is married, abortion is never practiced. If the teen is not married, she may seek an abortion in complete secrecy.

---

**NOTE TO THE HEALTH CARE PROVIDER**

Providers should discuss alternative methods to terminating pregnancy with great caution. They should determine if the accompanying family member is from the father's (in-law) side of the family or the mother's side. Though they may appear to have similar relationships, women may prefer to keep these delicate matters hidden from other than immediate family. Women will not volunteer information. Asking direct questions is best.

---

## Miscarriage

No data are available on the prevalence of miscarriage in this group. Women try very hard to preserve their pregnancies to term. They follow medical recommendations, and extended families provide support to prevent a miscarriage. Women are pampered, well fed, and provided with ample support to carry their babies to term. If miscarriage occurs, women are encouraged to try again. There is pressure to have women go on complete bed rest, avoid work outside the house, and refrain from carrying heavy loads and climbing stairs. These actions are believed to decrease the potential of having another miscarriage.

---

**NOTE TO THE HEALTH CARE PROVIDER**

The stress of immigration, the heavy demands on immigrant women, the lack of extended family support, the dearth of household help, and lifestyle changes may be risks for preterm birth or miscarriage. Careful history-taking may identify risks.

---

## Infertility

Egyptian families highly value having children, and not having children is a cause for divorce in rural areas. Urban couples with no children seek medical care to help them conceive. Women begin the process of seeking medical care and often take the blame for not becoming pregnant. Immigrant Egyptians spare no time, effort, or money to determine the cause of infertility, and they pursue medical treatment even if husbands are to be tested also.

## Pregnancy

**Activity Restrictions and Taboos.** Women are expected to curtail heavy lifting and physical activities during pregnancies for fear of miscarriage. They are also expected and advised to eat more to ensure a healthy baby. Cravings for certain foods during pregnancy are called *waham*. Expectant mothers are supposed to eat what they crave; otherwise, popular folklore suggests that the baby will be born with a birthmark reflecting the item craved.

Pregnant women in Egypt are treated gently and protected from painful experiences and seeing deformities or disabilities. Women are shielded from grief and mourning and, if possible, are not told of the death of a family member to protect them and their babies. Egyptian-American women living away from their extended families cannot and do not have these luxuries. They tend to follow recommendations for healthy mother and baby. They seek well-balanced food, but they tend to become inactive.

**Prenatal Care.** Women tend to seek prenatal care early in their pregnancy and to comply with recommendations for regular check-ups. They resist suggestions for alternative birthing or birthing without anesthesia, and they need to be coaxed to attend prenatal classes and to prepare the baby's room and layette. These women tend to avoid planning and preparation for fear of bringing a bad omen on their pregnancy.

## Birthing Process

**Home Versus Hospital Delivery.** Because of many myths about the process and pain of childbirth, pregnant women approach delivery with fear and apprehension. They prefer hospital deliveries and will not usually accept other than an obstetrician for prenatal care, delivery, and postpartum care. Egyptian Americans tend to have similar preferences.

**Cesarean Section Versus Vaginal Delivery.** While women prefer vaginal deliveries, they are not reluctant to have a cesarean section if there is any question that prolonged labor may harm the baby. They also prefer less pain and swifter labor and delivery, which a cesarean section usually guarantees.

**Labor Management.** Delivery and birth are the women's domain, and all expect a female from the birthing mother's family to be present during labor. Egyptian-American husbands are reluctant to participate in this process and have many apprehensions about being invited into the delivery room. This reluctance is lessening, however, as husbands become more involved in prenatal care and as they learn of the importance of their presence and coaching in the birthing process. In many cases, resistance transforms to total commitment.

---

**NOTE TO THE HEALTH CARE PROVIDER**
Egyptian-American women want to avoid pain and discomfort at any cost, so providers should offer pain medication during labor. They are less committed to medication-free delivery or to natural childbirth as are their American-born counterparts.

---

**Placenta.**   There are no special rituals for the disposal of the placenta among Egyptians in North America.

## Postpartum

The postpartum traditions that women experience in their home country are rarely available in North America. Prolonged bed rest, delegation of responsibility for the baby to a female relative, good nourishing meals, and being totally pampered are customs that they greatly miss. Women are advised to avoid bathing and exposure to drafts (cold breezes), and they are discouraged from leaving their homes for 40 days. These customs can be followed with extended family members in attendance, but increasing demands on women are contributing to the erosion of these practices. Because of this lack of attention, some women become depressed. Additionally, the postpartum transition may trigger early immigration transition traumas.

---

**NOTE TO THE HEALTH CARE PROVIDER**

Providers should avoid serving cold drinks or food to the postpartum woman. They should turn on the heater rather than the air conditioner and not open windows. Gentle discussion of regular showers or baths with newly immigrated women is helpful. A discussion about sources of support during the postpartum period may reveal the fears and anxiety about the absence of extended family.

---

## Newborn and Infant Care

**Breastfeeding Versus Bottle-Feeding.**   Bottle-feeding is preferred because of years of advertising campaigns promoting infant formula in the Middle East. Health care providers should initiate a discussion of breastfeeding versus bottle-feeding early in prenatal care. A common myth is that colostrum (first breast milk) is harmful for babies and should be discarded, which also discourages women from initiating breastfeeding. New mothers may become discouraged when milk flow is low, nipples are sore, and babies are crying. They tend to immediately resort to bottle-feeding. Coaching on how to burp the infant, on-demand feeding, and the timing of solid food for supplementation is in order.

**Infant Protection.**   New parents very strongly protect newborns from cold weather, drafts, the evil eye, and envy. They overdress their babies, do not bathe them regularly, shield them from open windows and fresh air, pin blue amulets (to prevent the evil eye) on their clothing, and are careful not to flaunt their beauty. The whole family becomes housebound. Taking an infant out is unusual during the first 40 days of the baby's life, but families will take the baby for a check-up. Symptoms associated with the evil eye are colds, rash, emergence of any abnormality, colic, and unmanageable crying. In the home country, women may boil mint or cumin leaves and give the colicky baby a teaspoon of the mixture to ease the pain. In North America, parents immediately seek medical care and will comply with suggestions for any symptoms. They are reluctant to use their ancestors' wisdom because they see North America as having the best medical care, and they prefer to take advantage of it.

**Primary Caregiver.**   Mothers are the primary caregivers, but Egyptian fathers in North America are becoming increasingly involved in raising their children. If present, extended family members provide support and baby-sitting. Parents do not trust outsiders to take care of their children; hence, the use of baby-sitters is minimal in this population. Unless they form a baby-caring co-op among their family and friends, parents will rarely go out without their children.

# Middle Age

## Cultural Attitudes and Expectations

Middle age is a time for women to feel entitled to the care, respect, and attention of their children. During this time, however, Egyptian mothers in North America feel deprived of their children's attention and attribute their children's focus on peers to westernization. Middle-aged women may consider this period as either a threat or a challenge. Those who see it as a threat may experience somatic symptoms that are difficult to diagnose. Those who perceive it as a challenge feel freer to befriend their children and adapt their expectations to fit those of their children. The strong connection between Egyptians and their extended families in Egypt is manifested more during the middle-age period. Movement between countries is more fluid, and extended family responsibilities increase during this time.

## Psychological Response

Middle-aged Egyptian-American women respond in one of two ways to middle age: they feel relief that they have accomplished the earlier responsibilities of childrearing or they feel threatened by their children's changing attitudes and lifestyle. Threats are related to children's educational achievements, occupational gains, and their own selection of partners. If the children have not met the education or career expectations of their parents or are not settled in an engagement or marriage that meets parental expectations, Egyptian mothers in North America may become anxious and depressed and may experience somatic symptoms.

### Menopause

**Onset and Duration.**   The average age for the onset of menopause is about 50 years. The Arabic word for menopause means "age of despair," an indication of how it is viewed in Egyptian folklore. Egyptian-American women, however, view menopause simply as the cessation of menstruation, not a long transition that includes both the perimenopausal and postmenopausal period. Data on the meaning and experience of menopause in Egyptian-American women are limited.

**Sexual Activity.**   Menopausal women remain sexually active; however, they experience decrease in their desires, needs, and ability to reach orgasm.

**Coping.** Egyptian women rarely discuss menopausal symptoms and sexual activities except among close friends and through rumor. If and when women experience hot flashes, dryness, and irritability, they request hormone replacement therapy (HRT). Trust in their health care providers supports their use of HRT, and use of alternative health care in this population is minimal.

Egyptian-American women cope with the changes in their bodies by becoming more involved in the lives of their adult children, friends, and extended family members. These individuals provide them with opportunities to discuss and receive advice on how to deal with health issues. While group support is essential for these women, most are reluctant to participate in support group activities that do not include their own friends and kin.

# Old Age

Growing old in North America is a fairly new experience for Egyptian-American women because most of them immigrated in the late 1950s and early 1960s. These groups are approaching the beginning of old age in the early 2000s. Life expectancy for Egyptian Americans is not known, although it may well exceed that of Egyptians in their own country, which is about 68 for women and 65 for men. Egyptian-American women are considered old when they reach the mid-60s, and younger people are expected to treat them with extra respect. Egyptian-American women also expect their children to care for them and, if widowed, to live with them. Even when women themselves do not expect to live with their children, strong extended family pressure and expectations prevent a living-alone arrangement. The norm is for family members to provide caregiving in old age, and retirement homes are frowned upon. It is acceptable to hire someone, if affordable, to care for the elder under the supervision of a family member.

Older women are revered by their Egyptian children. For children growing up in North America, however, these attitudes have changed drastically, much to the disappointment of older women. Being treated as a North American mother is the ultimate fear of an Egyptian woman. These women want to be totally involved in their adult children's lives, to be asked to care for grandchildren, and to participate in health care decisions for their children and grandchildren. They feel entitled to be taken care of when ill and during any health care issues or crises. If a partner is not available, they demand that their children step in and relieve them of the responsibility of caring for themselves.

# Death and Dying

## Cultural Attitudes and Beliefs

Egyptian cultural beliefs and behaviors related to the impending or actual death of a family member are based on pharaonic practices, Arab cultural heritage, and Christian and Muslim beliefs. Death is a topic that is avoided in conversation. When death is brought up, it should be followed by such a phrase as **Baad El Shaar**, which means "God forbid." The only planning for dying is ensuring a burial place that meets religious specifications. Beyond that, discussions about death or what might happen after a family member dies do not happen until after the family member dies.

There is resignation that death is governed by God's will; therefore, the health care professional's prognosis for dying is conceived as defying or disrespectful of God's will. The characteristics and context of the dying person, that is, the person's age, the length of his or her illness, and the suddenness of the death, may influence the family's responses. Death is never treated lightly, however, particularly by off-spring of the deceased.

### Rites and Rituals

Death is not to be prepared for, yet a burial place may be purchased. Muslims have many rituals that they must follow, preferably monitored by a family member, al-though a relative or specialist may perform such rituals. The naked body must be washed, and all orifices are cleaned and plugged with cotton or shreds of clothes to keep the spirit in or the insects out. The body is then wrapped in white muslin fab-ric and taken to the mosque for a final gathering and prayers. In some cities a mosque member may wash and prepare the body in a room attached to the mosque. Christians use mortuaries.

Burial is expected as soon as possible, and Egyptians in general resist autopsies. The rationale for autopsy needs to be carefully described to the significant others in North America. Some new practices, such as the family viewing the body, have been introduced into the Egyptian community.

The spirit of the deceased leaves the body at death and is tried for the sins com-mitted in his or her life. For Muslims, having the opportunity to listen to and to re-cite Koranic verses is expected to help the soul or spirit of the person in its peace-ful ascendance for the trial and a smooth passage to the heavens. Christians follow similar rituals for immediate burial; however, the body may be kept for a brief wake. Christian Egyptians in North America are increasingly using funeral homes to han-dle the burial process.

---

**NOTE TO THE HEALTH CARE PROVIDER**

Practitioners should provide the family with a room for privacy for discussion of how to handle the death and to allow them to wail and cry without disturbing others. Bringing a copy of the Koran or Bible to the bedside is regarded as culturally com-petent care.

---

### Mourning

**Cultural Expectations.** Egyptians tend to react to death instantly and dra-matically with audible wailing, crying, and even screaming. Mourning begins the moment their relative or friend dies and lasts a minimum of one year. A significant mourning ritual is gathering at home, in a mosque, or at a Muslim burial place to listen to the Koran and to drink black coffee. Egyptian-American women expect their friends and family members to participate in this ritual. The same ritual is repeated on the 7th day after death, two months of Thursdays, and on the 40th day, called **El Arbeen,** which literally means the 40th day after death. This day is a milestone that allows family members to reassume their daily routines. During the period of mourning, the immediate family wears black, silences radios and televisions, and does not participate in joyful activities. Family members also refrain from wearing make-up and jewelry. Those who come to pay respect to the family and to give con-dolences are expected to follow the same rules.

The milestones of the mourning transition (e.g., 7th day, two months of Thursdays, 40 days, and the first anniversary) bring intense grief reactions. Subsequent yearly anniversaries of the death **(El Sanaweya)** may also result in intense responses that tend to subside over the years. The length of stay in the United States tends to moderate these responses and rituals. Many Egyptian Americans, however, travel back to their home country to share their grief and mourning with extended family members.

Carrying out mourning rituals depends on whether the deceased is buried in North America or the country of origin. Some Muslim families insist on burying the deceased member in the family cemetery in Egypt. Increasingly, Muslims in North America are buying burial sites that meet religious criteria, and both Muslims and Christians tend to experience more anxiety about dying and burial processes than people of the dominant culture. Muslims and Christians believe that the deceased will go to heaven or hell based on his or her worldly actions, beliefs, and attention to religious rituals.

---

**NOTE TO THE HEALTH CARE PROVIDER**

Health care professionals will pick up on anxiety related to dying, but also on a peace in believers that reduces the survivors' fear and allows them to believe that they will join family members who preceded them. At the time of death (onset of mourning), health care providers need to anticipate and participate in such decisions as who will wash and wrap the body, who will transport it to the burial place, how long it takes to initiate religious rituals, and where the family can discuss these details in privacy. Avoiding discussion of death before it occurs may result in conflicts of opinion between members of the family after death.

---

**Coping.**    Family members cope with mourning through prayers, frequent rituals with religious readings, condolences from family members and friends, and opportunities to speak of the deceased person and to cry about the loss. Frequent visits to the burial site and faith in God help family members accept the death. The younger the age of the deceased (beyond infancy) and the closer the relationship, the more intense and the longer the grief will be; for example, losing a mother is especially hard on an Egyptian American.

---

**NOTE TO THE HEALTH CARE PROVIDER**

Practitioners should not judge intense grief responses and long mourning periods as being pathological. Mourning for Egyptian Americans must take its long course. Providers should encourage ritual observations, mobilize community support, and provide opportunities for privacy.

---

## IMPORTANT POINTS FOR PROVIDERS CARING FOR EGYPTIAN WOMEN

### The Medical Intake

#### Literacy and English Proficiency

The wave of immigration may have an influence on the woman's literacy and English proficiency. Many immigrants from the 1950s and 1960s were professionals and fluent in several languages. Those who arrived since the 1970s may have learned to communicate professionally in English, but they also tend to live in Egyptian communities and may speak less everyday English. Thus, the length of time in North America is not always an indication of proficiency in English, nor is spoken English always an indication of literacy level. Providers must try to judge the client's level of understanding before inviting an interpreter. Asking clients delicately about their preferences of having or not having an interpreter may help to avoid insulting their intelligence, literacy, and English proficiency. Health care providers should also use their clinical judgment as to whether to use a family member as an interpreter. Family members may intentionally mistranslate or leave out information to protect the patient from knowing the extent of her illness, which is culturally appropriate if the family chooses to moderate the effects of a grave diagnosis by introducing the news in stages. Questioning family members ahead of time about their intent, views, and plans for interpretation is advisable.

With regard to health care communication in general, providers should identify the advocate and the spokesperson for the Egyptian woman and develop a working relationship with this person. A personal and personable approach will help in developing a more effective relationship with the family.

## Status of the Provider

Egyptian Americans respect health care providers who were educated in North America. They have higher regard for those who are older, appear to have had more clinical experience, and are affiliated with universities. They tend to question those who are younger or appear to be more informal in their dealings with others.

## Communicating Illness and Symptoms

Egyptians best communicate their illness experience through narration and storytelling. They tend to describe symptoms within the context of events that may have occurred. If women are not given the time to build their illness stories, their answers are often too brief to give the total picture. Some women defer to their spouses or another family member to describe their illness. To get the full picture, the health care provider should take the time to listen to many sides of the presenting problem. In the long run, this time will be well invested in reaching an accurate diagnosis; otherwise, the story will unfold over several visits, leading to frustration for all involved. While Egyptian-American women are mostly well educated, beliefs about the evil eye and about hot and cold imbalances may still influence their views of health and illness. History of family and of relationships helps shape the responses and actions of Egyptian women in the health care system.

---

**NOTE TO THE HEALTH CARE PROVIDER**

Providers should ask questions related to sexuality in privacy. Asking the same questions several different ways can be helpful, as can asking questions related to grave stigmatizing diseases delicately and with compassion. Practitioners should not reveal a grave diagnosis or prognosis, or describe an illness as being terminal, without first consulting a significant family member. They should first build a personal trusting relationship.

---

## The Physical Examination

### Modesty and Touching

Egyptian-American women's levels of modesty depend on how religious they are. Highly religious Muslims or Christians are very modest. Providers should take special care not to offend them by uncovering and touching them unnecessarily. They must respect zones of touching allowed by the patient, particularly when a man is the examiner, and avoid male-to-female direct and continuous eye contact if the patient appears to be highly religious (covered hair, covered ankles, and covered wrists).

Health care providers should avoid exposing the whole body and should ask a female attendant to be present. Most Egyptian women accept male providers. Most women, even those who observe religious rituals, tend to differentiate between the necessity of cross-gender touching for health care and social touching. While they avoid the latter, they tend to accept the former. There are no taboos in same-gender touching.

### Expressing Pain

Egyptian-American women tend to be very expressive of pain, particularly labor pain. Moaning and crying are the most appropriate ways to demonstrate the level and intensity of their pain, which is not to be endured silently or alone. It is important to discuss pain with the woman when she is alone. Her description of the pain will differ from that of her family members, but both are accurate. Women feel free to openly express pain in the privacy of their families and tend to be more guarded when describing their pain to strangers (e.g., health care professionals). Clinical intervention should be congruent with the pain described by the patient and the involved family member.

## Prescribing Medications

Egyptian families tend to share medications. While they may not bring this practice with them to North America, it should be considered when prescribing medications. Health care providers should carefully assess medication use by asking questions about over-the-counter medications; those received from the home country; those that may be shared; and the use of herbs, vitamins, aspirin, anti-inflammatory medications, and medications related to the menstrual cycle. Some patients may not consider these medications to be of interest to health care providers.

### Drug Interactions

Recent immigrants tend to use herbal remedies and over-the-counter tranquilizers that they brought with them. Careful assessment will help uncover medications that may be potential sources of drug interactions.

### Medication Sharing

Self-diagnosis and shared processes of diagnosing tend to promote medication sharing. More significant is the liberty that some women may take in skipping a dose, doubling a dose, or discontinuing a medication when symptoms have disappeared.

Compliance

Egyptian-American women tend to follow a prescribed regimen as long as they trust the provider and understand the rationale for the particular intervention. Although Islam may promote fatalism, it also promotes taking care of the self. Taking advantage of scientific discoveries and advances in health care in North America prompts compliance with the health care provider's advice.

Follow-up Appointments

This population highly values the Western health care system. When the need for follow-up is carefully explained and if the economic situation is not a major deterrent, Egyptian women tend to follow up and maintain their appointments. Broken appointments usually result from other pressing priorities, probably involving their children. Providers should encourage them to reschedule.

Egyptian women tend to be present-oriented. Therefore, whatever is going on in their lives at the present time tends to distract them from future planning. Current problems, family needs, and social obligations may take precedence over future planning, which may hinder appointment-keeping. In general, however, Egyptian women follow "North American time" for appointments and are punctual.

Prevalent Diseases

Hypertension, breast cancer, colon cancer, colds, and influenza are reasons for which Egyptian women seek health care. No studies are available that show the incidence and prevalence of diseases in the immigrant population. While parasitic diseases are still prevalent in Egypt, lifestyle diseases are also on the rise. Egyptian women tend to have adopted Western standards in weight control and reduction of fat in diets; however, high-salt foods and sedentary lifestyles continue to prevail. Egyptian women tend to smoke more than those who have immigrated to North America.

## Health-Seeking Behaviors

These women usually seek medical attention early in any disease process. Egyptian women with health insurance tend to seek and receive medical care in a timely fashion. Because pain is to be avoided at all cost, these women usually attend to pain early. If a woman is experiencing a problem carrying out daily functions, she promptly seeks care.

### Preventive Health Care

Egyptian women are conscientious about seeking preventive health care as long as they have an insurance plan. There is some reluctance about intrusive preventive measures like Papanicolaou tests (Pap smear) and colonoscopies until the woman is given the rationale and the urgency for having them done. It is critical to provide these women with the necessary information.

### Self-Care of Minor Illness

Egyptian women do not tend to practice self-care. In their country of origin, they consult family members, pharmacists, and personal physicians. Lacking extended family members and knowledge of over-the-counter medications, they tend to seek health care for minor and major illnesses. They tend to take care of premenstrual discomfort, occasional stomachaches, and intestinal disturbances with over-the-counter medications after being in North America long enough to become acquainted with these remedies.

### Self-Care of Major Illness

An Egyptian woman expects to be totally relieved of all her daily responsibilities when she has a major illness. She also expects to be relieved from any responsibility related to decisions about the diagnosis and treatment of her illness. She expects immediate family members to step in to assume these responsibilities. Therefore, to health care providers, the woman may appear passive, dependent, and voiceless. Culturally, however, this behavior relates to the need to be protected and for her energy to be saved for healing and recovery.

### ⊕ BIBLIOGRAPHY

Hattar-Pollara, M., Meleis, A. I., & Hassanat, N. (2000). The spousal role of Egyptian women in clerical jobs. *Health Care for Women International*, 21, 303–317.

Keck, L. T. (1989). Egyptian Americans in the Washington, DC area. *Arab Studies Quarterly*, 11(2–3), 103–126.

Lane, S. D., & Meleis, A. I. (1991). Roles, work, health perceptions and health resources of women: A study in an Egyptian delta hamlet. *Western Science and Medicine*, 33(10), 1197–1208.

Meleis, A. I., & Meleis, M. (1998). Egyptians in America: Integrated and distinct. In L. D. Purnell & B. J. Paulanka (Eds.), *Transcultural health care: A culturally competent approach*. Philadelphia: F.A. Davis, pp. 217–244.

Morsy, S. A. (1993). *Gender, sickness, and healing in rural Egypt: Ethnography in historical context*. Boulder, CO: Westview Press.

# CHAPTER 10

# Ethiopians and Eritreans

## YEWOUBDAR BEYENE, PhD

### INTRODUCTION

### Who are the Ethiopian and Eritrean People?

Ethiopians and Eritreans come from the Horn of Africa, which is in the northeast part of the continent. The terms "Ethiopian" and "Eritrean" represent national and political entities but not separate cultural groups. Until May 1993, when a political resolution to a long-standing and bitter internal conflict divided the country, Ethiopia included Eritrea. All the existing literature treats Ethiopians and Eritreans as people from the same cultural group.

Both Ethiopia and Eritrea are multiethnic, multireligious nations with many different political factions and considerable regional variations. Despite tremendous diversity, similar core cultural values underlie the behavior of most Ethiopians and Eritreans. In addition, the people of northern Ethiopia and Eritrea speak the same language, and the cultural similarities are strong. Coptic Orthodox Christianity is the most predominant religion, but Catholics, Protestants and Muslims also live in Ethiopia and Eritrea. In North America there are Coptic Orthodox churches in several cities in which large numbers of Ethiopian and Eritrean immigrants live.

### Ethiopian and Eritreans in North America

Compared with other immigrant groups, the Ethiopian and Eritrean communities in North America are relatively new and small. The exact numbers are unknown because in the 1990 and 2000 U.S. Census counts Ethiopians and Eritreans were subsumed in the "other foreign born" category. In 1999, however, a joint report submitted by the Ethiopian and Eritrean Catholic Apostolate estimated that the entire population of Ethiopian and Eritreans in the United States is between 250,000 and 350,000. In Canada, as of the 1996 Census, the population numbered 21,178 people of Ethiopian or Eritrean ethnicity, of whom 46% are women.

Before 1974, of the estimated 3000 Ethiopians/Eritreans residing in the United States, 95% were students and expected to return to their home country after completing their studies. The other 5% were either diplomats or associated with various international organizations. In 1974, the rise to power of a Marxist government in

Ethiopia and brutal civil war in Eritrea and Tigray marked a watershed in the migration pattern of Ethiopians and Eritreans to North America. Many of those who already resided in North America decided not to return home, choosing instead to seek asylum. Since 1980, most Ethiopians and Eritreans have come as refugees. The U.S. Immigration Act of 1990 expanded the number and diversity of countries from which people were granted permanent visas to include Ethiopia and Eritrea, and many arriving since 1991 came under this program.

Most Ethiopian and Eritrean immigrants and refugees came from an urban background and live predominantly in major metropolitan U. S. cities: Washington, D.C., Los Angeles, San Francisco Bay Area, Chicago, Seattle, Houston, Atlanta, and New York. The Ethiopian and Eritrean communities are dominated by young single adults, of whom 66% are men and 34% are women. Seventy percent are younger than 40 years of age. The great majority of the Ethiopian/Eritrean Canadians live in Toronto.

## 🌍 BEING FEMALE IN ETHIOPIAN AND ERITREAN SOCIETY

A woman's "worth" is measured in terms of her role as a mother and wife. A high percentage of women who reside in rural areas in Ethiopia and Eritrea are engaged primarily in labor-intensive subsistence. Women traditionally have had fewer opportunities for personal growth, education, and employment outside of the house than men. Rights of property ownership and inheritance vary from one ethnic group to another. In the last 40 years, women in the rural areas have had more opportunity for education, health care, and employment outside the home.

## At Birth

### Preference for Sons

Families prefer their first-born to be a son, based on the expectation that the eldest son will be responsible for economically supporting his siblings and protecting the family's honor in case of the father's premature death. This cultural expectation does not make the birth of a baby girl any less important; indeed, mothers often state that they prefer daughters because daughters are emotionally closer and help with the household chores. The number and sex of children are believed to be God's will, and a woman is not looked on negatively if she bears only girls.

### Response to the Birth of a Female

Girls are loved and cared for, and there is no disregard or neglect of the female child. These societies have never practiced infanticide or abandonment of the female child. Descent in both Ethiopians and Eritreans is predominantly patrilineal, and children take the father's first name as their last name. A woman, however, never takes her husband's name.

### Birth Rituals

There is no special birth ritual for girls.

# Childhood and Youth

## Stages

Infancy is prolonged, and children are indulged and raised in a highly protective environment. From about 3 years of age, children are subjected to a regimen of discipline.

## Family Expectations

Obedience and politeness are the overriding goals of bringing up children. Physical aggression is discouraged; rather, a quiet and reserved manner of speaking is stressed. Children who are noisy and disrespectful are considered rude. In most families, especially less affluent ones, girls are assigned household chores as early as 7or 8 years of age. Boys have a longer childhood. Girls help their mother with cooking, childcare, and the like, while boys help the father in "masculine" work. Very strict gender roles are maintained, and boys are not expected to cook or do housework.

## Social Expectations

Social respectability and the importance of not "bringing shame" to the family's name is impressed on children, especially young girls. Anything the child may do outside the home that is deemed negative is believed to reflect badly on the family, and particularly on the parents.

## Importance of Education

In urban areas there is a strong emphasis on education; however, educational opportunity varies according to the family's social class and education level. Families with resources provide equal opportunities for boys and girls, but girls from less well-to-do families rarely have the opportunity for higher education.

# Pubescence

## Psychosexual Development

Girls are generally mature by 13 years of age, and breast development and the onset of menarche affirm maturity. Onset of menarche varies between girls from the highland and those from the lowland areas of the region. High altitude is known to delay growth; also, the climate and vegetation of the highlands differ. Thus, altitude and nutritional variation affect the onset of menarche.

There is a general cultural belief that hot foods, such as fresh chili peppers, and hot drinks trigger early onset of menarche and should be avoided.

## Rituals and Rites of Passage

There is no known ritual or celebration rite of passage for girls or boys in the mainstream cultural groups.

## Teen Sexuality

Dating, sexual activity, and childbearing during early adolescence are considered taboo, especially for young people from middle-class and upper-class families.

**Social Restrictions and Pressures.**   There are very strict rules and restrictions on women's public behavior, including that of young girls. Traditionally, girls were supposed to be very shy and feminine; wearing flashy colors and glaring jewelry is frowned upon. Conversation with males who are not immediate family members is totally discouraged. Although urban life and exposure to outside cultures have decreased some restrictions and modified dress codes, the "good families" still adhere to the strict rules. Traditionally, girls marry shortly after the onset of menarche, and this is still true in some rural areas. Age at marriage for girls in the urban area is delayed because of schooling. The majority of immigrants came from urban areas where the exposure to outside cultures is apparent. As a result, most Ethiopian and Eritrean women in North America appear more westernized; however, the very few elderly women prefer to wear their traditional outfits. Immigrants are generally shy and soft spoken, and values held by "good families" are still integral parts of the community.

**Teen Pregnancy.**   Dating and sexual activity before marriage are not allowed, and out-of-wedlock pregnancy brings tremendous shame on the family and the girl. If the pregnancy is discovered early, the girl's parents insist on marriage before the pregnancy becomes obvious. Use of contraception is not common among teens and young girls, and abortion is neither culturally nor legally acceptable.

Most immigrants came to North America as college students in their late teens or early twenties and very few have the supervision of close adult family members; therefore the traditional restrictions on dating and marriage are not reinforced, and use of contraception is common.

## Menstruation

**Relationship to Health.**   Menstruation is not openly discussed; however, heavy flow is a concern since losing too much blood is believed to affect a woman's health.

**Relationship to Fertility.**   Menstruation signifies fertility. Most women, however, consider it to be a nuisance. Hysterectomy is uncommon, but when it has been carried out, it is not associated with infertility since most women have by then already borne children. It does not make women less valued.

**Taboos and Restrictions During Menstruation.**   Traditionally, menstruation is considered unclean, and women are restricted from going to church during their menstrual periods. No other restrictions are placed on menstruating women, and they can socialize and be in the company of whomever they choose. The church restriction is changing in the urban areas.

**Dysmenorrhea.**   Missed periods are often first thought to be pregnancy, depending on the woman's age. In her early or late 40s, a missed period is an indication that the woman is approaching menopause. Clots are attributed to miscarriage or illness. For menstrual cramps, women use hot drinks made from toasted flax seeds or oats and are encouraged to rest; they avoid cold drinks and lifting heavy objects.

### Female Modesty and Touching

Both women and men are very modest. The Christian and Muslim religions both emphasize modesty for women; however, the level of modesty may vary by age and whether a woman's background is urban or rural.

---

**NOTE TO THE HEALTH CARE PROVIDER**

While modesty is very important for the group as a whole, touching in the context of medical examinations does not appear to cause problems. When possible, Ethiopian and Eritrean women prefer to be assigned to a female care provider. Modesty definitely affects women's willingness to obtain annual pelvic examinations, and such examinations are not customary. Again, this may vary by age and background.

---

# Adulthood

### Transition Rites and Rituals

Adulthood is socially defined. In rural areas, adulthood is defined by marriage, even for a 14-year-old girl. In urban areas, adulthood is also defined by age; for example, a girl is definitely an adult at 18 years of age. The only complete recognition of adulthood, however, is through marriage. There is no special celebration or rite of passage to mark the transition to adulthood.

### Social Expectations

Girls and young women who are not enrolled in higher education are expected to marry and start a family. Most stay close to their family in the same city. In urban settings, expectations vary by the social class and education level of parents. In North America, the majority of Ethiopian and Eritrean families highly emphasize education for both genders, and girls are encouraged to pursue higher education.

### Union Formation

**Union Types.**   Marriages in rural areas are commonly arranged, but in urban areas they are either arranged or the couple's personal choice. Polygamy is rare except in some Muslim groups. Most Ethiopian and Eritrean women in North America choose whom they want to marry.

**Social Sanctions for Failing to Enter into Union.**   Women have more pressure to marry than do men, although both men and women are expected to marry. In rural areas, arranged marriages enforce this expectation. The age for marriage varies, but it appears to be the early 20s in the rural areas. A common saying is, "Getting a husband is like catching cold," underscoring the expected norm that every woman will get married at some point in her life.

### Domestic Violence

Wife beating is a pervasive social problem. The laws in both Ethiopia and Eritrea provide for equality of women and a framework for improving the status of women; however, these laws are not applied in practice because of ingrained cultural attitudes. Much of society remains traditional and patriarchal. While women have recourse to the police and the courts, societal norms and a limited infrastructure inhibit many women from seeking legal redress, especially in remote areas. Thus, domestic violence is mostly addressed traditionally through the mediation of family and community elders. Although wife beating is common, it is considered shameful and reprehensible by the elders, and the husband is "fined," that is, expected to give his wife money or buy her jewelry. If the violence persists, the elders may decide to dissolve the marriage.

In the immigrant Ethiopian and Eritrean communities in North America, close friends usually mediate in cases of domestic violence. Women very rarely disclose domestic abuse to authorities because of shame and fear of disapproval within their community.

---

### NOTE TO THE HEALTH CARE PROVIDER

In cases of suspected domestic violence, providers must be cautious and bring up the topic gently, without being confrontational. It is very likely that the client will resist admitting to abuse, but it is nonetheless important to give her information on how to get help and reassure her of confidentiality.

---

### Rape

Both the Ethiopian and Eritrean societies consider rape shameful and an act that dishonors the woman and her family. It is kept secret. Although rape is punishable by law, social practices obstruct investigations into rape and the prosecution of the rapist. Moreover, many women are not aware of their rights under the law. For example, according to the 1999 Country Reports on Human Rights in Ethiopia, there were only an estimated 20 rape convictions per year, and rape sentences typically were much lighter than the 10 to 15 years prescribed by law.

Although illegal, abduction of women and girls as a form of marriage is still widely practiced in some rural areas and causes conflicts between families and communities. Abduction usually happens as a result of the girl's family feeling that a marriage proposal is an unacceptable match. The abductor gets away with his crime, traditional community elders mediate between the abductor and the girl's family, and the girl is forced to marry the man. Forced sexual relationships often accompany marriages by abduction, and women are abused physically during the abduction.

### Divorce

**Sociocultural Views.** Although the preferred norm is to remain married, a woman can divorce without social sanctions. Divorce is common in the home country, but no data on divorce in North America are available. A divorced woman can remarry with no sanctions or negative effects on her status in the community.

**Child Custody Practices.** Even in divorce, fathers remain close to the children. Marriage is the joining of two families rather than just that of two people. Even if the two parties form new families, the original families remain connected. In almost all cases, fathers take financial responsibility for and maintain close ties with their children.

### Fertility and Childbearing

**Family Size.** Ethiopian and Eritrean societies typically have large families, with an average of five children. The younger generation appears to be having fewer children, however, as the result of marriage delayed by education and nontraditional careers or in some cases the use of contraceptives.

**Contraceptive Practices.** In the rural areas, contraceptives are not used. Younger women in urban areas, however, are now using various types of contraceptives. In general, men resist using condoms. The only common indigenous methods of fertility control are abstinence and breastfeeding. There are no strong cultural or religious opinions on this topic.

---

**NOTE TO THE HEALTH CARE PROVIDER**

Contraception is not discussed openly. Therefore, it is difficult to assess the woman's knowledge, opinions, and concerns regarding the various contraceptive methods. However, immigrant women may express their opinions, depending on their age, length of stay in North America, and education level.

---

**Role of the Male in the Couple's Fertility Decision-Making.** The man has no role in deciding the type of contraception a woman should use. Children are gifts from God; therefore neither partner has any say in the number of children they should have. However, among educated urban couples and those who live in North America, the decision about the number of children is shared.

### Abortion

Abortion is not common, and miscarriage and abortion are perceived to be the same thing. In urban settings, abortions are discreetly performed in clinics and hospitals, but generally abortion is not an issue of concern in the society.

### Miscarriage

Miscarriage is common and is attributed to different causes, mainly physical labor, such as lifting heavy things, or accidents. Illness is assumed to be the cause of repeated miscarriages. Resting, avoiding heavy lifting, and eating well are the usual recommendations to prevent miscarriage.

### Infertility

Children are seen as being gifts from God; thus, infertility is seen as being God's will. The infertile woman is not treated with less respect than a fertile woman; rather, she is pitied. In these societies, a sister, or other relative, may offer one of her children to an infertile sibling to raise as her own. This is not the same as adoption in Western cultures because the legal system is not involved, and the child knows that an aunt is raising him or her. An infertile woman risks losing her husband to another woman, however, since it is considered to be important to have children. The husband may divorce her or just have another woman outside the marriage who bears children for him. This tradition is changing among the young urban generation.

### Pregnancy

**Activity Restrictions and Taboos.** The pregnant woman receives much attention from her family and others. She is supposed to avoid daily tasks that require bending and lifting, carrying heavy loads, climbing stairs, and exposure to emotional situations such as funerals, fights, and bad news. She is encouraged to eat well and get plenty of sleep. It is generally believed that unfulfilled cravings for special foods will cause miscarriage, so the woman is indulged. Traditionally, pregnancy is considered a dangerous state since the fetus could be easy prey for the Evil Eye, which is believed to cause miscarriage, premature delivery, and fetal malformations. Walking and moving around are encouraged as the due date gets closer.

**Dietary Practices and Observances.**   There are neither food taboos nor special foods required during pregnancy. Traditionally, however, a pregnant woman drinks a hot mixture of ground, toasted flax seed sweetened with honey or sugar. It is used as a laxative to clean the baby and the mother; it is also believed to ease labor.

**Prenatal Care.**   Rural women have no formal prenatal care. Affluent urban women may seek prenatal care from an obstetrician at a clinic or hospital, but there is no typical time for prenatal care to begin. Most immigrant women in North America seek prenatal care.

### Birthing Process

**Home Versus Hospital Delivery.**   Most rural deliveries are at home, assisted by a self-trained midwife or an older female family member. Urban women are accustomed to hospital delivery. Overall, women tolerate labor pain and prefer the presence of female family members and friends to provide comfort and to massage their backs and feet.

**Cesarean Section Versus Vaginal Delivery.**   Women prefer natural childbirth, and they are not accustomed to a cesarean section. Urban women do have the option of cesarean section, but only for difficult situations.

**Involvement of the Male Partner.**   Traditionally, the father and male members of the family were not allowed to be with the birthing woman. In North America, however, young fathers participate in Lamaze classes and stay close to their wives during delivery.

**Labor Management.**   The woman takes an active role during labor. Modesty is very important, so she must be kept covered. A low level of moaning or grunting is socially accepted; screaming is not. In rural settings, older women, mothers, and mothers-in-law coach the woman. The labor of the first-born is a cause for concern for most women; otherwise, labor, although considered dangerous, is assumed to be easy in subsequent pregnancies. After the rupture of the membranes, female family members attend the women, and the midwife is immediately called.

**Placenta.**   In home births, the placenta is buried in the family compound. It is believed to be part of the baby and is referred to as "the second child" since it has been with the fetus in the womb. In urban hospital births, however, this practice is no longer followed.

### Postpartum

The new mother is expected to be with the baby 24 hours a day. Female family members assist the mother in bathing and caring for the baby. Both mother and baby are considered delicate, and they are protected from diseases and harmful actions by at least 40 days of seclusion. The more affluent the family is, the longer the period of seclusion lasts. The mother is fed warm drinks and special warm foods, like porridge made from barley and other cereals, meat, and chicken stew. Childbirth is a joyful event celebrated by family and neighbors with food sharing and gift-giving to mother and baby.

Visitors who just arrived from a long trip or were exposed to the sun at length are feared to bring disease and should cool down before they enter the room where the baby and mother are staying. Mother and baby avoid wind and sunlight, based on the belief that direct sunlight or rays can affect the baby's sight and make him or her cross-eyed. The postpartum room is kept dim, and windows and doors are kept closed. Ethiopian and Eritrean women are surprised when North American women take their few-week-old infants outside or into public places. The baby's neck and head are considered especially delicate, and the neck and shoulders are supported until the baby can support its head.

---

**NOTE TO THE HEALTH CARE PROVIDER**
Postpartum women should not be given cold foods or liquids; their food and drinks must be warm. Providers must pay attention to how they handle the baby and make sure that the baby remains as covered as possible. They should keep the lights low and windows closed and limit the number of people who enter the room.

---

### Newborn and Infant Care

**Breastfeeding Versus Bottle-Feeding.** Traditionally, mothers breastfeed for an average of 23 months; there is no taboo on breastfeeding in public. Overall, women prefer breastfeeding. In North America, however, working mothers may supplement breastfeeding with formula. To increase their milk, women eat special foods and drink gruel made from oats, honey, and milk.

**Infant Protection.** Immunizations are encouraged in urban areas, but rural areas do not have access to preventive services. Ethiopians and Eritreans strongly believe in the Evil Eye, and they interpret fever, diarrhea, and colic as a sign of having been affected by it. In rural areas, the baby is covered with light gauzy material in public settings, and children wear special amulets for protection. Urban, young, educated people do not observe this practice.

**Primary Caregiver.** Mothers and female family members are the main caregivers of infants and toddlers, and extended family members also may assist in childcare. Caring for infants is the women's responsibility; husbands and male family members are not expected to care for infants, except during short periods of play. Young immigrant men in North America, however, often do share infant care responsibilities.

## Middle Age

### Cultural Attitudes and Expectations

Age is defined traditionally by the socially defined roles of being a wife, mother, and grandmother. Most women have only a very vague idea of their chronological age, which is a recent concept. A woman can be seen as being middle-aged when her children marry, but this chronological age varies by her own age at marriage and the age of her children. Birthday celebrations for adults are rare.

### Psychological Response

The nest is never empty for Ethiopian and Eritrean women because children remain deeply attached to their parents. There is no concept of expected crises at certain ages of a woman's life.

### Menopause

**Onset and Duration.**   It is assumed that menopause begins between 40 and 45 years of age, but some women give birth in their late 40s. Women do not talk about menopause and never refer to it as a time in which to worry about their health. For most women, menopause begins after they have fulfilled their reproductive responsibilities. Women may welcome menopause as the time when they feel free to attend religious duties with no restrictions.

**Sexual Activity.**   Menopause indicates that the woman no longer can have children. Being menopausal does not affect a woman's sexual relations with her husband, however. In some groups, widowed menopausal women play the role of sexual mentors for young males.

**Coping.**   Traditionally, no particular symptom is believed to be associated with menopause, so it is not a stage that requires coping strategies. This might change for some Westernized urban women whose lifestyle and reproductive patterns are very different from those of rural women. Menopause is not usually considered a crisis.

## Old Age

Life expectancy in Ethiopia and Eritrea is less than 50 years; it is slightly higher for women than for men. Because age is a social rather than a chronologic matter, most women do not know their age. Old age is described by the social role of grandmother and such physical characteristics as graying of one's hair and diminished physical abilities. Elderly women are respected and obeyed, and they are the main midwives and healers in their community. Elders are respected and looked after by their children, who remain deeply attached and are sensitive to the wishes of their parents. Children are responsible for caring for their old parents, who live mainly with the eldest child. The concept of nursing homes or rest homes is unknown. There are very few elders in North America, and the children are responsible for looking after them. The idea of putting a parent in a nursing home is unacceptable.

## Death and Dying

### Cultural Attitudes and Beliefs

Death is the most ritualized life stage in Ethiopian and Eritrean societies. It is believed that God gives and takes away life. Separation of a loved one by death, however, is bitterly grieved regardless of age or gender of the deceased. The death of a younger person with no offspring is lamented more. News of the death of a family member must be carefully communicated at an appropriate time and place and in an appropriate way. The news should be first disclosed to close friends so that they will be there to provide emotional support to the family members of the deceased.

### Rites and Rituals

Cremation is not acceptable. In rural areas, people die at home and burial is immediate, within a day or so. The situation in the major urban areas is changing because of deaths occurring in hospital rather than at home. Special prayers are performed at home, where the body lies and then at church before burial. Death rites and rituals do not vary by gender. Most Ethiopian and Eritrean communities in North

America have churches and native priests who carry out prayers and death rites. The priests are also willing to come to hospitals to provide services to a dying patient.

## Mourning

**Cultural Expectations.** People are brought up to restrain most emotional outbursts except at the death of loved ones, when great demonstrations of feeling are encouraged. They cry loudly and uncontrollably. Women tear their clothes and beat their chests to the point that they become sick with grief. Men are excused for crying out loud and shedding tears.

Religious prayers and gatherings mark the mourning period. Christian women wear black for one year when a close family member dies. Some shave their hair or cut it very short. Women take off their jewelry, and no make-up is allowed. Men wear black ties and grow beards as a sign of mourning. Close family and friends stay together for the first week, and food and drinks are brought to the family in mourning for a week or so. When a woman dies, the father automatically has custody of the children.

**Coping.** Women are expected to show strong emotion at the death of any family member—husband, children, and old or young family members. They express sorrow loudly and with tears. The task of mourning is to honor the departed family member and to express sorrow felt by those left behind. Men, women, children, and the aged are all mourned. Both men and women mourn; however, women are allowed to let their emotions overcome them.

---

**NOTE TO THE HEALTH CARE PROVIDER**

Practitioners must be very careful in disclosing the news of a death. They should never tell the female member of the family first. If the death occurs in the hospital, they should provide privacy for mourning and not attempt to quiet family members. They should not minimize or attempt to hasten the mourning period.

---

## IMPORTANT POINTS FOR HEALTH PROVIDERS CARING FOR ETHIOPIAN AND ERITREAN WOMEN

### The Medical Intake

#### Literacy and English Proficiency

Most Ethiopians and Eritreans in North America speak at least some English. One study showed that 81% had some skills, ranging from fluent to some English; however, 19% had absolutely no English skills. Ethiopians and Eritreans, particularly women, speak very softly. Elderly Ethiopians and Eritreans had minimal or no education in their own society and will need assistance in translation and the explanation of medical procedures.

#### Status of the Provider

People from this cultural group highly respect health care providers. They may make little eye contact when speaking with authority figures (doctors, nurses), although this behavior varies based on length of time in North America, level of education, age, and gender. They are typically very shy, polite, reserved, and nonconfrontational. Shouting at any time is frowned on. Patients and family members rarely disagree with treatment procedures if they have placed their trust in the health care provider.

## Communicating Illness and Symptoms

Personal information is not revealed at the first clinical encounter. People are socialized to assume that it is improper to reveal oneself fully or to disclose personal secrets to anyone other than a close friend. Privacy is further protected by the shared belief that others normally do not have a just claim to information about personal matters. Traditionally, such ailments as mental illness and epilepsy are routinely attributed to the action of evil spirits.

Communicating bad news, such as grave illness or the death of a family member, is very sensitive; and it should be done only in a carefully chosen and appropriate time, place, and way. Avoiding a sudden shock at all costs is essential, because of the harmful effects such shocks have on people with fragile emotional states. In case of serious illness, health care providers should communicate little information directly to patients. Whatever the diagnosis, they are expected to tell the bad news to a family member first. The family will judge how and when they want to let a patient know; this may vary with the patient's age, level of understanding, and emotional and physical condition. The family's importance takes precedence over the individual member's right to know.

Communicating openly about a patient's terminal illness evokes strong emotional reaction in the patient and family and may even interfere with the care of the dying. Ethiopians and Eritreans strongly believe in destiny and in God's power to influence events, especially health events. Their persistence in holding on to hope is tied to their religious belief in God's miraculous powers.

---

**NOTE TO THE HEALTH CARE PROVIDER**
Providers must reassure patients and families about the importance of personal information that is requested for a treatment plan and reassure them that such information will be kept confidential. Elderly patients will be accompanied by a family member, with whom the provider can discuss how to choose the appropriate approaches to probe for information from the patient. Health professionals must be selective in imparting a poor prognosis or death to family members; for example, avoid telling the mother or the wife because women are socialized to be fragile. To communicate bad news in the absence of an immediate family member, ask for a close friend. Friendship ties are strong among Ethiopians and Eritreans, and they are even stronger when they are away from their homeland. Friends substitute for the extended family.

---

## The Physical Examination

### Modesty and Touching

Christianity and Islam emphasize modesty for women. The level of modesty may vary by age and urban as opposed to rural background. The provider should offer a hospital robe to cover the gown. Elderly women prefer to wear a traditional cotton shawl on top of the gown at all times. Pelvic examinations are the most difficult and embarrassing; however, they are accepted in the context of medical examination.

### Expressing Pain

Ethiopians and Eritreans often do not explain symptoms clearly; they may express them very generally and cannot articulate specific sensations or organs. They have no understanding of the numerical scale of expressing pain. They do not like pain medication because they worry about addiction. Older women usually moan as a way of expressing pain. Women generally act very helpless and passive, consistent with the recognized sick role in these societies. The family and friends are expected to look after the sick, prepare their food, clean up after them, and pamper them. It is customary to bring home-cooked soothing foods for the patient. Family members alter their timetable to attend to the needs of the sick.

## Prescribing Medications

### Drug Interactions

There are no traditional Ethiopian/Eritrean healers in North America. The community consists mainly of young urban people, whereas the traditional healing is usually the domain of older people and religious leaders. The current popularity of herbal medicine in North America, however, is very appealing to these groups. Therefore, it would be wise to ask the patient if she is taking any herbal teas or other herbal substances.

### Medication Sharing

It is very likely that women share medication, such as antacids or skin ointments, for nonchronic conditions. Sharing medications for chronic conditions, such as diabetes or hypertension, is much less likely.

### Compliance

Traditionally, illness is identified by the presence of symptoms; wellness is measured by their absence. Illness conditions lacking symptoms are not well understood. Thus, it is important to emphasize the need to complete the full course of prescribed antibiotics and to explain that some conditions, such as hypertension, are risky even if they have no symptoms.

## Follow-up Appointments

These clients may take "feeling better" to mean cure and absence of any need to see a health care provider. Clients also may miss follow-up appointments because of employment constraints. A phone call or a post card may help to remind patients.

Ethiopians and Eritreans are usually tardy in social and business situations. This may be related to difficulty in judging distance and assessing traffic, public transportation schedules, and time needed to get from place to place. In social occasions, it is customary that the invitation will state 6:00 PM for an event that is planned to begin at 7:00 PM since the guests are expected to be at least one hour late. It is important to emphasize the importance of an appointment time as well as the medication schedule. Providers should specify the number of hours between medication doses, rather than telling patients to take their medication three or four times a day.

## Prevalent Diseases

Nothing is known about prevalent diseases in these groups in North America; however, these people come from sub-Saharan countries where infectious and parasitic diseases are common. In addition, it is very likely that the drastic lifestyle change from their country of origin would put them at risk for such diseases as hypertension, diabetes, and other stress-related illnesses, resulting from the immigration transition and everyday financial, educational, and social difficulties of living in a very different country.

## Health-Seeking Behaviors

In general, women delay seeking medical attention. They consult family and friends for major concerns before seeing a health care provider. Household self-care without the use of professional healers is common throughout Ethiopian and Eritrean communities. The pharmacopoeia is natural; for example, plants, grains, spices, oil seeds, herbs, and butter are used in home remedies. Popular remedies for headaches include drinking coffee and lemon tea or boiling or smelling eucalyptus leaves to treat colds. In North America, most Ethiopians/Eritreans rely on Western biomedicine. However, most women are reluctant to be screened for such diseases as cancer for fear of finding out that they have the problem. Prevention services and such practices as diet and exercise vary by age and level of education.

## 🌐 BIBLIOGRAPHY

Beyene, Y. (1992). Medical disclosure and refugees: telling bad news to Ethiopian patients. *Western Journal of Medicine, 157,* 328–332.

Kloos, H., & Zein, A. Z. (Eds.) (1993). *The ecology of health and disease in Ethiopia.* Boulder, CO: Westview Press.

Pankhurst, H. (1992). *Gender, development and identity: an Ethiopian study.* London: Zed Books.

Tronvoll, K. (1997). *Mai Weini: A small village in the highlands of Eritrea.* Trenton, NJ: The Red Sea Press.

Wilson, A. (1991). *Women and the Eritrean revolution. The challenge road.* Trenton, NJ: The Red Sea Press.

# CHAPTER 11

# Filipinos

JUDITH A. BERG, PhD, RNC, WHNP,
CAROLINA P. DE GUZMAN, MSN, CPAN, RN, and
DAISY M. RODRIGUEZ, MN, MPA, RN

## INTRODUCTION

### Who are the Filipino People?

Filipinos are immigrants to North America from the Philippines, an archipelago located slightly north of the equator between Taiwan and Malaysia. The Philippines consists of 7107 islands with a collective landmass slightly larger than Nevada. The three major island groups (Luzon, Visayas, and Mindanao) contain volcanic mountain ranges, some of which are active today. The tropical climate of the country promotes agriculture and fishing throughout the entire year, and natural resources are abundant.

Filipinos are of Malayan ancestry, with influences from regional neighbors (China, Japan, India, Indonesia, Malaysia, and Arab nations). Islam was introduced to the southern part of the archipelago in the 14th century, followed by Spanish colonization throughout the nation between 1521 and 1898. Spanish colonial rule transformed religious, cultural, economic, sociopolitical, and educational development. The Filipino Muslims of Mindanao, however, refused to embrace Catholicism and continue their Muslim traditions today. The Americanization of the Philippines began after the Spanish-American War (1898), which resulted in American-style education and military alliances.

### Filipinos in North America

The U.S. population of Filipinos was 1,850,314 in 2000 and is the fastest growing Asian group. About half live in California, and the next largest but considerably smaller populations live in Hawaii and Illinois. There were 242,880 Filipinos in Canada as of the 1996 Census, concentrated in Toronto, Vancouver, and Winnipeg. Women comprise 58% of the Canadian Filipino population.

Filipinos in North America speak more than 100 languages from an estimated 75 ethnolinguistic groups representing the Philippines. These groups reflect regional variations in belief systems, values, and behaviors; they have been identified with labels such as Tagalog, Ilocano, Bisaya, and Moro, among others.

Immigrants came in waves. The initial immigration occurred between 1903 and 1910. Immigrants in this first wave were sponsored by a U.S. government program that targeted bright, young Filipino men for attendance at American educational institutions. The second wave of immigration, after World War I, brought Filipino immigrants to the United States and Hawaii as workers in agriculture enterprises. These poorly educated men suffered discrimination and were prevented from owning property, becoming citizens, or intermarrying

The third wave of Filipino immigration began after the discontinuation of the U.S. quota system in 1965 and continues even now. This third wave has been comprised of well-educated, urban-dwelling people. Included were nurses whose recruitment to the United States was sponsored by the Rockefeller Foundation between 1945 and 1980 as a way to address the nursing shortage and who represent the "brain drain" from the Philippines. Women outnumbered men in the third wave, and they were mostly professionals in health care, education, and engineering who arranged employment and housing before immigrating. These immigrants depended less than their predecessors on the protection and support of family members, quickly established economic stability, and began to raise families. Many brought their aging parents to the United States under the family reunification provisions of the immigration law.

The declaration of martial law in 1972 in the Philippines precipitated migration of Filipinos to the United States and Canada with tourist, business, student, and refugee visas. Many were able to convert their temporary visas into long-term immigrant status and eventual citizenship.

## ⊕ BEING FEMALE IN FILIPINO SOCIETY

One distinguishing aspect of Philippine culture is the leading role that women play in both the family and society at large. These women are generally considered to be equal to men. Hispanic culture has influenced the traditional ideal for a female, which includes demureness, femininity, and modesty. While contemporary Filipinas in the Philippines maintain many of these traditional feminine traits, they also obtain formal education and pursue careers, as do Filipina Americans and Canadians. In fact, it is not unusual to find that women are better educated than are men.

## At Birth

### Preference for Sons

Cultural preference for sons is an influence from the Chinese. Chinese Filipinos have very strong feelings about this issue, while other families care less as long as they eventually have a male child who can carry on the family name. Often, a couple will continue to try to produce a male offspring. Sons have preferential treatment, especially in Chinese Filipino families.

### Response to the Birth of a Female

Failure to produce a male offspring affects Filipino men more than it does women. Children are considered a blessing (Catholic belief), and three consecutive children of the same sex are considered to be good luck.

Filipinos value all their children and do not neglect them because of gender. Whereas fathers may prefer boys to carry on the family name, mothers may prefer girls to have help with household chores.

## Birth Rituals

The child's gender does not change cultural observances. The umbilical cords of children are all buried in the same site to promote family unity and bonding among siblings.

# Childhood and Youth

## Stages

Boys and girls do not differ in their stages of development, and no official ceremony ushers them into adulthood. The exception is the debut of 18-year-old girls among well-to-do families. Families who cannot afford a lavish celebration usually plan some special event for the young girl's transition into womanhood.

Terms used to describe the stages of development differ from one region or dialect to another. Tagalog terms include **bata** (child), **binatilyo** or **dalagita** (young boy or girl), **binata** or **dalaga** (young adult unmarried man or woman), **kabataan** (youth), and **matandang dalaga** (spinster).

## Family Expectations

Family expectations differ somewhat according to gender. Boys are expected to help fathers earn a living, while girls are expected to help mothers with household chores. All children are expected to help with farm work in rural areas. Moreover, all children are expected to share part of their earnings, and in some instances to turn over all their earnings, to parents to help with household expenses and family support. The oldest child is expected to participate in disciplining younger siblings and to be a good role model in school.

Parents are strict with girls during pubescence with regard to their socializing with boys. Girls are to keep their distance from boys physically since Filipino society prohibits and rejects premarital sex. Although Filipinos in the United States and Canada have acculturated in many ways, they continue to follow Roman Catholic traditions, which frown on premarital sex.

## Importance of Education

Filipinas in North America are from families who value education, and most are encouraged to attend college. In fact, the education level of U.S. Filipinas exceeds that of the general U.S. population, with 41.4% of Filipinas graduating from college compared with 17.6% for all U.S. females. This high percentage reflects, in part, the immigration of health professionals, particularly nurses. As early as the beginning of the 20th century, education was valued and a family goal, and today families make great sacrifices to educate their children.

# Pubescence

## Psychosexual Development

At puberty, Filipinas are expected to be more modest in behavior and dress than they were as children. They are to avoid activities that will expose their bodies, especially in the presence or view of males. Young women are warned to avoid "touch" by other individuals, and they are discouraged from playing children's games.

Philippine culture, strongly influenced by Christianity, does not pressure females to marry early. Rather, modern women marry later because many have career aspirations and other goals. Parents usually encourage their children to "enjoy life," get a college degree, and embark on a career before contemplating marriage.

## Teen Pregnancy

In keeping with Roman Catholic tenets, a high value is placed on abstinence from premarital sex. Teenage dating is often not sanctioned, and first sexual experiences are typically reported to occur at the age of 18 years for both sexes. The only accepted and commonly used method of family planning is fertility awareness or "rhythm," which involves abstinence or withdrawal during the fertile period. Induced abortion is illegal in the Philippines, where Roman Catholicism dominates; however, women can obtain illegal abortions. In North America, more acculturated women access abortion services, most often without family knowledge or consent.

## Menstruation

**Relationship to Health.**   Filipinos view menstruation as a normal function for females. In the Philippines, however, some menstruation customs mark the symbolic end of girlhood and introduction to womanhood: (1) at menarche, wiping the face with the blood stained cloth or underwear is thought to give the young girl a pimple-free face; (2) the number of steps jumped down on a stairway will determine the number of days of the menstrual flow; (3) sitting on a banana leaf will prevent clothing from being stained with blood, even during the period's heaviest days; and (4) stepping on a blooming orchid three times while clutching a cotton ball will ensure that a menstruating woman will smell fragrant (the light and airiness of the cotton ball will prevent the feeling of being burdened during menstruation). These rituals are most commonly practiced in the more rural areas of the Philippines. More recent immigrants to North America are well-educated, urban dwelling individuals who are less likely to practice them.

The mother usually performs these rituals, and it is believed that they should be performed in silence to bolster effectiveness. The rituals are followed by a bath to ensure that the young girl can continue bathing during all future menstruations without getting sick. It is believed by some who live in rural areas that bathing during menstruation will make the woman insane.

**Relationship to Fertility.**   Regular menstruation signifies fertility in the Filipino culture. Yet women who do not menstruate are not valued less. A scant, irregular, or heavy menstrual flow raises a red flag to the woman, who then suspects some health problem.

**Taboos and Restrictions During Menstruation.**   Getting near flowering or fruit-bearing trees is discouraged during menses, as doing so is thought to disrupt blooming or fruit-bearing. Menstruating women, or any of their relatives, should not bet in a cockfight (a popular sport), as this is bad luck. Women are not prohibited from religious or social functions in the company of males during menstruation as long as they practice good hygiene. Menstrual odor is a source of embarrassment, yet some believe that taking a bath during the menstrual period is not good for health. Women usually refrain from strenuous activities for fear that this stress and increased intra-abdominal pressure might induce a heavier flow.

**Dysmenorrhea.** Missed periods, light or shortened menstrual periods, or the passage of clots can be attributed to medical problems. Treatments for dysmenorrhea include herbal remedies recommended by the *herbolario* (herbologist) in the form of external applications, herbal teas, or both to increase menstrual flow and relieve menstrual cramping. Sometimes knee/chest position exercises are recommended.

## Female Modesty and Touching

Female modesty is emphasized among traditional Filipinas. Female practitioners are preferred, and privacy of the woman's body is highly impressed on them. Exposure of the body is not an accepted practice. Annual pelvic examinations are not customary in the Philippines, and modesty may influence a woman's willingness to obtain one.

Breast and gynecologic examinations can be embarrassing experiences, even when they are part of an overall medical examination.

---

**NOTE TO THE HEALTH CARE PROVIDER**

Filipinas are inherently modest. Touching and exposing a young girl's or woman's body without prior explanation and client consent can be looked on as a sexual advance or utter disregard for privacy. Providers must explain the importance and necessity of the procedure carefully before doing any examination that will necessitate touching or exposing the woman's body.

---

## Adulthood

### Transition Rites and Rituals

At age 18, a young woman is considered a young adult, *dalaga* in Tagalog. This transition is important to most families; although some cannot celebrate it as lavishly as others, most families usually mark the milestone with a special family event.

### Social Expectations

Societal norms exhibited by traditional women include modesty, early preparation for motherhood through responsibility to siblings, and loyalty to spouses. Aggressiveness, which is considered manlike, is discouraged. The ultimate sign of respect is filial piety, which is honoring and respecting one's parents, and all are expected to adopt this philosophy.

Education is of paramount importance to the family and is seen as a mechanism for social and career advancement. In the Philippines, older children who have completed their education through the sacrifice and hard work of family members are obliged to help younger siblings with their education. In contemporary Filipino

American families, the pursuit of education continues to be a high priority, and women are not encouraged to marry until they have achieved their educational goals.

### Union Formation

**Union Types.**   Arranged marriages are now rare, but they were accepted in the past, particularly for single-male immigrants to the United States who were denied intermarriage with U.S. citizens. Contemporary society approves long courtship and engagement periods that culminate in marriage. This society frowns on living together before marriage and polygamy, owing primarily to the influence of Roman Catholicism. This disapproval applies only to women, however; Philippine society fosters a double standard that makes these situations acceptable for men. After age 18 (the legal age in the Philippines), marriage without parental consent is permitted.

**Social Sanctions for Failing to Enter into Union.**   Men are not ridiculed for failing to marry, although they are encouraged to do so to provide heirs to carry on their family names. Women are not encouraged to marry early either; however, in some areas, women who fail to marry or who marry at an advanced age are publicly denoted "old maids." It is common for women to be so denoted if they are unmarried after age 30 (interestingly, women who exhibit short tempers or irritability are also branded "old maids"). An unmarried pregnant woman faces social pressures to marry. It is immoral and considered a family shame **(hiya)** to be pregnant and unmarried. However, no pressure is placed on a man to marry the mother of a child he has fathered out of wedlock. Again, a double standard exists.

### Domestic Violence

Domestic violence is a significant problem, yet Filipinas are more accepting of violence directed toward them by their spouses than are North American women of European descent. Accurate statistics for the United States are not available because most counties and agencies put all Asian-Pacific Islanders in one group. Many abused women suffer in silence, which is most common among the less educated who do not know that their rights are being violated. They tolerate spousal abuse because they are poor and afraid, they fear that no one will believe their story, and they fear losing their children. Many do not know where to turn for help. The submissive role of women in the family is a Spanish-influenced phenomenon that contributes to the culture of silence regarding domestic violence. The culture of **hiya** (shame) could also be a factor.

### Rape

In the Philippines, rape is a crime and punishable by death. Statistics are very difficult to find for the United States and Canada. Women may not report rape if the rapist is someone known to them or is their spouse or significant other.

### Divorce

**Sociocultural Views.**   There is neither divorce nor divorce law in the Philippines, and the society rejects divorce, reflecting the strong influence of Roman Catholicism and the cultural values that foster **hiya** (shame) and **pakikisama** (getting along with others). Divorce is referred to in Tagalog as **diborsyo,** and "divorced" is **diborsyado.**

Separation and divorce are still not commonplace among immigrants, and yet, Filipino Americans do somewhat follow mainstream American practice, albeit to a lesser degree. In 1990, among foreign-born Filipino-American males 15 years or older, 4.8% were separated or divorced compared with 9.2% of American men; only 6.9% of women were separated or divorced compared with 11.9% of American women in general

**Women and Divorce.**   Women who are separated from their husbands and cohabit with other men are considered immoral and scorned in society. Since immigrants tend to follow mainstream North American practices, more of them are divorced or are living with partners to whom they are not married.

**Child Custody Practices.**   Following a divorce, the male partner is expected to maintain ties with the children. However, divorce is usually a result of hatred and great irreconcilable differences that lead to the parties avoiding each other. Sometimes the father will then abandon the family, move on, and perhaps establish a new family.

---

**NOTE TO THE HEALTH CARE PROVIDER**

A divorced woman can become sensitive because of self-pity, especially about issues that relate to sex. She may misinterpret behavior and speech with sexual undertones as flirtation or sexual abuse.

---

### Fertility and Childbearing

**Family Size.**   Large families are typical in the Philippines, six being the average number of offspring in a household. In rural areas where people are mostly farmers and generally poorer, recreational activities are few, and procreation is an important life focus. These factors, linked with Roman Catholic bans on contraceptive use, have contributed to large family size in contemporary Philippine society. The illegality of abortion and the unmet need for contraceptive services may also contribute to family size. Filipinos in the United States and Canada are more apt to mirror the family size of these countries, rather than that of the Philippines.

**Contraceptive Practices.**   Roman Catholic religious beliefs influence contraceptive norms and practices in Philippine society. Contraception, other than natural family planning (rhythm, fertility awareness), is frowned on. The natural methods are the most commonly used in the Philippines, although one in four contraceptive users uses a modern method, such as oral contraceptives, female sterilization, intrauterine devices, injectables, and condoms. Women who use these modern methods do not always continue their use. Reasons for discontinuation include side effects and health concerns relating to oral contraceptives; desire for more effective methods; inaccessibility or inconvenience; expense; and personal attitudes, such as husbands' disapproval or wives' belief that God determines how many children she will have. However, only 3% of couples use condoms, and the male sterilization rate is low. It has been reported that discontinuation rates for contraceptive users are high: one in three discontinued during the first year of use, with rates for condoms the highest (59%), followed by withdrawal (41%), and oral contraceptives (40%).

The degree to which a couple abides by Roman Catholicism significantly influences their decision to use contraceptives, as does their degree of acculturation. Such use is usually a mutual decision by couples, although women often initiate the conversation.

## Abortion

**Cultural Attitudes.** Abortion is not commonplace in the Philippines since it is illegal. Because the culture is child-centered, abortion evokes strong reactions even in liberal Filipino Americans. Some may support the right to get an abortion in the abstract but may experience difficulty and guilt about accessing this option for themselves.

**Sources of Abortions.** Abortion providers tend to be lay persons in the Philippines. Immigrants to North America who access abortion services do so from medical facilities and providers.

**Timing of Abortions.** There are no data on the stage of pregnancy during which abortion is accessed in the Philippines owing to the illegality of the procedure. Similarly, U.S. abortion data have not traditionally reported Filipina Americans as a subgroup.

**Complications.** Because abortions are illegal in the Philippines, statistics are not available about abortion-related complications or the demographic profile of women who access the procedure. However, excessive bleeding and infection are the complications most commonly noted by treating facilities.

---

**NOTE TO THE HEALTH CARE PROVIDER**
Women may have conflict about abortion decisions related to their Roman Catholic backgrounds. Thorough discussion of the pregnancy outcome options is essential for these women, who may have difficulty sharing their dilemma about the decision with family members or friends.

---

## Miscarriage

Some may believe miscarriage to be the work of evil spirits **(aswang)** or voodoo spells **(kulam)** cast by or for a jealous or disgruntled woman. Having a frightening experience is also believed to induce miscarriage.

## Infertility

Superstitious people may view infertility as a punishment for past sins. The special term for the infertile woman is **baog**. Filipinos are generally accepting of illnesses, genetic defects, and other disorders; thus, infertility tends to be accepted as the will of God.

**Role of the Male Partner in the Couple's Fertility Decision-Making.** Women are not mistreated for the inability to bear children nor are they particularly blamed for the infertility. However, men who are very anxious to have children do so with other women while remaining married to the infertile woman.

---

**NOTE TO THE HEALTH CARE PROVIDER**
Women may be open to infertility treatments; however, they may have approached herbolarios and faith healers before turning to medical consultation.

---

## Pregnancy

**Activity Restrictions and Taboos.**   In traditional families, pregnant women are discouraged from working outside the home, and they are afforded much attention. Pregnant women are encouraged to get ample sleep, eat well, and avoid staying in prolonged sitting or sleeping positions during the day to avoid water retention. Sexual intercourse is taboo during the last two months of pregnancy. Less acculturated people may believe that encounters with deformed or disabled people or specific animals that frighten the pregnant woman can affect the developing fetus. Women are encouraged but not required to stay indoors.

Pregnant women are afforded courtesies, such as a seat on the bus, are pampered by their mothers, and can demand attention during the pregnancy that they would not usually expect when not pregnant.

**Dietary Practices and Observances.**   Pregnant women are encouraged to eat well and are given choice foods whenever possible. Near term, the traditional woman is encouraged to eat fresh eggs (a slippery food) to facilitate easy delivery, the baby's "slipping" through the birth canal.

**Prenatal Care.**   In the Philippines, most pregnant women seek health care from providers trained in the Western medical tradition. Therefore, they receive prenatal care and monitoring by nurses, midwives, and community health nurses. Prenatal care among traditional Filipinas and Filipina Americans parallels that of Western women.

---

**NOTE TO THE HEALTH CARE PROVIDER**

Health care providers may not realize that a pregnant Filipina is expected to demand attention, pampering, and solicitude from her husband and family members. This behavior has been known to cause health care providers to perceive pregnant women as being lazy.

---

## Birthing Process

**Home Versus Hospital Delivery.**   Hospital deliveries are increasing in the Philippines. Most Filipinas still deliver at home, however, attended by experienced lay midwives called *hilot*. Most Filipina Americans deliver in the hospital.

**Cesarean Section Versus Vaginal Delivery.**   Vaginal delivery is preferred over cesarean section. Since women are respectful of medical providers, however, they will usually accept a medical decision to deliver via cesarean when necessary.

**Involvement of the Male Partner.**   Childbirth is a time for the family to focus on the delivering mother. Fathers generally play a passive role and are not present at the delivery unless Lamaze is being practiced. The soon-to-be-mother orchestrates her birth experience by commanding those present to attend to her needs.

**Labor Management.**   The laboring woman is generally accompanied by a female family member who is a mother as her labor coach. Some Filipinas believe that walking promotes dilation and will pace in the labor room until forbidden to do so by a person of medical authority. Noise and commotion are kept to a minimum since they are thought to increase labor pain.

**Placenta.**   Traditionally, the placenta is buried in a special place in the family yard. Placentas of all other children in the family are buried in the same place to keep close family ties. Today, only those who have home deliveries consider this important. Immigrants who deliver in the hospital do not expect to be given the placenta, and it is not an issue for them.

### Postpartum

Following delivery, the typical postpartum period is 10 days, during which the new mother is not allowed to take a bath and may only do light housework. Every day, the *hilot* visits the new mother to give a whole body massage, with special emphasis on the uterus.

During the postpartum period, the mother should avoid cold drinks and exposure to cold breezes. Her room window should be closed, and she should wear socks, a long skirt, and a long-sleeved shirt or sweater. Exposure to cold temperature is believed to predispose the mother to arthritic conditions. Perineal hygiene is supervised by the hilot, who uses a warm solution made from boiled guava leaves and ashes taken from the cooking stove.

---

**NOTE TO THE HEALTH CARE PROVIDER**
Serving cold drinks, requiring showers, and unnecessary exposure to cold weather are contradictory to the cultural practices in the Philippines for postpartal women.

---

### Newborn and Infant Care

**Breastfeeding Versus Bottle Feeding.** Filipinas are expected to breastfeed, sometimes until the child is a toddler. Working mothers breastfeed and supplement with formula for at least the first year. Colicky infants are treated by applying *aciete de manzanilla,* an oil-based liniment with special herbal components that is used to relieve aches and pains, to the abdomen.

**Infant Protection.** Filipino Americans access Western medical care and abide by prescribed immunizations and treatments. In remote rural areas in the Philippines, most children do not receive immunizations or regular health check-ups. One common practice to protect the baby from *usog* (the evil eye) is to pin a religious medal or tiger tooth made into a pendant on the baby's clothes. Incessant crying and unexplained fever are signs that the baby may have been a victim of usog. The mother may touch the child and say something to avert the interest of the evil eye should a compliment be given. Practitioners need not avoid giving compliments, as it is the mother's job to provide this protection.

**Primary Caregiver.** After the mother, the maid or nanny is the next most important caregiver to infants or toddlers. Women care for children and for the sick. Men make decisions and participate in discipline, but they do little physical care. Extended female family members who happen to live with a child's family usually assist with childcare.

## Middle Age

### Cultural Attitudes and Expectations

Women are considered middle-aged as they make the perimenopausal transition. No socially sanctioned behavioral or clothing restrictions are placed on middle-aged women. Women recognize a decline in sexual interest marked by menopause, but they do not believe that sexual relations cease at that time.

### Psychological Response

Filipinas tend to have a positive attitude toward menopause and aging, viewing perimenopause as a natural life stage. Many women enjoy the benefits of an "empty nest" and embark on new careers or return to previous jobs.

Filipinos widely believe that midlife women are "nervous" and "irritable." These conditions are treated lightly, however, and are thought to resolve themselves over time.

### Menopause

**Onset and Duration.** In a study of 165 midlife Filipina Americans, women varied in their beliefs about the average age of menopause. In actuality, the average age of menopause among women in the sample who were postmenopausal was 48.9 years for natural menopause and 42.2 years for surgical menopause.

**Coping.** Filipina Americans consider the perimenopausal transition to be a natural life stage. They report symptoms as minimal to mild in severity. Coping strategies include talking with friends (83%), prayer (78%), relaxation (66%), doing something else (29%), meditation (22%), visualization (19%), and affirmation (19%), as opposed to hormone replacement therapy (HRT) (28%). Interestingly, in the Philippines as well as in the United States, women report symptoms of nervousness or irritability more than hot flashes.

---

**NOTE TO THE HEALTH CARE PROVIDER**

Women are more likely to use self-initiated treatments than HRT for perimenopausal symptoms. Practitioners should recognize this preference and offer alternatives to HRT for perimenopausal symptoms.

---

# Old Age

### Cultural Attitudes and Beliefs

A woman older than age 65 years is considered old. The life expectancy of Filipinos ranges from 65.2 to 68.7 years, which is 17.3 years younger than the general U.S. population. This difference in life expectancy may be related to differences in nutritional status, disease control, health conditions, and level of available health services.

Respect for the older person is strong in the Filipino culture. Regional differences exist, however, as to how an older person is addressed. In the Tagalog region (Central Luzon area), elders are addressed with respect, using words like *po*, *opo*, or *ho*. Failure to use these terms is considered disrespectful. In the Visayan Islands and Mindanao areas, there are no similar words. Generally, older persons are not called directly by their first names. They are addressed with respectful terms such as *lola* (grandmother) or *lolo* (grandfather), *manong* (older man) or *manang* (older woman) even when they are not related to the person. A more formal address is Mr.____ or Mrs.____. Younger people give up their seats in public places to old women, serve them first in gatherings, and offer assistance if necessary.

An elderly woman usually lives with family members; she is viewed with pity if she lives by herself. Other family members or close friends are encouraged to live with her if she has no immediate family. A widowed woman usually lives with her children or extended family and helps take care of the young children. Because of the large extended family in the Filipino culture, a woman living alone is more an exception than the rule.

Elderly women who cannot care for themselves are usually cared for by other family members. Placing an elderly person in a nursing home is unacceptable and viewed as abandonment or lack of caring on the part of the family. The values of Filipinos in North America, however, are changing. Since both men and women most commonly work full time, caring for an elderly parent at home presents difficulties. Sometimes these adult children are forced to place their parents in skilled nursing facilities.

# Death and Dying

## Cultural Attitudes and Beliefs

The predominantly Catholic Filipino culture accepts death as part of God's divine plan. Views among various age groups, however, may differ. Regional differences in cultural practices related to death and dying may also exist. Many of these practices are influenced by the deeply religious nature of Filipinos. Most will freely accept the death of an elderly woman who has lived a productive life. Dying is considered "rest" and "being with God." Death of a midlife woman, however, is considered a loss. This woman had not reached the fullness of her life, and she may still have adult children to send to college or assist in some way. Death of a younger woman is considered a tragedy, since she may still be in her childbearing and childrearing years.

Catholics believe that most souls go to purgatory to cleanse their sins before going to heaven. Those who lived a good life are bound to go to heaven, while the evil go to hell. Souls or spirits of the dead are still around to watch over the family and guide them or help them with family problems.

## Rites and Rituals

A Catholic priest performs "Anointing of the Sick" or prays for the dying at the bedside of a dying person. Family members ask for forgiveness for any transgressions they may have committed and listen to the last wishes of the dying person. Someone with a disease or illness may ask the dying person to take the disease or illness with him or her to the final destination in the hope of being cured or healed.

Dying at home is preferred over dying in the hospital because the dying person prefers to be among loved ones and relatives. However, those dying in the hospital are often tended by family members, close friends, and a Catholic priest.

Rites and rituals do not vary by gender. Both men and women are accorded the same attention and regard.

### Mourning

One year is the official mourning period for the immediate family. The soul of the departed spirit is believed to linger, especially immediately after death. Sometimes these spirits show themselves as "ghosts" to family members or others. Those with unfulfilled wishes are believed to linger the longest.

The surviving spouse is to refrain from going to dances during the mourning period. Women in the immediate family are expected to wear black clothing, while each man wears a black ribbon pinned to his shirt. Later practices include wearing black and white apparel.

The sequence of the mourning period observed by most Catholics is the same. They say prayers for the souls in purgatory for three consecutive days and hold a feast on the third day. On the fourth day, the nine-day novena starts, and it is attended by groups of people participating in the nightly novenas. On the ninth day of the novena, a feast is again prepared for the mourners. Burial is usually scheduled around this time, if family resources permit; however, it may be scheduled earlier if agreed on by family members.

Remains of the dead are generally kept in the home during the wake; prayers are said, and offerings of food and flowers are made. Family members keep a 24-hour vigil to watch over the body. To some families, keeping the remains of their loved one in a funeral home during this time is considered uncaring or disrespectful. Contributions of cash, food, and other forms of assistance to the grieving family are made. This is a time when the community comes together in the spirit of **bayanihan** (a term loosely translated to mean "people helping each other").

If there are young children, the husband usually takes custody following death of the mother.

## IMPORTANT POINTS FOR PROVIDERS CARING FOR FILIPINO WOMEN

### The Medical Intake

#### Literacy and English Proficiency

English proficiency is unlikely to be an issue among younger Filipinas who have attended school in either the Philippines or the United States. The Philippine system of education is patterned after the American system, with English as the language of instruction. Although proficiency in English may be a problem for some elderly women who were educated during the Spanish regime, few of these women are still alive. More commonly, older women will understand English better than they can speak it. If English communication is a problem, however, a family member or friend is likely to accompany the woman to help as an interpreter or in filling out health-history forms.

#### Status of the Provider

Filipinos are respectful of their elders and of those in authority or higher positions. The health provider is viewed as a person of authority and so is given high respect. Every effort to help the woman is appreciated and considered a big favor **(utang na**

**loob**). Sometimes women show their gratefulness by giving the provider a small present.

Older or more traditional women are likely to be shy and modest and may refrain from making eye contact with unrelated men, including health care providers. These more traditional women can be nonverbal and passive. Younger generations are less likely to exhibit these characteristics.

### Communicating Illness and Symptoms

The shy Filipina may not volunteer significant medical history information, especially that which pertains to sexual practices. Sex is a topic that is embarrassing to talk about, and it is seldom discussed, even within the family. A Filipina may also be reluctant to discuss current symptoms or home remedies she is taking for an illness. The provider should be patient and take time to ask pertinent questions that help diagnose the medical condition.

Some Filipinos (mostly the less educated) strongly believe that "bad spirits" cause illnesses. Attendance at a clinic, however, signifies that the client does not think that bad spirits are causing present symptoms and that he or she is interested in Western medical treatment. Typically, a family member or friend accompanies the client and may help provide information regarding the illness. For conditions caused by bad spirits, people seek advice and treatment from **herbolarios** or **spiritistas** (faith healers).

## The Physical Examination

### Modesty and Touching

Filipinas may be very modest and shy about exposing their bodies. An explanation about the importance and need for the procedure that includes touching or exposure of the body is essential. Most women prefer a female health provider, reflecting their inherent modesty.

Touch by a nonfamily member is considered inappropriate. Indeed, without prior consent from the female client, she may misinterpret touch as sexual abuse. Also deemed inappropriate is touching the body of a female client when not essential to the consultation. During menses, most women do not want to be touched or close to others. The odor of menstrual blood is a source of embarrassment for Filipinas, who consider good hygiene difficult to maintain during their menstrual periods.

### Expressing Pain

Filipinas are thought to be somewhat stoic. They do not loudly complain of pain and may not want to take pain medications even during episodes of extreme pain. Many ascribe to the religious belief, "Suffer on earth and be rewarded in heaven."

## Prescribing Medications

### Drug Interaction

Herbal teas and roots as household remedies are still commonly used. Therefore, overdosing and drug interaction with prescribed medications pose a legitimate concern for health care providers. Clients may not volunteer information about medicinal herbs and home remedies being taken because of a lack of knowledge about potential interactions. The health care practitioner must ask specific questions about nonprescription treatments to elicit all pertinent data.

### Medication Sharing

Medication sharing is not customary, although some women may share leftover prescribed medications with family members or friends to avoid waste. Direct questioning about prior medication use and patient education that discourages medication sharing may be necessary.

Filipinas are not likely to hide information about medications that other health providers have prescribed. Careful, direct questioning about ALL current medication use, however, will avoid innocent and unintentional omissions.

### Compliance

Clients may have a tendency to not complete a full course of prescribed medication once symptoms disappear. Health care providers should be clear and emphatic about the importance of completing the full course.

## Follow-up Appointments

Filipina Americans are not known as having problems with keeping follow-up appointments. Family needs are given priority, however, and may interfere. It is not necessary to make a reminder telephone call, although such a call might be appreciated.

"Filipino time" means a culturally acceptable delay of 15 to 30 minutes past a set time. As this practice may be problematic in the health care setting, imposing penalties for being late (charging for missed appointments; rescheduling the visit for another date and time) may discourage it.

## Prevalent Diseases

The terrain and climate in the Philippines result in an increased prevalence of malaria, pneumonia, tuberculosis, and gastrointestinal diseases. The leading causes of mortality and morbidity are pneumonia, tuberculosis, heart disease, diarrhea, cancer, cerebrovascular accidents, traumatic accidents, bronchitis, and diseases associated with nutritional deficiencies. Among women, anemia is common in the elderly, infants, and pregnant and lactating women.

Among the few studies of the health of Filipino Americans, a cardiovascular risk study in California showed Filipinos as having a higher prevalence of hypertension than Chinese, Japanese, and other Asians. Results of another study suggest increased risks for developing coronary heart disease, hypertension, and diabetes at midlife and beyond. A study of 165 Filipina Americans found a low prevalence of chronic health problems compared with the general population. Prevalence of glucose-6-phosphate dehydrogenase deficiency, $\alpha$-thalassemia, and lactose intolerance and malabsorption is high in the Philippines, but these problems have not been studied in North American populations. A low intake of calcium-rich foods, however, might suggest the need for a study of osteoporosis in the elderly.

Filipinos experience lower incidence rates of cancers of the lung, skin, breast, corpus uteri, prostate, urinary bladder, and kidney than whites, but Filipina Americans have a higher incidence of cancer of the cervix uteri.

## Health-Seeking Behaviors

Typically, Filipinos do not seek medical attention at the first sign of illness. They try home remedies first for minor illnesses, as well as the services of ethnic and folk healers, such as **herbolarios** and faith healers. Only when these treatments are ineffective or the condition worsens do they seek medical consultation. Ethnic and folk healers are prevalent in the Philippines, but few are in North America.

Home remedies used for minor illnesses consist of herbal teas, massage, and external applications of heat and cold. When the illness is perceived as being major or life threatening, however, immediate medical attention is sought.

Filipinos in North America adopt health promotion and disease prevention behaviors to varying degrees. Midlife Filipina Americans have reported regular, moderate exercise; however, health promotion and prevention behaviors are not as prevalent among Filipino men. Gender differences are also found in the prevalence of risk behaviors known to threaten health, such as moderate to heavy alcohol consumption and smoking. Filipino men are known to drink more alcohol and are more likely to smoke than Filipino women in North America.

## 🌐 BIBLIOGRAPHY

Anderson, J. (1983). Health and illness in Pilipino immigrants. *Western Journal of Medicine*, 139(6), 811–819.

Berg, J., & Lipson, J. (1999). Information sources, menopause beliefs, and health complaints of midlife Filipinas. *Health Care for Women International*, 20, 81–92.

Berg, J., & Taylor, D. (1999). The symptom experience of Filipino American midlife women. *Menopause: Journal of the North American Menopause Society*, 6(2), 105–114.

Jenkins, C., & Kagawa-Singer, M. (1994). Cancer. In N. W. Zane, D. T. Takeuchi, & K. N. Young (Eds.), *Confronting critical health issues of Asian and Pacific Islander Americans*. Thousand Oaks, CA: Sage, pp. 105–147.

Lott, J. (1997). Demographic changes transforming the Filipino American community. In M. Root (Ed.), *Filipino Americans: Transformation and identity*. Thousand Oaks, CA: Sage.

# CHAPTER 12

# Haitians

JESSIE M. COLIN, PhD, RN, and
GHISLAINE PAPERWALLA, BSN, RN

## 🌐 INTRODUCTION

### Who are the Haitian People?

Haitians are largely an Afro-Caribbean people who inhabit the island nation of Haiti, one of the largest Caribbean islands (approximately 27,500 sq km or 10,714 sq miles), situated between Cuba and Puerto Rico. A French colony until 1804 (when Haiti broke the chain of slavery and gained its independence), much of Haitian culture has the underpinnings of a combined French and African heritage. In Haiti, the two official languages are French and Creole, which derives from a combination of French and an African dialect. Today, Creole is the national language spoken by 100% of the population, whereas French is spoken by only 10%. The dominant religions are Catholicism, Protestantism, and voodooism.

Haiti's population is about seven million. The skin colors of Haitians are of various shades, ranging from very light to very dark tones. This variation is partly because of intermarriage and the mixing of indigenous Indians with Europeans and African slaves brought to the island. **Mulattoes,** descendants of French colonists and African slaves, are one of these biracial groups. Like many Caribbean societies, Haitian societal identity has always been characterized by sharp class stratification and demarcation along color lines. Lighter-skinned people are treated better and given more privileges than darker-skinned people.

### Haitians in North America

Fleeing the suppressive government regime in Haiti, the first wave of Haitians to migrate to the United States occurred in the 1950s. The second wave arrived in the 1960s. Like their predecessors, this group consisted of skilled workers and professionals. In the 1980s, the third and largest influx of Haitians reached North American shores. The members of this group were primarily uneducated and unskilled rural residents escaping economic hardship.

At present, the Haitian population in the United States and Canada is neither well documented nor well known. A Haitian writer has pointed out that the exact size of this population will never be known since fear of deportation keeps most illegal residents from participating in any type of official tabulation or census recording. As of 1998, reports estimated about 503,000 living in the United States. Unofficial estimates by Haitian leaders and activists, however, suggest that there are about 1.2 million Haitians in the United States. Purportedly, 500,000 live in New York, 200,000 live in Florida, 150,000 are in both Boston and Chicago, and 100,000 live in California. Remaining communities of Haitians are believed to be scattered throughout the United States.

The 1996 Census enumerated 83,680 people of Haitian heritage in Canada, 53% of whom are women. The overwhelming majority live in Montreal.

## ⊛ BEING FEMALE IN HAITIAN SOCIETY

In the highly patriarchal Haitian society, men are expected to make family decisions. In reality, however, women appear to make many major family decisions. Functionally the "backbone" of the family (or **poto mitan caille** in Haitian Creole), the Haitian woman serves as the home economist, balances the family budget, and "makes do" with the limited money brought into the home. Additionally, she is expected to fulfill her roles of wife, mother, nurse, cook, and the like.

Societal and family expectations are that the woman must silently accept her partner's extramarital relationships. Until the early 1970s, women were not permitted to make major purchases or to own material goods except for property inherited, and even that property is considered communal within a legal marriage, the husband being the "administrator." The same rules follow for common-law marriages, which are quite common in this society and considered "legal" among those of the lower socioeconomic groups. In recent years, the plight of women has shown some promising signs of improvement with the involvement and election of a few women to high cabinet and ministry positions in the government.

## At Birth

### Preference for Sons

Haitian society highly values all children. In fact, parents usually perceive and describe a child's birth as **un cadeau du Bon Dieu** (a gift from God). There is still a preference for the first-born to be a boy. Indeed, the first-born being a girl may be interpreted to mean that the man is not sufficiently **"macho."** In Creole he is said to have **rein faible,** meaning that his sperm is weak. Apart from being teased by friends, this matter is very serious because without a son there is perceived to be no possibility of continuing the family name.

### Response to Birth of a Female

Although parents may not celebrate the birth of a female child in the same manner as they would following the birth of a son, it is not common for any child to be abandoned or made to feel unwanted within Haitian culture.

### Birth Rituals

No specific birth rituals or observances are common in this society. The new father may, however, invite some of his friends to the house to toast and celebrate the arrival of a son, which is seen as a reinforcement of his manhood.

# Childhood and Youth

## Stages

Haitian society does not clearly demarcate childhood developmental stages. Grounded in the traditional Haitian views about cognitive growth and development is the belief that the basic training of children—for hygiene, self-feeding, and toilet training—should begin at around 2 years of age. Individuals up to their mid-20s are considered **ti moun,** meaning child or children in Haitian Creole. **Ti moun** also applies to a young woman who remains unmarried or is still living with her parents regardless of marital status.

## Family Expectations

Parent-child roles are clearly defined, with limited tolerance for child self-expression. Children are expected to conform and obey parental rules. Corporal punishment is an accepted and frequent method of discipline in Haiti, being seen as an effective way to implement the parenting role. Because of laws protecting children from physical punishment at the hands of a parent, however, Haitian parents in North America report feeling lost and incapable of implementing their parenting role. Many of them perceive American or Canadian society as being too permissive, and they feel powerless in understanding how to raise their children within the Haitian tradition on North American soil.

## Social Expectations

Both boys and girls are expected to be competent, self-reliant, self-sufficient **(Sa ki lan men ou se li ki pa ou,** meaning, "What's in your hand is what you have"), and high achievers. They are expected to be obedient and respectful of parents and elders and to neither have nor express opinions because they are not believed to have enough life experience. Respect for elders is a serious matter. Haitians believe that misfortune will mar the future of a child who disrespects his or her elders. This phenomenon is known as **Madichon**. A child making eye contact with an adult is seen as challenging the adult. Bowing the head and avoiding eye contact demonstrate a respectful attitude.

## Importance of Education

Families hold extremely high expectations for their children in terms of academic achievement. Although the illiteracy rate is high, children are raised to believe that formal education is the key to their future. In the past, boys were educated with the expectation that they would become professionals and breadwinners for their future families. Today, the expectation seems to be the same for girls. The father, although in the home, is often not the prominent figure involved with the child's education, as is the mother. Instead, he functions more as a distant authority figure within this context.

# Pubescence

## Psychosexual Development

A child becomes a youth at puberty. A girl is considered to be entering womanhood once she has had her first menses and she is referred to as **demoiselle**. This occurs between the ages of 9 and 15. Boys, on the other hand, reach puberty between the ages of 15 and 17, typified by deepening of the voice.

## Rituals and Rites of Passage

Generally, no observed celebration or ritual marks a youngster's entrance into puberty. In fact, neither the teenage years nor adolescence is a truly recognized stage among Haitians.

## Teen Sexuality

**Social Restrictions and Pressures.**   Teenage girls are cautioned against engaging in sexual activity, which can result in pregnancy. Teenage boys, on the other hand, are given more freedom to explore and initiate sexual activity. With teenage girls, emphasis is placed on maintaining social respectability. Hence, social relationships of girls are closely supervised, and they are generally not permitted to go on unchaperoned dates until about age 18. With migration and acculturation of Haitians into North American societies, some of these attitudes are changing.

There are no social pressures on teenage girls to marry. The emphasis is on education, good behavior, and maintaining "purity" so that the girl can successfully marry later. Often there is subtle approval of a male "friend," especially if that person is from the same socioeconomic class as the girl and her family.

**Teen Pregnancy.**   Premarital sex is not sanctioned. It is viewed as a threat to the girl's future and a blemish on the family's prestige. If a girl becomes pregnant, parents will favor marriage over abortion, regardless of the situation. The parents view marriage in this case as a way of absolving disgrace (**sove façade,** meaning "to save face"). Rural residents place far fewer restrictions on teenage girls. Out of economic necessity, these girls are more likely to enter into unions with older men to bring economic stability to themselves and their families.

## Menstruation

**Relationship to Health.**   Generally, parents do not discuss the subject of menstruation with their daughters. Only if there are medical problems (such as dysmenorhea or amenorrhea) will the parent seek medical advice. During menstruation, the girl is encouraged to report "overflows" (very heavy flow) to her mother so that she can be assisted with folk remedies and have her diet adjusted. Haitian women consider reporting overflows particularly important to avoid anemia, known as "thin blood."

**Relationship to Fertility.**   When a girl has her first period, it is customary for her mother or an older sibling to caution her about her now-fertile state and the fact that having sex could result in pregnancy. Amenorrhea (failure to menstruate or missed period) is taken seriously and is perceived as the result of a poor diet, pregnancy, or anemia.

**Taboos and Restrictions During Menstruation.**   There are no restrictions or taboos during the menstrual period; however, cleanliness is emphasized. **Pedi san** refers to the loss of blood through menstruation, and menstrual irregularities are referred to as **san kap boulvese**.

**Dysmenorrhea.**   Dysmenorrhea is very common among Haitian teenagers for reasons unknown. Herbal medicines in the form of tea are typically used for this condition. The youngster is encouraged to rest, to apply warm compresses to her lower abdomen, and even to stay home from school. She is also cautioned not to use "cold" substances or sit on cold surfaces, which are believed to increase the discomfort. Also discouraged is the ingestion of such acidic foods as pineapple juice and orange juice because acidic foods are believed to cause severe menstrual cramping and clots. For very severe dysmenorrhea, a physician may be consulted.

## Female Modesty and Touching

Touching, kissing, and embracing are standard ways of interacting with and greeting family and friends. Typically, men will not kiss or embrace women unless they are very close friends or relatives. In Haitian society, a woman's body is considered "precious" and to be touched only by her partner. As to interactions between women, it was quite common until recently to see two Haitian women walking hand in hand as a demonstration of their friendship. This trend is disappearing, however, because of concerns about possible connotations of homosexuality, which is considered taboo in Haiti.

Although modest, most Haitian women will not object to being touched by a male practitioner for therapeutic reasons. Haitians are accustomed to being treated by male physicians since men predominate in the practice of medicine in their country. Young Haitian girls, however, do not undergo routine pelvic examinations. In the case of illness, the young girl's mother or a female member of the family is present during any examination.

---

**NOTE TO THE HEALTH CARE PROVIDER**
This culture emphasizes female modesty. Women are hesitant about touching or inspecting their bodies, which can be an impediment, if not a barrier, to health teaching and performing breast self-examinations. Also, economic concerns take precedence over preventive health practices.

---

# Adulthood

## Transition Rites and Rituals

There are no special rites of passage for entering adulthood. Generally, a young woman is considered an adult when she marries and leaves her parents' home or moves to live abroad independently. Although a young woman may be an adult chronologically, she is not treated as an adult as long as she remains in her parents' home.

## Social Expectations

Traditionally, young women were prepared for marriage and starting a family. Today, with the emphasis on education and career, far less pressure is placed on a young woman to marry. If at home, she is expected to assist with the care of younger siblings; and if there are elderly parents or grandparents, she is expected to participate in their care as well.

### Union Formation

**Union Types.** The vast majority of Haitians follow the marital pattern of *plaçage* (common-law unions). The term *femme caille* describes the woman who shares her home with a man in a common-law arrangement. Traditionally, among the lower classes and rural residents, polygamous unions are frequent; the man generally engages in extramarital relationships with several different women at the same time. Under this arrangement, the woman who is the mother of some of the man's children but with whom he does not share a household is referred to as *man-man petite*. Members of the middle and upper classes, on the other hand, engage primarily in monogamous marriages. In North America, traditional gender roles may change as a result of women working outside the home and gaining greater autonomy, perceivably a source of conflict.

**Social Sanctions for Failing to Enter into Union.** A woman who fails to enter into union is not publicly ridiculed. If unmarried by age 30, however, she is referred to as *vieille fille* (old girl), which does have some negative connotations.

### Domestic Violence

There is no term for "domestic violence" in the Haitian vocabulary. Relations between a man and a woman are generally considered a personal matter. Since the man often assumes authority over the family, including his wife, it is not considered abuse for him to batter her physically. To date, Haitian society remains silent about domestic violence, although its occurrence is believed to be widespread. The society also provides little or no support for an abused woman; indeed, she may be viewed as having been at fault or responsible for the abuse.

Today, even though there is some discussion about women's rights in Haiti, battered women (aware of the lack of available support) are still very reluctant to report abuse to the Department of Social Service **(Bien Etre Social).** The only time this behavior or criminal conduct is taken seriously is when a woman is murdered.

Among more recent Haitian immigrants and refugees, there may still be a hesitance to report domestic violence or even view it as a crime. Haitians who have lived longer in North America, on the other hand, may be more inclined to seek help and avail themselves of the resources available to battered women.

---

**NOTE TO THE HEALTH CARE PROVIDER**

Haitian women who have recently arrived in North America are not likely to admit abuse. If it is suspected, providers must broach the subject cautiously with the client and try to establish a trusting relationship before discussing it. They need to consider the real possibility that the woman who is dependent on the abuser may not even recognize her situation as abusive.

---

### Rape

In Haiti, there is not a high incidence of rape as it is known in North America. There is, however, a high incidence of "veiled" rape, known as **restavec.** Restavec occurs to young girls, aged 10 or even younger, who are adopted by family members or privileged families with the expectation that, in exchange for room, board, and the chance for a better education, the child will assist with household chores or simply be a playmate for the family's biologic child. Often, a male member of the hosting family molests and rapes the adopted child. This type of rape (restavec) occurs frequently but is not discussed or admitted in Haitian society. To avoid being returned to her family, who is likely to chastise the girl for causing this "lost opportunity," the young girl often must accept this abuse without complaint. Although the local service agency **(Bien Etre Social)** could be used to report these offenses, most families do not do so because of the shame and secrecy that surrounds restavec.

Although support systems are in place in North America to help rape victims, the stigma and shame that are culturally attached to rape may still prevent many Haitian victims from coming forward, reporting the crime, and seeking help. Haitians living in North America for longer periods and who have assimilated more American/Canadian belief systems and views may, however, be more inclined to report this crime.

### Divorce

**Sociocultural Views.** Strongly influenced by the tenets of the Catholic Church, Haitians view divorce as a social disgrace and failure. Although divorce is common among Haitians, before it becomes final, family members, friends, the church, and elders generally try to counsel the couple to stay together.

**Women and Divorce.** In the past, a divorced woman was considered to have lost her place and status in society, which she regained only upon remarriage. Today, with the influence of migration and more liberal views about relationships, Haitian women no longer abide by these cultural rules and standards.

**Child Custody Practice.** Following a divorce the children are generally the woman's responsibility. The man is expected to maintain ties with his children, but no laws force men to care for their children. Typically, the man is inclined to move on and establish a new family unit. In the United States, if not forced to do so in court proceedings, Haitian men also tend to avoid child support payments.

---

**NOTE TO THE HEALTH CARE PROVIDER**
Providers should approach the issue of divorce with care and sensitivity and establish a trusting relationship before raising the issue.

---

### Fertility and Childbearing

**Family Size.** By North American standards, the average family, consisting of six or more children, is large. Haitians have demonstrated far higher rates of fertility than American Caucasian women. In North America, however, there are social and economic pressures to limit family size, including the absence of the extended family once available in Haiti to assist with childcare.

**Contraceptive Practices.** Largely because of the strong religious influences of the Catholic Church, Haitian society neither encourages nor openly discusses contraceptive use. Privately, however, Haitians (especially upper- and middle-class groups) who can afford the high cost of modern contraception (often beyond the means of the average Haitian) will use it. Nonetheless, although the acceptance and use of modern contraception by Haitians in North America has improved, the level of such use remains far below that of American Caucasian women. Although condoms are the simplest form of contraception, Haitian men strongly resist their use, believing that condoms impair "sensation during intercourse."

**Role of the Male in the Couple's Fertility Decision-Making.** Because of the
many loose union formations and common-law marriages that typify Haitian society,
the responsibility for contraceptive use generally falls squarely on the woman's shoulders. At the same time, findings from a recent study suggest that much contraceptive
behavior demonstrated by refugee Haitian women in the United States, particularly
their limited or non-use of contraception, is largely influenced by their male partners'
negative views. For example, a woman may refuse to use a diaphragm because of her
male partner's complaints about its interference with his sexual pleasure.

## Abortion

Abortion is not an accepted practice in the eyes of most Haitians. In the event of an
accidental pregnancy resulting from incest or rape, however, the stigma attached to
abortion has perceivably decreased. While most abortions in Haiti, especially
among the wealthy, are performed in a clinical setting, the use of herbal abortifacients remains a viable source for those of lesser means. The herbal teas are given
during the first trimester of pregnancy, when inducing an abortion is safest. In North
America, these herbs and plants are readily available in botanical stores to Haitians
wishing to use them. **Boule ti mas** is an example of one herb from which a tea is
made that has anticoagulant and abortifacient properties.

**Teen Abortion.** Abortion is a very sensitive subject, almost never openly discussed, whether in relation to a teenager or an adult. Although it is not socially sanctioned, it is not unusual for members of the upper and middle classes to allow their
daughters to have a secret abortion to "save face" and avoid the shame and disgrace
that a teenage pregnancy would bring to the family. Rural residents, on the other
hand, strapped with fewer social mores, are less inclined to seek a teen abortion.

## Miscarriage

A miscarriage is a very traumatic event likely to be interpreted, especially among
lesser-educated and rural residents, as a punishment from God or a curse placed on
the woman by a rival or jealous neighbor. The Haitian belief in the curative powers
of voodooism strongly influences the course of action taken. Women seek biomedical help, the help of a voodoo priest **(hougan** or **mambo)**, or both. A woman who has
frequently miscarried will generally be cared for and pampered during the course of
her pregnancy.

## Infertility

Haitian women often perceive childbearing as an obligation or role fulfillment as well as the means by which to establish social respectability. Infertility has a negative impact on the woman. Many see the infertile woman as having been cursed and label her **"mulette"** (mule) because mules do not reproduce. A man who can have children with a mistress will often seize this opportunity to prove his masculinity, that is, his ability to father children. The infertile woman, on the other hand, is powerless and must accept this arrangement since she is presumed to be the "guilty party," unable to conceive.

---

**NOTE TO THE HEALTH CARE PROVIDER**
Although a woman may be receptive to infertility treatments, her male partner may be less eager to participate. The cost of infertility treatments may also be a barrier. Providers need to be supportive and explore viable treatment options with the client and her partner.

---

## Pregnancy

Haiti reportedly has one of the highest rates of maternal mortality in the Caribbean. Nonetheless, pregnancy is a perceived "normal" and healthy state and a time of joy for the entire family. Because of this perception, Haitian women often will not seek prenatal care. To improve pregnancy outcome, however, a pregnant woman is discouraged from eating spicy foods for fear of irritating the fetus. Conversely, she is encouraged to eat vegetables and red fruits because these foods are believed to be capable of improving fetal blood. Likewise, she is fed large quantities of food since she is said to be "eating for two." Other measures taken to protect the developing fetus from harm include never awakening the pregnant woman for fear that doing so will interrupt normal fetal growth and protecting or shielding the pregnant woman from situations in which she may be frightened by an animal or deformed individual, believed to negatively affect or "mark" the baby.

**Prenatal Care.**   Preventative healthcare, including prenatal care, is not a priority for most Haitians because of major economic constraints. Pregnancy does not relieve the expectant mother from her day-to-day work and employment responsibilities. While some Haitian women may seek prenatal care at their physician's office or neighborhood clinic, a great many never do so. Believing that pregnancy is not a disease state, they see little if any need to be distracted from regular responsibilities to seek prenatal and follow-up care.

---

**NOTE TO THE HEALTH CARE PROVIDER**
Practitioners should stress the importance of early and continued prenatal care as a means of improving pregnancy outcomes.

---

## Birthing Process

**Home Versus Hospital Delivery.**   Most deliveries take place in the hospital or at specific maternity hospitals; home delivery is less frequent. Generally, Haitian women favor natural childbirth, and often they will not request analgesia. To detract from the discomfort of labor, a rural woman may sing or chant in an effort to attain the strength to endure the discomfort. Haitians in North America, however, are more inclined to request analgesics when labor contractions become closer and stronger.

To hasten the delivery process, it is customary for the woman to pace, walk, sit, squat, and rub her belly, unless she has been placed on strict bed rest. Customarily, the Haitian man does not participate in the birthing process, believing that childbirth is a private event best handled by the woman and her mother.

**Cesarean Section Versus Vaginal Delivery.**    Vaginal delivery is the most frequent mode of delivery. A cesarean section is most feared and avoided by Haitians, except in extreme cases, because it entails abdominal surgery which is perceived as dangerous and possibly a threat to one's life.

**Labor Management.**    A Haitian woman is very vocal and animated during labor. She is likely to respond to painful contractions with loud screams and cries; sometimes, she may even become hysterical. Women who have had multiple pregnancies, however, tend to be stoic, only moaning or grunting in response to heightened contractions.

**Placenta.**    No special cultural meanings, significance, or practices surround disposal of the placenta.

### Postpartum

Perceiving the postpartum period to be crucial in the birthing process, the new mother avoids white foods such as lima beans, okra, and mushrooms, because they are believed to increase vaginal discharge. After birth, Haitians also believe that the woman's bones are "open" and that she should stay in bed during the first two to three days to allow her bones to close. The postpartum woman assumes an active role in her care and takes the necessary measures to ensure that she dresses warmly and remains healthy. One of these measures is wearing an abdominal binder to facilitate closure of the bones and provide support.

Postpartum women also engage in a practice called "three baths," which occurs over a period of one month and is believed to enhance and tighten the internal muscles. During the first three days postpartum, the mother bathes in hot water made from special leaves; she also drinks teas made from those leaves. During the next three days, she takes a bath prepared with leaves in water warmed in the sun. The mother also takes vapor baths with boiled orange leaves. At the end of the third to fourth week, she takes the third bath, which is a cold bath. This being the final step of the process, the woman may now drink cold water and resume her normal activities.

---

**NOTE TO THE HEALTH CARE PROVIDER**
Acknowledge and respect the woman's culturally observed postpartum practices. Do not serve cold drinks and take this opportunity to instruct on the importance of early ambulation postdelivery.

---

### Newborn and Infant Care

**Breastfeeding Versus Bottle-Feeding.**    Traditionally, breastfeeding has been the preferred method of nourishing babies, given its convenience and economy. Today, however, bottle-feeding has taken precedence because more Haitian women, in both Haiti and North America, work outside the home. The use of herbal teas is also an integral part of the infant's feeding. For example, herbs such as **marjorlene** tea are routinely fed to a colicky infant.

> **NOTE TO THE HEALTH CARE PROVIDER**
> Encourage and support breastfeeding and underscore the health benefits of breast milk to the infant. Teaching the client to pump and store breast milk for infant feedings while she is away from home is also a useful intervention.

**Infant Protection.** The infant mortality rate in Haiti is high, 102.6 per 1,000 live births as reported in the 2000 World Population Report. To date, immunization and preventive infant care are limited in the urban areas of Haiti and practically nonexistent in rural communities. Although health care, especially preventive health care, assumes a low priority when compared with economic concerns for most Haitians, immigrant Haitians will take advantage of health education programs and preventive infant care services when made available and accessible to them.

On a more personal level, parents will often take extra steps to protect their infants from evil spirits and harm from the environment by attaching religious artifacts such as blessed medals or neck chains to the infant. An example is the **ouari** seed, which is used as a charm, attached to a chain and placed around the child's neck. Signs and symptoms of a child who has been afflicted by the evil eye or witchcraft include failure to thrive, colic, diarrhea, and sickliness for no apparent reason.

> **NOTE TO THE HEALTH CARE PROVIDER**
> If practitioners find any cultural (nontraditional) items on the infant's clothing or around the arms or neck, they must be respectful and nonjudgmental. Assess for tightness and the tendency for these items to cause strangulation as the infant grows but do so in a caring and diplomatic manner.

**Primary Caregiver.** Although the mother or grandmother is usually the primary care provider, given the importance of and extraordinary support systems provided by the extended family, childrearing does, in fact, become a "family affair." Godparents, although often not blood relatives, are considered members of the family, and they also play a central role in childrearing. In the event that the parents suffer misfortune, the godparents often will assume full responsibility for bringing up the child.

## Middle Age

### Cultural Attitudes and Expectations

Women 40 to 50 years of age are considered middle-aged. At this time, the woman is expected to dress more conservatively and conduct herself in a "mature" manner. For many Haitian women (especially rural ones), extending childbearing well into midlife is not unusual.

### Psychological Response

For most Haitian women the concept of "midlife crisis" holds little meaning because, unlike women in North America who think in terms of "self," they think more in terms of "family" and their roles as wife, mother, and grandmother. Moreover, since their relationships with the tightly knit extended family remains the same or becomes stronger, Haitian women typically experience no negative consequences at midlife.

#### Menopause

**Onset and Duration.** The onset of menopause or *rete* (stop) occurs, on average, between 40 and the mid-50s. Most Haitians view menopause as a natural phenomenon, and the age of onset is believed to be genetically influenced.

**Sexual Activity.** Many Haitian women welcome menopause, which they view as a liberator from future pregnancies. At this midlife junction, however, many women may also become frustrated with their partner's many extramarital affairs and divorce or separation looms as a real possibility for the couple at this point.

**Coping.** Individual strategies are applied in coping with the discomforts of menopause. Generally, however, the consumption of various herbal teas remains an integral part of the treatment for hot flashes. In North America, Haitian women are, for the most part, receptive to the use of hormone replacement therapy (HRT) if they receive appropriate patient education.

---

**NOTE TO THE HEALTH CARE PROVIDER**
Carefully assess herbal teas consumed for possible drug interactions with other medications being used.

---

## Old Age

Haiti is considered the poorest country in the Western Hemisphere. The life expectancy of Haitians is 47 years for males and 51 years for females, compared with 74 and 79 years in the United States. Haitian society considers a woman "old" when she is in her late 50s. A man is not viewed as "old" until his mid-70s. With old age comes respect; this culture views an older woman as being mature and wise. Elders are considered the family advisors, babysitters, and historians.

Elderly and widowed women do not live alone; rather, their children are expected to care and provide for them. Migration to North America, however, has created certain challenges regarding caring for elders when one has to work outside the home. Recently, a small percentage of Haitians in North America have started reluctantly placing their elders in nursing home facilities.

## Death and Dying

### Cultural Attitudes and Beliefs

Haitians often misunderstand and fear the concepts of death and dying. While the death of an older woman is viewed as more acceptable because it is felt that she has "lived her life," the death of a young or middle-aged woman is much more difficult to accept. It is felt that she has not yet "lived her life" or "accomplished her mission."

### Rites and Rituals

After death, Haitians believe that the departed spirit needs nurturing; if it is not at peace, it will wander and become restless. Usually there is a special prayer service called **dernie priye,** which consists of seven consecutive days of prayer. This service usually takes place in the home, and its purpose is to facilitate the passage of the soul from this world to the next. On the seventh day, a mass called **prise de deuill** begins the official mourning process.

### Mourning

**Cultural Expectations.** The traditional period of mourning in Haiti, although less closely followed today, varies depending on whose death is being observed. Mourning for a mother is two years, while it is one year for a father or husband. During the mourning period, women are generally expected to wear black. When mourning the death of a child, however, mothers typically wear white. Other family members are expected to refrain from wearing brightly colored clothing and to limit the amount of makeup. A mother who loses a child also refrains from going to the cemetery because it is believed that if she has other children, she is casting doom and possibly bringing death closer to them.

---

**NOTE TO THE HEALTH CARE PROVIDER**

Providers must be supportive and respectful of what may seem a prolonged mourning period. Referral to grief counseling may be in order.

---

**Coping.** After the death of a mother, the father or grandparents assume responsibility for the care of minor children. Godparents also play an important role in caring for orphaned children.

## IMPORTANT POINTS FOR PROVIDERS CARING FOR HAITIAN WOMEN

### The Medical Intake

#### Literacy and Medical Proficiency

Illiteracy and lack of English proficiency are likely problems for Haitian clients. Hence, they may need help to complete forms, and Creole-speaking interpreters may be needed to assist with explaining procedures. Usually, for reasons of confidentiality, most Haitian clients prefer using family members instead of official interpreters. If no family member is available, clients would much prefer having a professional interpreter whom they will likely never see again and with whom they have no relationship. When dealing with a sensitive topic such as sexual matters or issues pertaining to the female genitalia, a female interpreter will be much more acceptable to the client.

### Status of the Provider

Haitian clients hold health providers in high esteem. Women are extremely modest, project a timid attitude, and smile a lot. Less-educated people avoid eye contact as much as possible, especially with those in positions of authority.

### Communicating Illness and Symptoms

Generally, a woman will not readily volunteer information about her perceptions of illness or its cause, symptoms she has experienced, or home remedies being used. These women believe some illnesses to be of a spiritual nature. If the practitioner probes, the woman is apt to state that her disease does not have a natural cause.

---

**NOTE TO THE HEALTH CARE PROVIDER**

Do not appear intolerant of the woman's perception of the disease and resist being judgmental. Take this opportunity to educate the client, at an appropriate level, on the pathogenesis of the disease and its treatment regimen.

---

## The Physical Examination

### Modesty and Touching

Women are extremely modest and unlikely to perform monthly breast self-examinations. They are not likely to seek Papanicolaou's tests or mammograms, which they perceive as invasive and likely to cause anxiety. For intimate procedures, these women usually prefer a female health care provider.

### Expression of Pain

Haitian women are stoic and frequently will not express pain or request analgesics. This is especially true for recent immigrants and refugees. When pain becomes intense or unbearable, however, the woman's demeanor is likely to change. She may become very irritated and cry and scream loudly and seemingly uncontrollably. Pain management should include careful pain assessment and intervention at an early stage.

## Prescribing Medications

### Drug Interaction

Risk for drug interaction (synergism or antagonism) is very high, given the common use of herbs and home remedies.

### Medication Sharing

The sharing of leftover medications with family and friends is customary, as is using another person's health experiences as a barometer for assessing one's own health. For example, if a friend or family member experienced dizziness, lightheadedness, blurred vision, and headaches and was diagnosed with hypertension, another woman with some of the same symptoms is likely to identify herself as also being hypertensive. The lack of access to health care, coupled with the high cost of pharmaceutical drugs, may be partly responsible for the practice of medication sharing and self-diagnosing.

### Compliance

Compliance with treatment regimens may be problematic. Most Haitians perceive one course of a treatment or medication dose as sufficient to cure the offending disease, even hypertension or diabetes. The same is true for the treatment of infections. Generally, these clients will take two to three days' of antibiotics, after which they will discontinue the medication as symptoms subside. The practitioner should explain and stress the importance of complying with the full course of treatments, especially antibiotics.

## Follow-up Appointments

Typically, preventative health care and follow-up care are not priorities. This has much to do with Haitian perception of health and illness and a higher priority on working to meet financial obligations rather than taking time off to keep appointments. Unless health-care services are made accessible (for example, by increasing the flexibility of clinic hours), clients are unlikely to return for follow-up care.

### Orientation to Time

Adherence to strict schedules and appointments is inconsistent with the Haitian cultural pattern of doing things at one's own pace, which is much slower than that practiced in North America. Arriving late for appointments is not seen as being impolite. Health care practitioners should be mindful of this time orientation by making reminder calls for appointments and respectfully encouraging clients about the importance of timeliness.

## Prevalent Diseases

Prevalent diseases among immigrants and refugees include hepatitis, tuberculosis, acquired immunodeficiency syndrome (AIDS), venereal diseases, and parasitosis from inadequate potable water sources in Haiti. Additionally, Haitian populations report a high incidence of hypertension and diabetes, believed to be caused by both dietary practices and genetics. The high incidence and poor outcomes of breast and uterine cancer may, on the other hand, be largely attributed to women's failure to practice early detection measures.

## Health-Seeking Behaviors

It is not unusual for clients to present in the clinic setting at an advanced stage in the disease process. Often, they use symptom management (with self-care) followed by spiritual care. They will use the same home remedies for both minor and major illnesses. Such remedies often consist of herbs, teas, folk medicine, and massage. In North America, spiritual healers and voodoo priests and priestesses (*mambo* or *hougan*) are readily available to believers wishing to worship spirits to relieve their illness. Both groups' perception of health and illness and their response to illness pose increased health risks. At the same time, such health promotion activities as regular exercise and closely monitoring one's food choices are not typical for this population. Foods high in carbohydrates, fried foods, and a significant amount of red meat tend to comprise the typical Haitian diet, as with most Caribbean people.

##  BIBLIOGRAPHY

Bibb, A., & Casimir, G. (1996). Haitian families. In M. McGoldrick, J. Giodano, & J. K. Pearce (Eds.). *Ethnicity & family therapy*. New York: The Guilford Press, pp. 97–111.

Colin, J., & Paperwalla, G. (1996). Haitians. In J. G. Lipson, S. L. Dibble, & P. A. Minarik (Eds.). *Culture & nursing care: A pocket guide*. San Francisco: University of California, San Francisco Nursing Press, pp. 139–154.

Corrine, L., Bailey, V., Valentin, M., Mortantus, E., & Shirley, L. (1992). The unheard voices of women: Spiritual interventions in maternal-child health. *Maternal Child Nursing*, 17, 141–145.

Harris, K. (1997). Beliefs and practices among Haitians American women in relation to childbearing. *Journal of Nurse Midwifery*, 3(32), 149–155.

Laguerre, M. S. (1981). Haitian Americans. In A. Harwood (Ed.). *Ethnicity and medical care*. Cambridge, MA: Harvard University Press, pp. 172–210.

Stepick, A. (1982). *Haitian refugees in the* US. London: Minority Rights Group.

# CHAPTER 13

# Japanese

## YUKO MATSUMOTO LEONG, RN, MS

### INTRODUCTION

### Who are the Japanese People?

Although the Japanese are often considered a single ethnic or monolithic group, in reality Japanese culture includes elements of Chinese, Korean, and other Asian and Western cultures. In recent years the number of foreigners or **Gaijin** (outsiders) in Japan has increased. Although interracial marriage has become more common, it is still not fully accepted; and some interracial couples leave Japan in search of a better future for their children. No one religion is dominant; Shintoism, Buddhism, and Christianity coexist. For example, an ordinary Japanese may, without much conflict, go to a Shinto shrine for blessing of a baby, go to a Christian church for a wedding, and be buried in a cemetery at a Buddhist temple.

The Japanese language includes Chinese characters and the Japanese alphabets (**Hiragana** and **Katakana**). Children whose parents lived overseas (**Kikokushijo**) and children of immigrants find it a challenge to master Japanese communication skills, both the language itself and restraining themselves from sharing their opinions freely with others. English is taught at secondary schools for high school entrance examinations, rather than as a way in which to communicate with others. Some Japanese read English, but they may have a hard time understanding spoken English.

### Japanese in North America

About 500,000 Japanese emigrated to the United States between 1820 and 1996. The largest immigrant communities are in Hawaii, the U. S. West Coast (Los Angeles, the San Francisco Bay Area, and Seattle), New York, and Detroit; younger Japanese Americans are scattered throughout the United States. As of 2000, the number of Japanese living in the United States was 796,700. As of the 1996 Census, 77,130 people of Japanese heritage live in Canada. The largest number live in Vancouver, followed by Toronto.

Japanese-Americans identify themselves by generation to distinguish their experience and values: **Issei** (first generation), **Nisei** (second generation), **Sansei** (third generation), **Yonsei** (fourth generation), and **Gosei** (fifth generation). For example, Issei and Nisei tend to be more traumatized, and Sansei have tried to help them by establishing culturally appropriate health and social services, such as senior centers and long-term care or home support services. While Sansei, Yonsei, and Gosei may maintain their ethnic identity, they are much like the dominant American group in lifestyle, health beliefs, and values. Those who may have difficulty in the health-care system are Issei, Nisei, and Japanese students and visitors.

The first wave of immigrants came to Hawaii and the Pacific Coast before World War II. Executive Order 9066 in 1942, which forced all West Coast Japanese Americans to move to "relocation camps," traumatized many Japanese Americans and left lasting psychological scars in this group.

The second wave (1947 to the late 1960's) consisted of more than 60,000 women married to American citizens, many of whom were U. S. servicemen stationed in Japan. Their adjustment was as difficult as that of Issei women, but they had no social support from people who shared Japanese culture, language, and values. They were almost completely dependent on their spouses and often chose to **gaman** (endure) and suffer in silence. For the sake of their children, however, some women became "strong" and divorced, relocated, and sought jobs despite their limited English skills. They often have American surnames, and their children may not have a strong sense of Japanese identity.

The third wave (late 1960s to present) has consisted of 4000 to 7000 immigrants annually. Some came as students and decided to stay. They may call themselves "newcomer" or "new Issei," and many are educated professionals who live in large metropolitan areas. They are quite different from Issei who arrived decades ago.

Many Japanese newcomers in the United States do not intend to settle permanently, planning to return to Japan in the future. They may maintain a strong connection with Japan, visiting frequently to attend to the needs of aging relatives.

## 🌐 BEING FEMALE IN JAPANESE CULTURE

In Japan, the woman's role has changed from participating in a multigenerational family household to managing a small nuclear household. The traditional ideal of womanhood, **ryosai kenbo** (good wife and wise mother), is still highly valued. Career and self-expression are regarded less highly than is being a good mother, and the woman's major role is nurturing her children. Many women attend college to attain a good marriage rather than prepare for a good job and financial independence. Women are expected to maintain the house and to care for children, husband, and the elderly, even when they have jobs. Most women now work part time or in temporary jobs to supplement their spouses' income.

In North America, adherence to ryosai kenbo varies; some women find it difficult to be a "good mother and a wise wife" without extended family or a Japanese community.

## At Birth

### Preference for Sons

In the past, sons were strongly preferred. The first son inherited all family assets, along with the responsibilities of caring for elderly parents, unmarried siblings, and other needy relatives. If a family had only female children, the family often adopted a **yooshi,** a daughter's husband, to carry on the family name. After World War II, family-law changes gave equal family assets to each sibling, and the number of children decreased.

### Response to the Birth of a Female

Japanese families will be concerned about who will carry on the family name, take care of the family grave, and conduct the **Obon** ceremony (annual Buddhist ceremony for family ancestors) if no male child is in the family. Although parents may be concerned about the cost of weddings for daughters, it is not a social pressure. Many women now work to pay some of their own wedding expenses.

There is no neglect of daughters in the current context of small families.

### Birth Rituals

A special celebration is held, not at the time of birth, but in the following year, on March 3rd **(momo no sekku)** for a girl and May 5th **(tango no sekku)** for a boy. The first-born girl receives a set of ancient dolls **(ohina-sama)**; the first-born boy receives several 10-foot-long fish-shaped kites **(koinobori)** made of cloth that are hung outside on tall poles to publicly announce the arrival of a son. Sons also receive a set of samurai figure dolls. Special foods are prepared for each occasion. The boys' day (May 5th) is designated "children's day," a national holiday in Japan.

## Childhood and Youth

### Stages

No special term differentiates child and youth; however, many small celebrations recognize a child's milestones. Some celebrations have become quite commercialized and expensive, for example, **hichi-go-san** (7–5–3). In this celebration, held on November 15th, 3-year-old and 7-year-old girls and 5-year-old boys are taken to Shinto temples in their traditional kimonos to be presented for blessings.

### Family Expectations

Children of both sexes do schoolwork and share house chores. School-aged children, especially boys, are often busy with homework and attend extra outside school classes **(juku)**. Thus, parents usually expect boys to perform fewer house chores.

### Social Expectations

The young girl is expected to be a successful wife and mother when she grows up. Instead of going to juku, some girls take classes in **okeiko-goto** (traditional Japanese arts, such as flower arrangement, tea ceremony, calligraphy, and music lessons).

### Importance of Education

Formal education is very important. Less than 0.7% of the Japanese population is illiterate. In Japan, there are few opportunities to change careers or retrain for new skills; therefore, receiving a "good education" is a crucial element of Japanese society. Although this aspect of employment is changing in some Japanese workplaces, many jobs are still open only to new graduates. Employers often view and treat men as life-long committed workers, while they consider women to be temporary workers.

High school is not compulsory, and students must take an entrance examination. Parental pressure to get into a "good" high school is very strong because high school is seen as a step to a "good" college and then to a "good" life-long job. Some families prefer to send their children to private school from kindergarten through college. Parents usually do not encourage girls to study as hard as they do boys, and family resources may not be available for girls to attend a juku.

## Pubescence

### Psychosexual Development

Adolescence is called **shishun-ki** (time of thoughts about spring). The onset of female puberty is seen as the beginning of menstruation, which may occur between 8 and 15 years of age. Reaching the height of 146 to 148 cm indicates that onset of the menstrual cycle should be expected.

### Rituals and Rites of Passage

Some families prepare **osekihan** (sweet rice with red bean) to celebrate the onset of menstruation. Turning 20 years old has a special meaning, and the second Sunday of January is a national holiday called **Seijin-no-hi,** the day of reaching adulthood. Women often wear traditional kimono to attend the ceremony and are professionally photographed.

### Teen Sexuality

**Social Restrictions and Pressures.**   Modest appearance is encouraged, and many secondary schools require uniforms. At the secondary-school level, adult expectations change for boys and girls; for example, boys are allowed more freedom to be with friends, while girls are expected to be home early. Pubescent girls are not pressured to marry, but parents and society may pressure them to marry after age 20.

**Teen Pregnancy.**   Teen dating is allowed, but it varies for each family. The family may not openly discuss sexuality, and sexual activities are not encouraged. Teenage pregnancy and abortion are nonetheless increasing in Japan, and the need for family planning education for teens is also growing, including information regarding sexually transmitted diseases (STDs). If a teen is married, however, pregnancy is not stigmatized.

### Menstruation

**Relationship to Health.**   Menstruation and the menstrual flow have no special significance in Japan.

**Relationship to Fertility.**   Regular menstruation signifies fertility. A woman may need to reveal and discuss her perceived potential for fertility or infertility with a prospective future husband before engagement.

**Taboos and Restrictions During Menstruation.**   There are no restrictions or taboos during menstruation, except that a woman may be restricted from Shinto ceremonies.

**Dysmenorrhea.**   Missed periods, light or shortened menstrual periods, or the passage of clots are attributed to stress, heavy lifting, or too many activities. A

Japanese law states that women can request a day off from work for menstrual cramps. Some women seek treatment, such as Chinese herbs, for this condition.

## Female Modesty and Touching

Modesty is emphasized, especially in the presence of elders and teachers. This provision is based on Confucian teachings emphasizing respect.

**Relationship to Health Care.**   Women can be appropriately treated by either a female or male health provider. Some older women postpone or totally avoid such examinations because of embarrassment, but this is changing for younger women in Japan. Immigrant women and Japanese Americans tend to obtain regular pelvic examinations and mammograms.

Physical contact is minimized in physical examinations, and the focus is on the particular part of the body being examined. In outpatient offices or clinics, patients wear their own clothing rather than changing into examination gowns.

---

**NOTE TO THE HEALTH CARE PROVIDER**

For a pelvic examination, some practitioners in Japan use a curtain hung over the examination table between the woman's head and the practitioner. Having eye contact or carrying on a conversation during the examination is not usual. Providers should explain the procedure before the examination and converse only when necessary.

---

# Adulthood

## Transition Rites and Rituals

At age 20 years, a woman is considered an adult. No specific word describes this transition. The only ceremony is "the Day of Reaching Adulthood" (see previous).

## Social Expectations

Japanese women are expected to marry. In the past, women were expected to be able to cook, do flower arrangements, and conduct the tea ceremony; they were not expected to be educated. These expectations have changed. Younger women value independence and often seek full-time jobs after completing their education at the junior college level. Many employers view women as temporary workers who will resign when they marry or have a child. Some career women have difficulty in breaking through the thick "glass ceiling" to reach management positions in the traditionally male-dominated business world.

## Union Formation

**Union Types.**   Relationships are monogamous by law. Some couples are casually introduced as prospective marriage candidates by their relatives and friends, who consider their family backgrounds, suitability, finances, and the like. Sansei and later generations in the United States meet one another as do any other Americans and, not infrequently, marry interethnically.

**Social Sanctions for Failing to Enter into Union.**   Young women and men are encouraged and may be pressured to marry before they are 30. In 1950, the average marriage age of women was 23; in 1999, it was almost 27. In 1950, the average male marriage age was 26, increasing to 28 by 1993.

If a woman remains single or marries at an advanced age, she may be ridiculed by being called *ikazugoke* (widow without marriage) or *ikiokure* (late to go). Some single women now support themselves and live independently. If a single woman lives with her parents and her brother plans to marry and bring his wife to live with the parents in a multigenerational household, the single woman may need to move out and establish her own household. This practice is declining because some families wish to avoid "in-law conflicts." The percentage of three-generation households was 10.5% of all households in 1995, down from 16.1% in 1970.

### Domestic Violence

Some young women who come to the United States end up in violent relationships, with or without children. This may occur because of a lack of knowledge about the potential for such problems, and the woman may not know what to do once the violence starts. In Japan, women who experience domestic violence used to be taken care of, but now they are more isolated as a result of changes in family and community structure. In North America, there are a few services (e.g., an Asian woman's shelter in San Francisco), but women who use them may still feel that they have betrayed the expectation of holding the family together. The prevalence of domestic violence is unknown. A few women with temporary status (married to U.S. citizens less than five years) report domestic violence to obtain asylum and a permanent green card.

### Rape

Date rape among younger Japanese women exists. The most frequently raped women are young, single immigrants who may be very naive, and do not know about STDs. In Japan, if a woman becomes pregnant from date rape, her family may persuade her to marry the man.

A woman who is raped by a stranger is often blamed for the incident, and she may not report it to avoid embarrassment.

### Divorce

**Sociocultural Views.**   Divorce is not encouraged, especially if one or more children are involved. Many divorced women have difficulty establishing an independent life without financial support from their parents. Some such women may be called **demodori** (returned to home). In Japan, the divorce rate has increased in recent years, although it is still far lower than in North America. For example, in 1993 it was 1.52 per 1000 persons, in contrast to 4.33 (1996) in the United States. Twenty-seven percent of divorces involved couples married more than 15 years. No statistics are available regarding the divorce rate of Japanese Americans.

**Women and Divorce.**   A divorced woman is generally not treated with respect, although it depends to some extent on why she divorced. For example, if she divorced her husband because of his drinking or gambling problems, she will receive much sympathy. She may not receive sympathy, however, if the reason for divorce was pursuit of her own career. Remarriage is acceptable, but the law prohibits a divorced woman from remarrying during the year following the divorce.

**Child Custody Practices.**   In the past, divorce meant that the woman had to leave the household and children behind. Although each case varies, more than 70% of divorced mothers are now granted custody of the children.

## Fertility and Childbearing

**Family Size.** Small family size is typical. The number of children has decreased in recent years; in 1999, the average was 1.34. Many families have difficulty affording educational and marriage expenses, which are seen as the responsibility of the parents even after their children reach adulthood. Therefore, more women than in the past work outside the home to supplement their spouses' incomes.

**Contraceptive Practices.** In Japan, condoms are the most popular means of preventing conception. In June 1999, a low-dose version of the contraceptive pill was finally approved in Japan. Japanese strongly fear using what they view as unnatural, and some believe that the pills interfere with women's natural hormonal cycles.

---

**NOTE TO THE HEALTH CARE PROVIDER**

Explain different contraceptive methods and monitor immigrant Japanese women closely, since they are unfamiliar with some methods, especially the benefits and risks of oral contraceptives. To increase effective counseling, provide written materials with pictures about contraception, but make sure the material does not directly refer to the topic on the brochure cover.

---

**Role of the Male in the Couple's Fertility Decision-Making Process.** In general, the man's decision significantly affects the woman's decision regarding use of contraception. Some men object to using condoms, preferring instead that women tell them when conception is less likely, that is, "the safe time" (rhythm method).

## Abortion

**Cultural Attitudes.** In 1995, 42,229 abortions were performed in Japan. Women who have abortions are not stigmatized. Some abortions are viewed as medical necessities, but others are performed for unplanned pregnancies or family planning (an additional source of birth control). No strong anti-abortion movement based on religion exists in Japan, and abortion is not considered a sin. So that the soul of an unborn child can rest, women may put a little stone statue of a Buddha with a little red bib (**mizuko,** a water child) in the cemetery of a temple; this practice comforts some women.

**Teen Abortion.** The teen abortion rate is increasing, although most abortions are performed on married women ranging in age from 30 to 44 years. Teen pregnancy may be acceptable for teens who are engaged to marry. Such teens are not necessarily considered "troubled" youths.

**Sources of Abortions.** Women generally obtain abortions safely and legally in private physicians' offices or clinics. In North America, women seek abortions from recognized clinics or private offices. Few, if any, herbs are used as abortifacients in Japanese culture.

**Complications.** Abortion-related complications and deaths are rare in Japan because abortions are legal and provided by licensed physicians. Abortions are likely to be sought early in pregnancy; in 1993, 94% were performed within 11 weeks of gestation.

## Miscarriage

The causes of miscarriage are seen as medical, not magical or spiritual; but women may be blamed for not taking care of their own bodies. Precautions to prevent miscarriage include avoiding heavy lifting, traveling, and drastic changes in lifestyle. Women are also advised to pay attention to diet, to rest, and to keep warm, especially their abdomen and feet.

## Infertility

Infertility tends to be viewed as the woman's fault. The infertile woman is not publicly ostracized, but she may be privately called an **umazume** (stone woman). No cultural norms influence how the man treats his infertile wife, but the woman may feel strong pressure to seek medical fertility treatment and bear a child. High-tech fertility treatment is illegal in Japan, but Japanese immigrants or visitors may seek it in North America.

## Pregnancy

**Activity Restrictions and Taboos.** Miscarriage in Japan may be related to strenuous or difficult shift work. By law, a pregnant, working woman may request a different job assignment, involving less standing, lifting, or night shifts. This situation is ideal; however, it may not be possible to arrange it in many work settings. Women can continue to do all the same daily activities at home as before the pregnancy. They are not required to stay inside, but they are encouraged to avoid stressful conditions.

**Taikyo** (education in the womb) is a traditional belief in Japan in which pregnant women are encouraged to stay positive and engage in cognitive thinking, reading, and listening to music to enhance the development of the fetus.

Pregnant women are generally treated with great respect. They may not be treated well, however, if the pregnancy occurs outside marriage.

**Dietary Practices and Observances.**   Dietary beliefs revolve around avoiding cold, as do pregnancy beliefs in general. The woman should avoid "cooling" the abdomen, which can result from going barefoot, not covering the abdomen, or drinking cold drinks. Some women, depending on the generation, avoid cold foods such as watermelon and eggplant. Sansei women do not observe this practice. Women do not eat nonfood items (pica) during pregnancy.

**Prenatal Care.**   A woman seeks prenatal care at a medical clinic when she misses her period and receives a certificate of pregnancy from her physician. She brings the certificate to a public health department office, where she receives a "maternal-child handbook" that she takes to each prenatal visit for recording her progress.

Some women celebrate their pregnancy at the time they first feel the movement of the baby. In the fifth month of pregnancy, on the *day of the dog* (dogs are believed to have easy labor), a woman may be given a special cotton sash to wrap around her abdomen, and she may start wearing maternity clothes.

## Birthing Process

**Home Versus Hospital Delivery.**   Most deliveries occur in a hospital, attended by a nurse-midwife and physician.

**Cesarean Section Versus Vaginal Delivery.**   Women in Japan attend natural childbirth classes, and vaginal deliveries are most common, usually without anesthesia. A cesarean section is accepted if it is a medical necessity.

**Involvement of the Male Partner.**   Fathers are more involved than in the past, and some relatives may visit a short time to assist the new mother. Among new immigrants, the man may not have time to be involved or participate in the birth process because of his work or study commitments. The partners of Sansei or Yonsei women, or of those who married non-Japanese men, are typically involved in the birth in the same way as their dominant-culture peers.

**Labor Management.**   The natural progress of labor is encouraged, with little intervention. Bed rest is recommended following rupture of the membranes. Immigrant women may request an epidural, however, based on their respect for North American technology.

**Placenta.**   No spiritual practices surround the placenta. Many mothers save the dried umbilical cord in a special small wooden box. Many women also save the first hair of their baby.

## Postpartum

In Japan, women stay in the hospital for one week after vaginal delivery and two weeks after cesarean section. The typical postpartum recovery period is one month. Traditionally, the new mother is expected to rest and breastfeed, and her relatives cook and clean for her.

In Japanese hospitals, new mothers are served hot water, not ice water. It is common to see a thermos of hot water on the bedside table. Women avoid cold water in general, as well as washing the dishes and wet hair, in the belief that if the body surface becomes cold, it will cause postpartum complications (e.g., the cervix will not close). Health providers should respect these beliefs and provide hot water instead of ice water.

### Newborn and Infant Care

**Breastfeeding Versus Bottle-Feeding.**  The preferred method of infant feeding is breastfeeding. Japanese mothers believe in the importance of breastfeeding for bonding, immune systems, and infant nutrition. There is some concern, however, about dioxin contamination of mothers' milk. New mothers are encouraged to drink fluids and eat non-spicy and light food to avoid upsetting the baby.

**Infant Protection.**  Infants and toddlers receive regular immunizations and checkups in public health department offices, where their growth and development are monitored and recorded in the maternal-child handbook and on clinic charts. There are no cultural beliefs or practices to protect the child from evil. There are reports of sudden infant death syndrome even though babies always sleep on their backs in Japan. There is also concern about increasing child abuse by family members.

**Primary Caregiver.**  Mothers are primary caregivers, although fathers may contribute. Traditionally, the family unit consisted of parents, their oldest son, and his wife and children. Many young people now move to urban areas to seek better jobs. Some new mothers may return to their parents' house before the labor and remain for one month after the birth of the child. Conversely, other women will visit and help their daughter or daughter-in-law with the new grandchild.

---

**NOTE TO THE HEALTH CARE PROVIDER**

Immigrant parents may find early discharge from a hospital traumatic, especially if they have never taken care of a newborn and have no close family or friends on whom to rely.

---

## Middle Age

### Cultural Attitudes and Expectations

Women are considered to be middle-aged at 50. Midlife women do not have any clothing or other restrictions, but they prefer a modest appearance.

### Psychological Response

There are some reports of the "empty-nest" syndrome in middle-aged women whose children have gone to college or married. Some women start to take classes (**okeiko-goto**), seek employment, or both.

The number of divorces among middle-aged couples who have been married more than 15 years is increasing. Some women desire to start a new life or career, having spent many years bearing and raising their children. More women than men initiate divorce, even though age discrimination in Japan is considerable, and few jobs for women older than age 35 are available. Sansei midlife behavior reflects that of the dominant culture.

### Menopause

**Onset and Duration.**  The word for menopause is **heikei,** which means the closing of the cycle. The average age of menopause is 51 years, onset usually occurring between ages 43 and 55, except in the case of surgery.

**Sexual Activity.** Menopause is regarded as a normal life transition. Sexual relations continue during and after menopause.

**Coping.** Some women may experience distress from hot flashes and emotional changes and may seek medical treatment (e.g., with Chinese herbs). The menopausal transition, however, is not usually a big issue for Japanese women. Fewer symptoms may be associated with a diet lower in fat and higher in soy products than typical North American diets. Usually, women are knowledgeable and open about discussing menopause with a trusted practitioner.

# Old Age

## Cultural Attitudes

The average life expectancy of Japanese women was 83.99 years in 1999, while it was 79.4 years for U. S. women in 1997. The longer life expectancy may be genetic, or it may result from diet and self-care practices.

A woman is considered old if she is older than 65. September 15th is the Japanese national holiday to celebrate respect of elders. Respect of elders continues through the Sansei and Yonsei generations in North America, despite the lack of opportunity for elderly women to pass on family history and wisdom to younger generations.

In Japan, families are also losing the sense of extended family, especially in urban areas, with a steady decline in the number of three-generation households to 20%. Nursing homes are used in both Japan and the United States when adult children cannot care for their parents at home. Most families try to care for the elderly at home as long as possible. Sansei have been active in developing culturally appropriate, long-term care or day programs for Japanese elderly in the United States.

# Death and Dying

## Cultural Attitudes and Beliefs

Many Japanese wish to die at home, saying, "I want to die on a **tatami"** (Japanese straw floor mat). Death often occurs in institutions, however, especially in the case of terminal illness. In 1993, more than 70% of deaths from terminal illness occurred in institutions. The concept and actuality of hospice care is still new, especially in home settings.

Death is not discussed openly. Revealing the prognosis of terminal illness is a new concept among both patients and health care providers. The death of an elderly woman can be viewed as a celebration for her completion of a full life, but death of a young woman, especially one leaving small children, is seen as a tragedy.

According to Buddhist beliefs, the human soul should go to **gokuraku** (heaven), but some souls cannot go to gokuraku and remain among humans if the deceased person still worries about people left behind. It is the family's duty to make sure that the soul does not remain in the human world and can go to gokuraku. The family ancestor's soul will visit the family and stay with the family each year during **Obon,** and the family will prepare a welcoming and farewell ceremony for the occasion.

## Rites and Rituals

The family covers the face of the deceased with a white cloth, turns the head toward the north, and wets the lips with water. The family stays all night to make sure that the incense continues to burn to guide the soul to heaven. There are no gender differences in practices for the deceased.

### Mourning

**Cultural Expectations.**   Buddhist rituals include 7th- and 49th-day ceremonies after death, and then 1-, 3-, and 10-year anniversary ceremonies (some do more). Family, friends, and neighbors attend these ceremonies. The appropriate mourning period is one year. Mourners wear black and white clothing; generally, they do not change their hairstyles or other appearance.

When the deceased person is the mother of young children, a family conference is held to make required decisions as to child custody, which will depend on the ages of the children and the father's circumstances. Most children remain with their fathers, but some stay with grandparents. Among Japanese Americans, it depends on the generation.

**Coping.**   There are no typical mourning or coping strategies for Japanese wives. Following the death of a spouse, many women face a drastic change in their lifestyles. Some may even face eviction since many companies and government offices provide housing for their employees. Again, coping difficulties depend on generation; for example, Nissei women in their 60s or 70s have a particularly difficult time since they were protected by their spouses and never learned such skills as driving or using a checkbook.

## ⊕ IMPORTANT POINTS FOR PROVIDERS CARING FOR JAPANESE WOMEN

### The Medical Intake

Understanding the health-care system and accessing appropriate services may be difficult. Japanese women in North America are spread across the spectrum of acculturation, and navigating the system and communicating with health care providers is very challenging. Many women appear to be passive, polite, and competent to hide their fears or true feelings. They frequently report somatic symptoms and physical distress when they are under psychological and interpersonal stress. With careful and sensitive communication, the client may share her real concerns; thus, a sensitive interpreter among non-English speaking women is very important.

Bringing their family members or friends to interpret can be difficult, especially for elderly war brides, who might not have their extended family nearby to help. Women who marry non-Japanese may also have few family members to assist them and may be unwilling or unable to ask a friend for help.

---

**NOTE TO THE HEALTH CARE PROVIDER**

Japanese women have many "private" topics that they do not wish to willingly volunteer to health providers, particularly any history of diseases that are considered "bad" such as STDs, mental illness, and communicable diseases, such as tuberculosis. Many women are reluctant to tell what they consider family secrets.

---

# The Physical Examination

## Modesty and Touching

Issues regarding modesty and covering the woman's body vary depending on women's acculturation and knowledge of North American health-care practices. Health care providers do not have to worry about specific taboos about touch as long as it is medically necessary or necessary for care, and the procedure is explained in advance.

## Expressing Pain

Complaining about pain is not well accepted; instead, women endure in silence **(gaman).**

# Prescribing Medications

## Drug Interaction

It is possible that some women keep many medicines and home remedies from Japan; examples are pain remedies used for stomachaches, headaches, and toothaches. Immigrant women may use these remedies along with prescribed allopathic medications.

## Medication Sharing

It is not customary to share leftover prescribed medications with family members.

The health care provider can address the issue of a woman taking concurrent medications prescribed by others by asking her to bring all the medicines she is currently taking when she comes to the appointment. The provider should explain the importance of managing prescribed medications and obtain her permission to communicate with other providers.

## Compliance

Compliance issues may include not coming to an appointment, even though the woman says that she will be there. Compliance is generally very good if the woman is happy with her health provider; she will go along with his or her suggestions. If the woman is not comfortable with the provider, however, she is apt not to comply and yet say nothing.

Japan has a well-established public health system that prevents many communicable diseases. A particular issue for Japanese immigrants is testing for tuberculosis exposure (PPD) required for school entrance. They find it difficult to accept preventive tuberculosis treatment for a positive PPD test because Japanese school-aged children have annual PPD screening and are given bacilli Calmette-Guérin (BCG) boosters that cause PPD positive results. The practitioner should update information on communicable disease with clients to encourage partnership in treatment.

## Follow-up Appointments

Some women miss follow-up medical appointments and others do not; this is an individual rather than a cultural characteristic. A reminder postcard might be helpful and appreciated.

### Orientation to Time

Japanese people are generally future oriented, but they also revisit their past and evaluate it in light of improving their future. They subscribe to clock time and are mostly punctual.

## Prevalent Diseases

Cancer (stomach, colon, and breast cancer) and cardiovascular and pulmonary diseases are major causes of mortality. They are more prevalent in Japan than they are in North America. Suicide is the most prevalent cause of death for women in the 25 to 29 age range; it is the second greatest cause of death for women 20–24 and 30–39 years. As for women of all ages, 11.1 per 100,000 committed suicide in Japan in 1993, compared to 4.8 per 100,000 American women in 1990. Reasons for suicide include physical and mental illness, and family, financial, and job-related problems.

## Health-Seeking Behaviors

Some Japanese people seek medical attention in a timely manner, but it depends on their knowledge, reliable friends, financial circumstances, and immigration status. Some women have a primary care provider and schedule annual check-ups, but others may use the emergency department rather than making a clinic appointment. Japanese immigrants and Japanese Americans are quite health conscious, although they frequently use family remedies and self-care before seeking medical attention.

There are no specific ethnic or folk healers, but in Japan, people will go to temples and pray for many different life and health conditions.

Stress-reduction techniques, exercise, massage, acupuncture, and herbs are often used in self-care. People monitor diet and their activities, and manage symptoms with home remedies and over-the-counter medicines along with prescribed medication.

## 🌐 BIBLIOGRAPHY

Ishida, D, & Inouye, J. (1999). Japanese Americans. In J. Giger & R. Davidhizar (Eds.). *Transcultural nursing: Assessment and Intervention* (3rd ed.). St. Louis: Mosby.

Kim, B.-L. C. (1977). Asian wives of U. S. servicemen: women in shadows. *Amereia*, 4, 91–115.

Marsella, A. J. (1993). Counseling and psychotherapy with Japanese Americans: Cross-cultural considerations, *American Journal of Orthopsychiatry*, 63(2).

True, R. H. (1995). Mental health issues of Asian/Pacific Island women. In D. L. Adams (Ed.). *Health Issues for women of color*. Thousand Oaks: Sage Publications, pp. 89–111.

White, M. L. (1987). *The Japanese educational challenge: A commitment to children*. New York: The Free Press.

# Koreans

## EUN-OK IM, PhD, MPH, RN, CNS

## 🌐 INTRODUCTION

### Who are the Korean People?

Korea is surrounded by China (north), the former Soviet Union (northeast), the Yellow Sea (west), and the Sea of Japan (east). At the end of World War II it was divided into two nations: the Republic of Korea (South Korea) and the People's Republic of Korea (North Korea).

Koreans are an ethnically homogeneous Mongoloid people who have shared a common history, language, and culture since the seventh century AD. The Korean alphabet, **han'gul**, was developed in the 15th century by King **Sejong**. The Korean language belongs to the Altaic language family, which includes Turkic, Mongolian, and Tungusic. There are no specific dialects, but slang varies by region. Four levels of speech characterize the degree of intimacy between speakers. These levels reflect inequalities in social status based on gender, age, and social position. Using an inappropriate level of speech is unacceptable and interpreted as intended informality, disrespect, or contempt to a social superior. Religions include Confucianism, Buddhism, Shamanism, and Christianity.

### Koreans in North America

Most Korean immigrants came from South Korea. Koreans are a rapidly increasing group in the United States, comprising one in three immigrants from East Asia. Korean immigration began in 1903. By 1905, when the Korean government prohibited further emigration, about 10,000 Koreans had entered Hawaii and 1000 had reached the mainland. The 1924 U.S. Immigration Act virtually ended further immigration from Korea until it was amended in 1965, after which most Korean immigration occurred. Between 1970 and 1980, the number of Koreans in the United States increased from approximately 70,000 to 354,529. In 1997 alone, 14,239 Koreans were admitted to the United States. Although they are dispersed throughout the United States, more than 20% of the total Korean population in the United States is located in Los Angeles and Orange Counties (California). New York has a large population as well. The 1996 Census lists 66,655 people of Korean origin in Canada. The largest number of Koreans live in Toronto and Vancouver.

Although many are college educated and held white-collar jobs in Korea, it is difficult for immigrants to obtain work commensurate with their experience. Language difficulties, restricted access to the corporate sector, and unfamiliarity with American culture are all contributing factors.

Among recent immigrants, women outnumber men by three to two because a large number of women came as wives of U.S. servicemen or as adopted children. Recently Korean-American men are bringing spouses from Korea, but acculturated women rarely bring immigrant spouses because the society is still overwhelmingly male-dominant. In Canada, 52% of those of Korean heritage are women.

Recent immigrants are largely young couples with children, with the most populous age groups being 25 to 39 years and younger than 10 years. Most Korean-Americans younger than 20 years were born in the United States, and only 3% of the population is elderly. Slightly less than half the women are employed, but their employment is often unstable and concentrated in small ethnic or family businesses; for example, sewing work constituted 22% of the total jobs held by working wives, many of whom were college graduates.

## 🌐 BEING FEMALE IN KOREAN SOCIETY

Korean culture is largely based on patriarchal and Confucian norms that subordinate women. In the traditional Korean family, the wife is confined to the home and bears the major responsibility for household tasks; the husband is the breadwinner. Since wives do not share household tasks with their husbands in traditional families, they tend to be physically overloaded and psychologically distressed. Their exploitation is hidden under Confucian norms that praise women who sacrifice themselves for their families and nation.

Immigrant women hold the family together and play a vital role in building an economic base for the family and community. For example, a typical immigrant woman works 10 to 15 hours a day, 7 days a week, with few vacations. She may have started as a cleaning woman or seamstress, then worked at a fast-food restaurant, and then in a small shop co-owned with her husband.

Women are aggressively dedicated to the welfare of their husbands and children. Despite women's financial contributions to the family, their husbands still occupy center stage, exercise the authority, and make the major family decisions. They expect their wives to work full-time outside the home but also to take care of the housekeeping and childrearing. In recent years, some women have broken away from male domination by divorce, marrying non-Koreans, or remaining single with professional careers. Most women, however, quietly endure a triple burden without complaint for the sake of the family and the future of their children.

## At Birth

### Preference for Sons

The preference for sons is openly acknowledged, and son preference in South Korea is stronger than anywhere else in the world. Families regard the first son as a continuation of family lineage. Once the family has a son, it welcomes the first-born daughter as an important resource for the household. If a family has limited resources, the family will provide health care for sons rather than daughters, and husbands rather than wives. Despite considerable recent social change in Korea, gender discrimination in health care remains.

### Birth Rituals

When a baby is born, the family protects the child by allowing only close relatives to visit. They hang red peppers under the roof of the house to show that the family has a newborn son. Parents hold a celebration for family members, close relatives, and friends when the baby is 100 days old. Guests bring such gifts as gold rings, baby clothes, and baby toys. At one year, parents have another big celebration, called a *dol* party. The baby wears Korean traditional clothes and is asked to choose one thing from a bowl, which tells the baby's fortune.

## Childhood and Youth

### Stages

There are no clearly delineated stages of childhood; but up to the age of 18 years, individuals are considered children (*adong, aiee, aurinee*) and are expected to behave as such.

### Family Expectations

Most families have extremely high standards and expectations for their children. "Giving a whip to a beloved child" is the basis for discipline. Children and adolescents are pressured to do well in school and enter a highly ranked university. There are rules such as "girls should not sit with boys after seven years." Most families are not happy with very masculine girls or very feminine boys.

### Social Expectations

Korean traditional culture had a strict authoritarian system based on a rigid hierarchical order. Every human relationship was governed by this hierarchical order, determined by social class, sex, generation, and age. For example, older people have a higher social position than younger people, and men are considered higher than women. This hierarchical social order is emphasized in children's education, in which children are taught to respect their parents, elder siblings, grandparents, and teachers. Social respectability is emphasized, and children are not to "bring shame" to the family by doing anything perceived as negative outside the home that may reflect badly on the family, especially the parents.

### Importance of Education

Families strongly emphasize education, and Koreans believe that all human beings should be educated. Children tend to be extremely competitive in school and are often pressured to excel, so as not to bring shame on their families. Girls are encouraged to compete equally with boys. When resources are limited, however, families tend to educate sons rather than daughters because sons will be the heads of their households.

# Pubescence

## Psychosexual Development

The Korean word for adolescence is **sachunki,** which means the time when children begin to think about spring. Girls start their sachunki earlier than do boys, and the onset of puberty of girls in Korean culture is usually between 10 and 13 years. No special rituals are held to celebrate puberty.

## Teen Sexuality

Dating is allowed, but adolescent girls are usually not allowed to spend the night at their friends' houses. Virginity is emphasized, and sexual activities and pregnancy at puberty are considered to stigmatize the family, regardless of social class. Talking about sexuality, contraception, or pregnancy in public is taboo, but close girlfriends exchange information on these topics or get their information from women's magazines.

## Menstruation

The five words for menstruation are **wulkyung** (monthly unchangeable principle), **saengri** (physiology), **mens** (from menstruation), **kyungsoo** (water from an unchangeable principle), and **kyungdo** (the degree of unchangeable principle). These terms refer to menstruation indirectly in terms of its physiologicand biologic aspects. Women also refer to menstruation by such other ambiguous terms as **geugu** (this or that), **sonnym** (guest), and **wolrehengsa** (monthly event).

**Relationship to Health and Fertility.** Koreans have ambivalent feelings about menstruation. Menstrual blood is considered a sign of good health and a symbol of reproductive ability, but it is also seen as being dirty, messy, disgusting, unsanitary, and uncomfortable. Menstruation brings about feelings of cleanliness and being refreshed after it is over. Yet many women complain about discomfort and psychological or physical difficulties related to menstruation.

There are no specific restrictions and taboos during the period, but women generally believe that vigorous physical activity during that time is not good for their health.

**Dysmenorrhea.** Dysmenorrhea is generally considered a sign of bad health, although it is viewed as being normal when a girl first begins to menstruate. In contrast, heavy menstruation is considered a sign of good health. Rather than going to a Western doctor, women seek help for dysmenorrhea from Korean traditional doctors **(haneui),** who provide herbal medicines that balance **um** and **yang*** to resolve dysmenorrhea.

---

*In Korean traditional medicine, signs and symptoms are interpreted and treated in a cosmology that centers on the concepts of **um (yin** in Chinese medicine) and **yang** and the five elements (fire, earth, metal, water, and wood). Nature acts through two opposing and unifying forces, um and yang. Um represents the female aspect of nature (negative pole) and encompasses darkness, cold, and emptiness. Yang, or male force (positive pole), is characterized by fullness, light, and warmth. Various parts of the human body correspond to um and yang; for example, the inside of the body is um, while the surface is yang; the liver, heart, spleen, lungs, and kidney are um; and the gallbladder, stomach, large intestine, small intestine, bladder, and lymph systems are yang. Diseases of winter and spring are um, and those of summer and fall are yang. When um and yang are balanced, the person has a peaceful interaction of mind and body; an imbalance creates illness.

### Female Modesty and Touching

Confucianism, which has heavily influenced Korean culture, emphasizes women's modesty and virginity. Traditionally, women were not allowed to see men before their marriage, and outside activities of middle-class and upper-class women were limited. Thus, Korean women are unwilling to have male health providers do pelvic examinations. They are also unwilling to expose their bodies for physical, breast, and gynecologic examinations.

---

**NOTE TO THE HEALTH CARE PROVIDER**

Consider allowing a girl's mother, sister, or female relative to stay with her when she is having a physical, breast, or gynecologic examination. Keeping her covered as much as possible should help reduce anxiety.

---

## Adulthood

### Transition Rites and Rituals

A young woman is legally considered an adult when she turns 20. Culturally, she is considered an adult when she marries. The word **ureun** signifies this transition.

### Social Expectations

A young woman is now considered a responsible adult who can become pregnant; take care of children, the elderly, and her household; and have legal rights in every aspect of daily life (e.g., voting, being elected, working). In reality, however, legal rights do not mean equal rights. For example, a young woman with the same qualifications as a young man cannot earn the same income.

### Union Formation

In traditional culture, marriages were arranged. Current marriage practices can vary according to socioeconomic class, from more common law unions in the lower class, family ceremonies in the middle class, and more luxurious wedding ceremonies among upper class.

Matchmaking is common for meeting the opposite sex. Young women are socially pressured to marry before they turn 30. Single women older than 30 bring stigma on their families, because parents take responsibility for their daughters' marriages. In contrast, single men older than 30, though considered "late for marriage," can still marry women in their 20s. Women who fail to marry are publicly ridiculed; the word for a woman who remains single after 30 is **nochunyu** (old single woman).

### Domestic Violence

In Korea, domestic violence laws came into being in the early 1990s, and while they are better enforced now, they are less strict than such laws in North America. Few report violence between husbands and wives to the police, considering it to be meddling with their private life. Simple quarrels accompanied by a little physical abuse are frequent, and husbands always make excuses (e.g., she came home late, a child got hurt because she wasn't watching, she spent too much money, she did not care enough about parents-in-law, she did not do her work as a wife and mother

sufficiently). Most men think that the husband is always right and that the wife must obey her husband's orders without questioning. In North America, however, men find it difficult to control their wives, which in turn is associated with more serious violence between husbands and wives. Many men ignore domestic violence laws and do not care that domestic violence is considered serious. New immigrants in particular think that beating their own wives is acceptable.

The father is the head of the family, and family members are expected to obey his orders. With acculturation of family members, however, many immigrant men have lost their control over their family, especially children raised in North America. Intergenerational cultural differences may lead to domestic violence. Immigrants may order second-generation Korean-Americans to learn Korean culture and expect them to behave "traditionally." Many second-generation people rebel against this control, which causes frequent quarrels that at times involve physical abuse.

---

**NOTE TO THE HEALTH CARE PROVIDER**
Korean women, especially immigrant women, are unlikely to report or admit to being victims of domestic abuse. In cases of suspected domestic abuse or violence, practitioners should be very tactful and supportive when addressing the subject. If not, the woman is likely to shut down previously established communication.

---

## Rape

Sexual violence, including rape, is an unspeakable crime surrounded by secrecy among Korean Americans. Both the rapist and the rape victim are blamed. In traditional Korean culture, rape victims were encouraged to commit suicide so as not to bring shame to their families. Even now, victims tend to be blamed for immodesty and seduction, and their families feel shame and guilt. Because of the stigma attached to rape, victims are unlikely to report it to the proper authorities; this is especially true of those who are undocumented immigrants or have recently migrated.

## Divorce

Confucian cultural roots emphasize the importance of family. Therefore, divorce is viewed as social failure and a stigma to avoid because divorced men or women are seen as breaking up their families. Recently, however, with the increase in the divorce rate, traditional views of divorce are changing. While it is viewed as the best choice in unavoidable situations, it is still considered a social stigma, and divorced women are viewed and treated negatively. Korean immigrants maintain a traditional view of divorce. Remarriage is acceptable, but women usually cannot take their children to their new families when they remarry. Following divorce, the male partner is typically responsible for maintaining ties with the children, actively participating in their upbringing, and providing financial support.

## Fertility and Childbearing

The national family planning program of South Korea, initiated in 1962, has lowered the fertility rate, as have the increasing age of marriage for women (fewer younger married women to reproduce) and the popularity of abortion. The typical family size is now two parents and two children.

**Contraceptive Practices.**  Women are responsible for contraception. When it fails, pregnancy is regarded as the woman's responsibility. Most women use modern biomedical methods, oral pills being the usual choice because of convenience. The male partner plays an important role in deciding the number and spacing of children, but he does not determine the use or type of contraception.

## Abortion

Since abortion was legalized in Korea in 1973, it has become widespread and available at moderate cost in most private obstetric-gynecologic clinics. Women have a positive attitude about abortion, and they know that they can use it when needed. The preference for sons has caused a high number of abortions of girls.

Abortions may be perceived to be similar to menstrual periods, and some women do not get adequate rest and food. They may immediately resume their usual activities without complaining, although some feel guilty. In contrast, some upper-class or middle-class women view abortion as affecting the body in a manner similar to childbirth; they may use such "postpartum" measures as resting, eating seaweed soup, and warmly covering their bodies.

**Teen Abortion.**  With rapid economic growth and industrialization, Korea's cultural transition has created social conflict and confusion. Many teenagers and single women are sexually active despite Confucianism's prohibition of open discussion or dealing with these issues. Because of the cultural stigma attached to pregnancy in single women and teens, these women hide their pregnancies and may have unsafe abortions.

While many women obtain abortions in medical clinics, both in South Korea and North America, those with limited finances may obtain cheap illegal abortions that may be followed by complications such as hemorrhage, infection, and inflammation.

## Miscarriage

No statistics on miscarriage rates in Korean-American women are available. Miscarriage is usually regarded as a misfortune and as happening to pregnant women in stressful situations. Sometimes it is regarded as a punishment for not observing **tae-kyo** (special traditional care of the fetus), and women themselves are blamed.

## Infertility

An infertile woman is referred to as **suknyu** (woman made of stone). Traditional Korean culture regarded production of sons as the woman's obligation to her family. An infertile woman had no right to remain in her family, and her husband was free to take a new wife who could produce sons. Even when the husband discarded his wife, however, society did not blame him.

**Naeng** (cold or chill) is seen as a cause of infertility. Infertility is a cold state (loss of yang), and hysterectomies are seen to produce a state of permanent cold. Even though girls and unmarried women are not given explicit information about menstruation, sex, and gynecologic complaints, they are cautioned from an early age against the dangers of catching naeng. They are taught to keep the bottom half of their body warm and are warned that perpetually cold feet will produce leg aches, headaches, arthritis, and sterility.

To correct the cold state (loss of yang), women sometimes take dog meat soup, herbal brews, or both to enhance warming, potent yang conditions.

---

**NOTE TO THE HEALTH CARE PROVIDER**
Be aware of the possibility that men may hesitate to participate in infertility diagnosis and treatment because women are usually blamed for infertility.

---

## Pregnancy

Pregnancy is an important and welcomed family event, accompanied by practices to ensure healthy babies (*tae kyo*) before childbirth. Although pregnancy taboos protect the woman from danger, they may also keep her from getting essential nutrients or cause feelings of isolation and depression. Korean folk beliefs prescribe specific instructions for food consumption during pregnancy. Primigravidas may avoid eating as many as 20 different foods. Duck, eggs, crabs, and rabbit are believed to affect the infant's appearance or character. Seaweed soup is good for anemia and bleeding.

*Tae mong* (a dream about conception experienced by the relatives of the pregnant women) is an important practice in pregnancy. It predetermines the future of the expected baby. For example, if a mother dreams tae mong of a dragon, the baby will become a great person with money and success.

Immigrant pregnant women maintain their cultural values, attitudes, and practices in pregnancy, but they use Western prenatal care. For example, they may concentrate on remaining calm and thinking about the good things in life to influence the baby. Women tend to seek prenatal care during the first trimester of pregnancy. Nothing special is used to enhance the delivery in the weeks or days prior to delivery.

## Birthing Process

**Home Delivery Versus Hospital Delivery.** Traditionally, babies were delivered at home. Since the introduction of Western biomedicine, however, babies are usually delivered in hospitals.

**Cesarean Section Versus Vaginal Delivery.** Vaginal delivery is usually encouraged; but in recent years, some women choose a cesarean section so they can select the exact date and time of birth, based on the belief that the birth date, hour, and minute will determine the baby's destiny. Health care professionals do the delivery. In recent years, the father is encouraged to be involved.

**Labor Management.** Western biomedicine has standardized labor management.

**The Placenta.** In Korea, the placenta is sometimes viewed as good medication for specific types of cancer and restoration of *ki* (vital energy) of old people.

## Postpartum

In the past, women were expected to stay in bed for 21 days, not bathe, and eat lots of seaweed soup. They may not be able to stay in bed now, but six to eight weeks is the typical postpartum period. Postpartal women are prevented from being exposed to cold air, water, and foods. They usually do not take baths for several weeks to prevent exposure to cold air and water.

## Newborn and Infant Care

Korean mothers tend to view infants as being passive and dependent; they do not encourage autonomy as do European-American mothers. Korean culture is highly ritualistic, and mothering is molded more by societal rules than by individual desires or choice. Women seek less professional advice and more folk information on taking care of the infant.

**Breastfeeding Versus Bottle-Feeding.** Traditionally, breastfeeding was the only method for infant feeding. After Western medicine was introduced, women began to use bottle-feeding, and in recent years, it has come to be preferred, especially among working women.

**Infant Protection.** In the past, infants and toddlers did not receive regular check-ups, and their families monitored their growth and development. Since the introduction of Western biomedicine, infants and toddlers are immunized, and health providers monitor their growth and development on a regular basis.

**Primary Caregiver.** Mothers are usually the primary caregivers of infants and toddlers. Traditionally, childcare was the responsibility of women and men were not involved. More recently, however, many more men significantly contribute to childcare.

## Middle Age

### Cultural Attitudes and Expectations

Women from 40 to 60 years are considered middle-aged. Middle-aged Korean women tend to be free from social restrictions on behavior or clothing. Becoming a mother-in-law and grandmother signifies a change of status from a low position in the family to a position of power and control over family members. Traditionally, middle-aged women were regarded as less ego-centered, more concerned with others, and wiser. They were respected and served by their children, and aging was positively viewed. Today, with modernization and industrialization, attitudes toward aging people have become more negative. The wisdom of maturity may be seen as irrelevant or useless in the context of current and materialist values. Immigrants live in this context of materialism and negative perceptions of aging.

### Psychological Response

Korean women perceive the social meaning of menopause as a loss of attractiveness and becoming useless. Menopause means "the evening twilight of life," and current social conditions reinforce loss of power in the family and feelings of uselessness, loneliness, and isolation. Most middle-aged women regard their children as the purpose, fruition, and meaning of their lives, and many sacrificed themselves for childrearing. Thus, most have problems allowing their children to become independent, and most adapt poorly when their children leave the nest, feeling loss, depression, anxiety, and sadness or other physical and psychological symptoms.

### Menopause

**Onset and Duration.**   The average onset of menopause among Korean immigrant women is 49 years. Two terms are used for the menopausal transition, but they imply different dimensions. **Gangnyunki** means the change of one's life, the time when a woman's life starts again, emphasizing the social meaning of menopause. **Pekyungki** is the time when menstruation ceases to flow, emphasizing a time-limited biological event, "closing menstruation."

**Sexual Activity.**   **Pekyung** (end of menstruation) is usually perceived as a sign of aging and the end of womanhood, which also means the end of sexual activity. Fertility is associated with sexuality, and culturally it is thought that sexual desire and activity should end with the cessation of fertility. It is also believed that sexual activity should be minimized to preserve health.

**Coping.**   Korean women have more positive attitudes about the physiology of menopause than Western women do, viewing it as a normal developmental process that does not require special coping mechanisms. Studies show that Japanese, Chinese, and Thai women are less likely than Western women to experience vasomotor symptoms like hot flashes and night sweats. This experience also holds true for Korean women, who report low levels of hot flashes (12%), dizziness (10%), and night sweating (8%).

Women use multiple strategies to manage their symptoms. Such strategies include over-the-counter medicine; medical care; dilatation and curettage or hysterectomy; physical therapy; vitamins and minerals; Korean traditional herbal medicine; acupuncture; exercise; rest; making changes at work; changing their diet; using such tools as fans, massagers, hot packs, or heaters; and simply living with the symptoms.

# Old Age

### Cultural Attitudes

Confucianism emphasizes respect for the elderly and familial bonds. Korean culture is rooted in filial piety, in which care for the elderly from family and kin is a customary and normal duty. Elderly and widowed women usually live with their adult children and grandchildren, especially the first sons, who are responsible for taking care of them. If elderly women and men can no longer care for themselves, family members care for them. Koreans are hesitant to place their old parents in nursing homes except in unavoidable situations.

A landmark of reaching old age is the 60th birthday, which is called **hwangap.** The children and grandchildren of a person who reaches that age celebrate the birthday with their relatives and close friends. Koreans have traditionally used the lunar calendar and currently use both the lunar and Gregorian calendars. Based on the lunar calendar having 60 cycles, the age of 60 years means that the person is starting the calendar cycle over again. This celebration was more significant in the past when life expectancy in Korea was much lower than it is today. Koreans also celebrate the 70th birthday for the person's longevity, which is called *jingap*.

## Death and Dying

### Cultural Attitudes and Beliefs

Although people are hesitant to talk about death, a peaceful death is considered to be one of the five blessings in life (the others are longevity, wealth, health, and virtue). A peaceful death is the result of a blessed life and places no undue emotional burden on the children. The death of unwed men, women, or children is considered shameful.

Shamanism, Confucianism, Buddhism, and Christianity mingle together in Korean culture, influencing people's attitudes toward death. Christians believe that dead persons go to heaven or hell; Buddhists believe that dead persons will be reborn somewhere else; and Shamanists believe that souls either wander the earth and can harm survivors or settle down in heaven, depending on the individual or death situation.

### Rites and Rituals

The ancestor commemoration ceremony is a specific ritual related to death that may have significant therapeutic value. When a person dies, all family members, relatives, and friends are informed of the death and invited to the funeral, the ritual that ensures safe passage of the deceased into the afterlife. Each mourner brings a white envelope containing money for the family. At the funeral, each mourner picks a white chrysanthemum and stands in line to offer final respects to the deceased. Together, the mourners kneel on a mat to pray for the family. The mourners place the chrysanthemums in a vase beside a picture of the deceased (the body of the deceased is behind a screen). After bowing and paying their respects, mourners are received by the eldest son and daughter, which is followed by refreshments. Cremation is a family choice, but it is generally practiced for those who have no family or who die at a young age.

### Mourning

The principles of Confucianism, Buddhism, and Christianity strongly influence many aspects of daily living, including bereavement, in which dignity and harmony are integral. The surviving spouse and family members wear white clothes and a white pin for 100 days after the death; although in the past, the mourning period was three years. Koreans also have an annual ceremony to honor the dead.

Following the death of a mother, the father takes the custody of young children, but if the father also dies, the grandparents take custody. If the grandparents have already died, uncles or aunts take custody, depending on the situation.

**Coping.**  A natural death is accepted more easily than an unnatural one, such as a murder or suicide. If anyone in the family dies within the first three years of marriage, the wife is believed to have caused the misfortune. She may be made to feel guilty for the rest of her life. Men can remarry without recrimination, even during mourning. In the past, widows were not allowed to remarry during the mourning period. Currently, although widows may remarry, they often do not because of the traditional view on women's remarriage.

## IMPORTANT POINTS FOR PROVIDERS CARING FOR KOREAN WOMEN

### The Medical Intake

#### Literacy and English Proficiency

Korean immigrants have acculturated slowly, and very few use English at home. In 1990, approximately half of the respondents in one study had English problems and did not read printed media in English. The first generation uses **Han'gul,** the Korean language. Patients frequently need an interpreter and help with filling out forms. Family members are likely to accompany children, women, and elderly people to health-care encounters to assist.

#### Status of the Provider

Since immigrants tend to work in self-owned businesses, they tend not to have health-care insurance and frequently cannot afford medical visits. If their financial status allows it, however, they tend to visit Western medical doctors for acute illnesses and emergencies. Because health care providers are viewed as authorities and are highly respected, they will be listened to and generally obeyed even when they treat the clients insensitively. Women, in particular, tend to be shy, modest, nonverbal, and passive, and to refrain from making eye contact.

#### Communicating Illness and Symptoms

Women are unlikely to openly volunteer significant medical history, current symptoms, and home remedies taken for an illness. They tend to be brief when they describe their illness. More information may be forthcoming if the provider asks specific open-ended questions with a courteous attitude. Families usually actively participate in patient care, including giving information. This is not true in psychiatric settings, however. When family members are asked to reveal details of a patient's disorder, they usually cover up the extent of the illness to save face, because mental illness is highly stigmatized or they use traditional healing modes for mental illness.

---

**NOTE TO THE HEALTH CARE PROVIDER**

Providers should not use direct terms referring to sexual organs to avoid embarrassing the patient. Instead, they should use general terms like "the privates," "down there," and "the bottom."

---

## The Physical Examination

In traditional Korean medicine, diagnoses are made based on making visual observations, obtaining a history, listening to the patient's voice, and taking the patient's pulse. Traditional doctors can often make a diagnosis from the pulse alone. For example, among the 24 types of pulse are floating, sunken, smooth, accelerated, vacant, real, diminished, thin, soft, weak, and slow. Therefore, Koreans expect a correct diagnosis in one clinical visit. When they are further asked about their symptoms and additional tests are ordered, they tend to perceive the health care providers as being novices or incompetent.

### Modesty and Touching

Modesty is a major issue for women, and many do not participate in breast cancer screening because of modesty issues. Korean women are much more comfortable with female health providers, particularly for obstetric and gynecologic problems.

---

**NOTE TO THE HEALTH CARE PROVIDER**

Make sure the woman has a gown and do not ask her to uncover body parts that are not being examined. It is helpful to allow a female family member or the woman's husband to stay with her during the examination.

---

### Expressing Pain

In general, Koreans are stoic with respect to pain. Complaining is perceived as a sign of impatience, a negative characteristic. Women tend to describe pain in detail, but they usually do not receive adequate medication, especially when family resources are limited. Men tend to be more tolerant of pain and do not verbalize it.

## Prescribing Medications

### Drug Interactions

Harmful effects of traditional herbal medicine **(hanyak),** such as lead and arsenic poisoning, are frequently reported. The concurrent use of traditional and Western medicines may result in overdose or adverse reactions, as traditional herbal prescriptions frequently contain the same chemical ingredients that are used in Western medicine.

---

**NOTE TO THE HEALTH CARE PROVIDER**

The issue of overmedication is real. Traditional Korean medicine and other Asian medicines should not be considered to be "just herbs" and therefore harmless. Herbs can be very potent and can interact with Western medications. Providers must do close follow-up with Korean clients when traditional medicines are being used, and educate the clients about the synergistic and antagonistic effects of Western and herbal medicines. Explain why it is important to be aware of all medications the woman is currently taking.

---

### Medication Sharing

Over-the-counter medications are frequently used. Until 2001, many drugs available in the United States only by prescription (e.g., antibiotics, anti-inflammatory and cardiac medications, and certain pain control medications) were sold over-the-counter in Korea. Thus, immigrants could easily get many prescription drugs through their relatives in Korea. Also, Korean Americans sometimes share leftover prescribed medications with family members or friends who have similar symptoms and diseases. They also may not tell the provider about medications prescribed by other health providers because they are afraid to show "disrespect."

### Compliance

When symptoms subside, Koreans have a tendency not to complete the full course of prescribed medications. When prescribing a medication, it is important to explain the importance of completing the full course and the possible adverse effects of discontinuing the medication before the bottle is empty.

## Follow-up Appointments

Making appointments for follow-up clinical visits is not familiar behavior to immigrants, and they may not see the point of going to an appointment when symptoms have subsided. It is important to call the day before the appointment to remind patients.

### Orientation to Time

Koreans use clock time, yet they tend not to be punctual in general. They may joke among themselves about appearing 30 minutes after an appointed time. Yet immigrants' conception of time depends on the circumstances. Clinical appointments and work are recognized as situations in which punctuality is necessary. However, they may arrive at parties and visits to family and friends within 30 minutes of the agreed-on time, which is socially acceptable.

## Prevalent Diseases

Korean women have more stomach cancer, liver cancer, and stroke, but less heart disease and breast cancer than do women in the U.S. general population. Stomach cancer, liver cancer, and stroke are reported to be associated with genetic, environmental, and lifestyle factors such as dietary habits, heavy alcohol consumption, and smoking (22.5% of adults). Other prevalent conditions include lactose intolerance among older Korean immigrants, dental hygiene problems and gum disease, and high rates of hypertension.

With regard to mental health, one study showed that Korean immigrants who are married, highly educated, and currently employed in high-status occupations had better subjective mental health than those who were not. Work-related variables correlated most strongly with mental health in men, while family life satisfaction and several ethnic attachment variables were related to women's mental health.

# Health-Seeking Behaviors

Health is based on harmonious relationships in the human and supernatural worlds, as well as in the universe in general. The key is maintaining *ki* (vital energy) balance in all parts of one's life, and in particular for health and illness, balancing um and yang in diet and other areas of life. For example, one might eat "hot" foods for a "cold" condition or eat dog meat soup to build strength (supplement ki) and decrease sweat in hot weather (sweat is seen as depleting energy, ki). For example, an excess of heat is dangerous, causing fever, boils, and convulsions.

Illness care is characterized by pluralism, including western medicine, traditional medicine, and Shamanistic approaches. This combination varies with age, sex, education, and socioeconomic status. Some immigrants have fully adopted Western medicine, while others, even younger immigrants who were educated and spent most of their lives in the United States, continue their traditional health care practices.

Koreans usually use both traditional medicine and Western medicine simultaneously for acute illness, hoping for a cure from one or both; but in chronic or terminal illness, they depend more on traditional medicine or the Shamanistic approach, not trusting Western medicine to cure the condition. Traditional medicine (*hanbang*) is thought to be especially effective for certain incurable or chronic diseases that other treatments have not helped.

Hanbang includes four common treatment methods: *chi'm* (acupuncture), *hanyak* (traditional herbal medication), *d'um* (moxabustion), and *buhwang* (cupping). For example, hanyak is used to produce harmony in the individual within a larger harmonious cosmology; it includes the use of tonics made from ginseng, deer horn, or bear gallbladder. The Shamanistic approach is based on the belief that restless ancestors, ghosts, and angry household gods bring to the home such afflictions as illness, financial loss, and domestic strife. For prevention, men honor the family's ancestors (*chesa*), and women make periodic offerings to the household gods (*kosa*). Sometimes, illness attributed to hovering ghosts can be cleaned up with a simple exorcism by housewives, without consulting a shaman.

Lack of health insurance is associated with lack of preventive screening tests, and immigrant women rarely participate in Papanicolaou's test (Pap test) or breast screening tests because of a cultural emphasis on women's modesty and their busy schedules.

Most women have a holistic view of physical activity, considering such physiologic functions as breathing, heartbeat, digestion, thinking, and their jobs as physical activity. In contrast, women perceive that exercise involves only particular parts of the body and is a way to engage in social relations and entertainment. Their busy schedules lead to exercise being viewed as a luxury and they tend not to exercise regularly.

In the past, fatness was considered beautiful and associated with prosperity and good health. Currently, under the influence of Western culture and rapid economic growth, even the elderly now view growing fat as unhealthy and slenderness as the ideal. Immigrant women, especially young women, are now striving to lose weight using diet control and exercise, but only among middle and high socioeconomic class women.

# 🌐 BIBLIOGRAPHY

Im, E. O., & Meleis, A. I. (2000). Meanings of menopause to low income Korean immigrant women. *Western Journal of Nursing Research*, 22, 84–102.

Kim, Y., & Grant, D. (1997). Immigration patterns, social support, and adaptation among Korean immigrant women and Korean American women. *Cultural Diversity in Mental Health*, 3, 235–245.

Light, I., & Bonacich, E. (1988). *Immigrant entrepreneurs: Koreans in Los Angeles 1965–1982*. Berkeley: University of California Press.

Pang, K. Y. (1989). The practice of traditional Korean medicine in Washington, DC. *Social Science and Medicine*, 28(8), 875–884.

Yu, E. Y., & Phillips, E. H. (1987). *Korean women in transition: At home and abroad*. Los Angeles: Center for Korean-American and Korean Studies, California State University, Los Angeles.

# CHAPTER 15

# Mexican Americans

## KATHLEEN LAGANÁ, PhD, RN, and
## LETICIA GONZALEZ-RAMIREZ, BSN, RN

### 🌐 INTRODUCTION

### Who are the Mexican-American People?

Mexican Americans are a very heterogeneous cultural group. Diversity in cultural be-liefs and practices is influenced by level of education, socioeconomic status, gener-ation, time spent in North America, and degree of attachment to tradition. Through the process of acculturation and assimilation, Mexican Americans selectively main-tain or assume a variety of cultural traits, rendering it difficult to make generaliza-tions. Nonetheless, most are the descendants of Spanish Mexican colonists from the 17th and 18th centuries. Historically, some have self-identified as Hispanic whites or Spanish Americans, in part to avoid perceived discrimination against Mex-icans in the United States. Many recent Mexican immigrants are *mestizos* (blend of Mexican Indian and Spanish cultures).

The primary language of Mexico is Spanish. With the exception of newer immi-grants, Mexican Americans are bilingual and many are monolingual in English. Among Spanish speakers, formal Spanish is required in non-intimate relation-ships. Mexican culture is collectivist and emphasizes the needs of the extended family group. *Familismo* or *familism* calls for a strong, reciprocal relationship with and loyalty to the family, which contrasts with North American cultures that focus predominantly on the rights and choices of the individual. Mexican culture also has a more distinct delineation between social classes. It is considered inappro-priate (and perhaps unsafe) to challenge authority figures (e.g., doctors, police, teachers, elders).

For purposes of this chapter, a Mexican-American is anyone who has cultural roots in Mexico and is a citizen or permanent resident of the United States or Canada. Much of the following discussion relates to traditional culture but with the assumption that individuals may subscribe to all, some, or even none of these be-liefs and practices. Although the majority are Catholics, some Mexicans have be-come Pentecostals, Baptists, Seventh-Day Adventists, or Mormons.

## Mexicans In North America

Much of the Southwestern United States was Mexican territory until Mexico lost it in 1848. Economic opportunity and family reunification are the main reasons for immigration. As of 1999, the Hispanic population in the United States was estimated at 11.7% (31.7 million) of the total U. S. population, and those of Mexican origin account for 65.2% of all Hispanics.

There were 23,295 people of Mexican origin counted by the 1996 Canadian Census.

Mexicans are the largest immigrant group in the United States, accounting for 28% (7 million) of the foreign-born population. The Immigration and Naturalization Service (INS) estimates that between 1982 and 1996 another 2.7 million undocumented Mexican immigrants took up permanent residency. Thirty-three percent of Mexican Americans are younger than 15 years, which is nearly three times the percentage of children in the general population.

There is great disparity in income among Mexican Americans, possibly related to immigrant status, time in North America, and education level. In 1999, family income ranged from less than $5000 per year (5.1%) to more than $50,000 (20.5%).

In Canada, the largest numbers live in Montreal, Toronto, and Vancouver, but Mexicans are more widely distributed across Canada than are many other ethnic groups. In the United States, the states with the largest numbers of immigrants are California, Texas, and Illinois, all of which encourage cultural preservation. Texas and California share borders with Mexico, facilitating movement between the two countries. The Illinois population is based on early movements of laborers to work on the railroad.

### Demographics of Mexican-American Women in the United States

Of the 20.7 million persons of Mexican origin in the United States (1999 Census Population Survey), approximately half are women. More than 90% of these women live in the West (5.7 million) and South (3.5 million). There are gender differences in income, with twice as many men as women earning $25,000 or more per year.

More than 50% of Mexican-American women are employed, with approximately one-third in semiskilled, non-professional jobs. Nearly 53% of these women, however, are in white-collar jobs, with 15.6% working in professional specialties or executive/administrative positions. In contrast, only 21.7% of Mexican-American men have white-collar occupations (8.9% in professional and executive/administrative positions).

### 🌐 BEING FEMALE IN MEXICAN-AMERICAN SOCIETY

Traditionally, female roles are well delineated in the private sector of home and family. Motherhood is highly valued. Some believe females to be the "weaker sex," and modesty and passiveness are expected social behavior. Twenty percent of families have female heads of household with no spouse present.

The more educated, urbanized, or acculturated the woman is, the more likely she is to move into the public sector of work to contribute economically to the family. This move does not excuse her from her responsibilities to the family, however.

## At Birth

### Preference for Sons

There is a strong cultural preference for sons, especially the first born. Some women perceive rejection from the father of the baby for failing to provide a son. The birth of a daughter is well received, however, and generally children are loved and well cared for. Still, male children are highly esteemed and may be given preferential treatment. Sons are expected to stay close to home to work and assist in providing for the extended family; whereas women are expected to follow their husbands.

### Response to the Birth of a Female

Families do not neglect or abandon girls. Daughters are loved and protected within the family. Female newborns commonly are dressed with adornments in the hair and clothing with feminine frills.

### Birth Rituals

Among Catholics and Christians, baptism (*baptismo*) is expected, generally by the time the infant is 6- to 8-weeks-old. Birth of a new baby is a time for public celebration for the family. Friends and family visit the household, bringing gifts and food. Generally, the baptism is a time when the infant is introduced more formally to the community. Traditionally, male babies were not circumcised; however, circumcision may be done to make sure the boy resembles his non-Mexican peers. Baby girls often have their ears pierced shortly after birth.

## Childhood and Youth

### Stages

While there are recognized stages in childhood, the transition between these stages is gradual. With infants, for example, transition into childhood occurs at about 2 years of age. Boys between age 2 and puberty are referred to as *niños* or *muchachos;* while young girls are referred to as *niñas*. At physiologic puberty, a boy is considered a *hombresito,* or little man. Similarly, a young girl at menses is referred to as a *señorita.* For the girl, these stages are marked by increasing responsibility to the family until she marries.

### Family Expectations

A boy is treated as "the man of the house" and is exposed to male role modeling through participation in activities with adult men. These activities may involve work or socializing. As the boy moves closer to adolescence, he has increased responsibility for protecting the honor and well being of females in the family. Girls, on the other hand, are expected to assist with housework, including starting dinner, organizing the house, and completing assigned chores. They are also often expected to supervise the younger children and "cater" to the men in the house. All these responsibilities are designed to prepare the girl for her future role as wife and mother. Because of these responsibilities, girls tend to participate less in peer groups or school extracurricular activities than do boys.

## Social Expectations

Females are expected to become "good" wives and mothers. They are the "nurturers." Their public behavior is expected to be modest and chaste. They are expected to show respect for parents and other elders.

## Importance of Education

Traditionally, girls are not required to pursue education because of the expectation of a "home-based" existence. Completion of primary school is becoming more common in Mexico because of public education efforts; however, completion of high school is less common and regarded as a major accomplishment. Illiteracy is still quite common and may present more problems for immigrant women from rural areas than for those coming from urban centers, who have higher levels of education and language literacy. Many women who immigrated as children or are children of immigrants view education as the key to success, pursuing it themselves and encouraging it in their daughters. In the United States, 49.7% of those of Mexican origin have a high school degree or higher, and 7.1% have bachelor's degrees or higher. The comparable figures in the non-Hispanic white population are 87.7% and 27.7%.

# Pubescence

## Psychosexual Development

The average age of onset of puberty in girls is 10 to 11 years of age, which is earlier than for boys (12 to 13 years). There is some concern among mothers that inadequacies in the U.S. diet may lead to menses at a much younger age than is customary. A so-called "generation gap" often exists between immigrant parents and their offspring as social pressures contribute to a desire among teens for a less traditional lifestyle. This gap appears to be larger in the more acculturated youths who either were born in North America or immigrated at a very young age than in those born in Mexico. A breakdown in parent/teen relationships can contribute to risk-taking behavior among teens.

## Rituals and Rites of Passage

At age 15, a girl makes the transition into womanhood through a ceremony called the **quinceañera.** It begins with a formal mass in the Catholic Church. At this ceremony, attended by parents and godparents **(padrinos)** and community members, 14 hombresitos and 14 señoritas are chosen to accompany the young woman. Mass is followed by a **fiesta** with food, drink, music, and dancing. Families may spend a great deal for this celebration, which may be as elaborate as a wedding; it introduces the daughter to the community as now being of courting age. The quinceañera is celebrated in North America by families who are trying to maintain or rediscover traditional roots. Today, this tradition is becoming less common in Mexico, probably related to cost and changing roles of women. The quinceañera has assumed the less serious nature of a debutante party among well-to-do Mexicans. Families of lower socioeconomic status may find the ceremony cost prohibitive.

### Teen Sexuality

**Social Restrictions and Pressures.**   Girls are expected to remain virgins until they marry. Modesty and conservative behavior are expected, and unsupervised interaction with boys is strongly discouraged. There is a general perception that, because pregnancy is possible, it is best to stay away from boys. Because of geographic separation from extended family and because most women in North America work, supervision of young women is often unavailable. Traditionally, women marry in their late teens after a period of courtship. Early marriages are more common than in the general U.S. population, but more acculturated families discourage marriage until the girl has completed high school or, in some cases, college.

**Teen Pregnancy.**   Maternal age is less important than being married when pregnancy occurs. Many families however, see early marriage and motherhood as deterrents to the daughter's education. Because of the strong influence of Catholicism, birth control is neither taught nor encouraged. Abstinence is expected and abortion is taboo. This traditional value of chastity in unmarried women persists in more acculturated families. If a girl is sexually active, she keeps this information from parents and other family members.

Pregnancy at any age becomes the responsibility of the family. Traditionally, marriage is expected if a young woman becomes pregnant. In North America, however, it is becoming more common for unmarried, pregnant, teenage daughters to stay with their parents and complete schooling, while the parents assist with the care of the child.

### Menstruation

**Relationship to Health.**   Menstruation is generally perceived as a sign of health and potential fertility; its absence signifies possible illness. Because of general modesty in women, menstruation is not discussed with men and is even a very sensitive topic among women. Discussions about menstruation and the use of tampons may often be a source of embarrassment.

**Relationship to Fertility.**   First menstruation is associated with female fertility. Good food and rest are recommended during this period.

**Taboos and Restrictions During Menstruation.**   Menstruation is a time of increased modesty and privacy, and women generally avoid or defer sexual intercourse. It is commonly believed that the menstrual period increases the woman's susceptibility to illnesses, so she is forbidden to view or touch the dead. Exercise is discouraged for fear of increased bleeding. Eating certain fruits, such as lemons and bananas, is also discouraged.

**Dysmenorrhea.**   Menstrual symptoms such as cramping are considered normal but requiring rest. Tea made of oregano and the head of a carrot is believed to decrease menstrual cramps. Missed periods are believed to represent illness or pregnancy, and women will wait to rule out pregnancy, seeking medical care only if symptoms interfere with functioning.

### Female Modesty and Touching

Female modesty is emphasized; nakedness is embarrassing and avoided, even with close family members. While touch, embracing, and even holding hands while walking (all signs of a close relationship) are very common between same-gender friends and family members, being touched by strangers, including health care providers (if judged inappropriate) can be embarrassing or even offensive. Handshaking is a much more acceptable greeting.

**Relationship to Health Care.**   Women generally prefer to be treated by a female practitioner, if possible. Seldom, however, will the woman's reluctance to have her nude body viewed by a strange man (male practitioner) deter her from seeking medical care, including physical and pelvic examinations. Breast self-examinations are also embarrassing, but they are done by more acculturated women.

---

**NOTE TO THE HEALTH CARE PROVIDER**
Avoid performing pelvic examinations unless they are determined to be absolutely necessary. An adolescent girl's mother or female relative should attend physical examinations. Education about breast self-examination may be more acceptable in the form of practice with breast models in private, by videotapes, or with written literature rather than actual demonstration by the health care provider.

---

## Adulthood

### Transition Rites and Rituals

The traditional quinceañera marks the girl's transition into womanhood. However, she may still experience restrictions on dating or extracurricular school activities. Motherhood, on the other hand, signifies the completion of the transition to adulthood. All married women (or any woman who is a mother, even if not married) should be referred to as *señora.*

### Social Expectations

Women are responsible for passing on cultural information and observances to the next generation, which is of extreme importance for those with children born in North America. Cultural memory (the maintenance of traditional beliefs) is believed to depend on this all-important female role. Women are expected to marry and bear children. Today, although it is common for a woman to work outside the home, her career or work is usually viewed as secondary to that of her husband's, and it does not relieve her of her duties as mother and wife. Although better-educated husbands tend to be more flexible regarding gender roles, women working outside the home still assume multiple roles with associated stress. Unmarried women are expected to stay with the parents and provide care for the extended family.

### Union Formation

**Union Types.**   Consensual or common-law marriages are the most common type of union formation, even for Mexicans living in North America. Often, couples are introduced and approved by family members. Although polygamy is not sanctioned, it is not uncommon for an immigrant man to have a wife and children both in Mexico and North America. This pattern may be related to the difficulty of moving back and forth across the border, as well as to the lack of acceptance of divorce in Catholic Mexico.

**Social Sanctions for Failing to Enter into Union.**   It is expected that a woman will marry in her 20s, and a single woman is referred to as *soltera* or *solterona* after she reaches the age of 20. After 30, an unmarried woman is considered a spinster.

Men prefer to marry younger women and may be teased for showing serious interest in an older woman. A young man is not pressured to marry early unless it is to the woman with whom he has been intimate.

Women who become pregnant and do not marry are considered to have damaged the family's reputation. Such a woman may experience much shame from the family, especially from her father, and may be ostracized. Depression is common among unmarried, non-partnered pregnant women.

### Domestic Violence

According to the Instituto de la Mujer del Distrito Federal in Mexico, 70% of women suffer violence at the hands of their partners. Increased risk of domestic violence is attributed to rigid gender relationships between men and women and **machismo.** Machismo is the cultural expectation that men must be strong, in control, and the providers for their families. Women, in turn, are expected to tend to the needs of the spouse (and the family) at home, even if they work outside the home. Insistence by the male partner that the woman meet these expectations at all costs may be perceived as emotional abuse.

A 1995 study in California found that 48% of Latina women reported domestic violence. However, women tend to be silent about it because of family values or fear of deportation. Domestic violence appears in all socioeconomic and educational levels. In North America, women are often family providers (or co-providers); as they assume more public and independent social roles, the man's perception of control over his family erodes. As control is a key motivation in batterers, the man's loss of control may put the woman at increased risk for battering. For example, battered women living in a shelter reported that the desire for family planning and contraceptive use contributed to episodic battering by their male partners.

**Familismo** also contributes to decreased reporting of domestic violence. Loyalty and dependence on family members for most social support needs mean that family problems are not shared with outsiders. Family members sometimes intervene in domestic violence situations but, on occasion, hold the woman responsible for the battering. Authorities are not trusted and are usually not notified. Women have been known to leave their male partners and return to their families in Mexico if supported to do so. In extreme situations, they will use shelters. Mexican-American women report controlling behavior from partners and battering as reasons for divorcing their husbands.

### Rape

Little is known about the incidence of rape among Mexican-American women. Conjugal relations are expected of wives. What is reported as partner rape in other cultural groups may be perceived as spousal duty among Mexican Americans.

Rape is not condoned. Statutory rape traditionally led to a marriage to save the honor of the young woman. Male family members would take revenge on anyone who "dishonored" a female in the family. The protective nature of machismo appears less prevalent in more acculturated Mexican-American families. When rape occurs, the woman and her family are usually too ashamed to report or prosecute. In some states, partner rape and domestic violence are crimes against the state and out of the hands of the victim. As a result, women may be fearful of family breakup and loss of financial resources and, accordingly, report less often.

To avoid attracting sexual predators, women are expected to behave and dress modestly in public. There is little sympathy for women who experience problems if they have violated the rule of modesty.

### Divorce

Divorce is becoming more common in both North America and Mexico, although it is viewed negatively because of the strong influence of the Catholic Church. There are no reliable statistics on divorce rates.

**Women and Divorce.**    Women are generally expected to tolerate a difficult marriage. Divorced women may be scorned or ostracized. ***Abandonadas*** or ***dejadas*** are two colloquial words referring to divorced women. A divorced woman is not viewed as an optimal marriage partner. For more acculturated women in North America, there is less stigma, and divorced women are less likely to lose family support.

**Child Custody Practices.**    Following divorce, children usually stay with their mothers. Men are expected to contribute financially, but they seldom do and rarely maintain close relations with the family. If the woman remarries or, more commonly, takes a new partner but does not marry, the children of the first marriage may not be accepted by the new partner or his family. Some women report disdain for blended families but less so in more acculturated families.

---

**NOTE TO THE HEALTH CARE PROVIDER**
Practitioners should anticipate insufficient social support systems, feelings of inadequacy, and shame. Divorced women may be initially resistant to referral to group therapy or counseling. They need gentle persuasion and support.

---

### Fertility and Childbearing

**Family Size.**    Large families are becoming less common, especially among younger Mexicans in North America. Three children are more typical now. Others may make negative comments about large families or close spacing of pregnancies.

**Contraceptive Practices.**    Eighty-three percent of the immigrant or Mexican-American population is of childbearing age or younger; yet contraceptive use is limited, discouraged by the Catholic Church. Depo-Provera, a long-acting progesterone, is often the contraceptive of choice since it only involves an injection once every three months at the provider's office. This method is easy to conceal from others, involves less frequent "sin" than daily forms of birth control (such as oral contraceptive pills), and is relatively effective. Condom use is not well accepted among male partners, who complain that condoms decrease sexual sensation. Also, women who ask their partners to use condoms risk being viewed as "loose" or inappropriately open about sex as well as resistant to having the man's child. Women who request that their partners use condoms are believed to be at an increased risk for domestic violence. Infidelity in the partner is a common complaint voiced by young women, increasing the risk for the spread of sexually transmitted diseases (STDs).

---

**NOTE TO THE HEALTH CARE PROVIDER**
Inclusion of the male partner in family planning education is likely to result in more effective contraceptive use. Secure the woman's permission before including the male. Include the topic of STDs in patient education.

---

## Abortion

Abortion is culturally taboo, even among acculturated Mexican Americans. While reliable statistics on abortion rates are unavailable, unplanned pregnancies are usually carried to term and the family cares for the child. Anecdotal evidence suggests that more acculturated single women with educational and career plans are more likely to terminate unplanned pregnancies. This information is not shared with the social network, however, putting women at increased risk for emotional trauma following an abortion. Rape is the one condition under which abortion is more tolerated.

**Teen Abortion.** Teen pregnancy is not socially sanctioned except among married teens. Abortions are more common among upper-class families; although even in this group, abortion is rarely disclosed outside the family.

**Sources of Abortions.** In North America, women use established providers for abortion. Private clinics are considered more confidential than public clinics. For financial reasons, abortion is more common in the upper classes. Because abortions are illegal in Mexico, the use of substandard providers in that country is greater. The associated risks leads to relatively lower rates of abortion in Mexico. If a woman seeks an abortion, it is usually very early in the pregnancy.

---

**NOTE TO THE HEALTH CARE PROVIDER**

A great deal of guilt and shame is associated with having an abortion. Practitioners should take extreme care to ensure the client's privacy and anonymity. A woman may be reluctant to disclose this history to providers and may describe it as a "miscarriage." "Social primips" are women who socially deny a previous pregnancy.

---

## Miscarriage

Miscarriage is often seen as divine intervention, taking a fetus that is ill or has a birth defect. Following a miscarriage, rest and good nutrition are encouraged. A woman who has recurrent miscarriages may, like an infertile woman, be perceived as being less of a woman. Traditional women may pray to the Virgin of Guadalupe for personal strength in the presence of personal suffering. More acculturated women, especially those with health insurance, seek medical attention.

---

**NOTE TO THE HEALTH CARE PROVIDER**

Following miscarriage, the woman is likely to display anxiety and feelings of low self-esteem. Practitioners should evaluate available social support systems, make referrals as necessary, and be sensitive.

---

## Infertility

Consistent with the ascribed woman's role as wife and mother, infertility leads to lowered self-esteem. Society views the infertile woman as being incomplete or "less of a woman" and men may view their infertile wives as weak or incompetent. It is socially expected that all married women bear children and failure puts the woman at risk for social isolation and abandonment, making infertility a family tragedy. Many see infertility as a curse bestowed on the woman for some misdeed. For example, a woman who undergoes an abortion is likely to attribute this perceived sin as the cause of her later infertility problems. Similarly, the inability to bear children is often attributed to substance abuse, including alcohol use or smoking, which are also considered harmful and disgraceful behaviors. One coping strategy for the reported suffering associated with infertility and infertility treatment is to pray to the Virgin of Guadalupe, who is perceived as a survivor of great suffering.

---

**NOTE TO THE HEALTH CARE PROVIDER**
Although acculturated women are likely to be proactive in seeking medical assistance for their infertility, practitioners should not assume that these women have spousal support. Male partners are unlikely to be willing participants and may even resist screening for male infertility.

---

### Pregnancy

**Activity Restrictions and Taboos.** Pregnancy is a vulnerable time during which women return to more traditional health practices to protect the developing fetus. Female relatives, who are often most instrumental in pregnancy support, encourage rest, sound nutrition, and avoidance of stress and worry. A healthy diet is believed to be a prerequisite for a healthy fetus. Warm, natural foods are recommended; processed foods are discouraged. Food cravings **(antojos)** must be satisfied to avoid adverse effects on the fetus. For example, ignoring a craving for strawberries is believed to contribute to birthmarks on the infant.

Traditional diet includes fresh-boiled beans and corn tortillas. Generally, women do not practice pica (eat non-food items, including clay, chalk, and dirt). Herbal teas are sometimes recommended as a general tonic **(yerba buena** or spearmint tea) or for stress and stomach upset **(manzanilla** or chamomile).

Lifting, bending, and vigorous exercise are discouraged. Some activities, such as hanging clothes (lifting the arms above the head), are traditionally believed to cause the umbilical cord to wrap around the unborn baby's neck. Gentle activity, such as walking, is encouraged. It is believed by some to avoid a folk condition in which the fetus sticks **(se pega)** to the side of the uterus as a result of too much bed rest. There are other traditional beliefs about vulnerability to external forces, such as the moon and other celestial bodies, the evil intentions of others **(mal ojo** or evil eye), the spirit world, and certain foods. **Susto,** a folk illness that means "fright," occurs when a portion of the person's soul escapes and cannot return. This can occur in pregnant women who attend funerals or are traumatized in other ways. Susto leads to general poor health. It is considered a very serious and potentially life-threatening illness that requires diagnosis and treatment by a practitioner of folk medicine.

---

**NOTE TO THE HEALTH CARE PROVIDER**
Fearing the perceived ill effects of "too much" bed rest, clients with high-risk pregnancies may resist or fail to comply with orders for "total bed rest."

---

**Societal View of Motherhood.** Motherhood is highly esteemed in Mexican culture. Bringing a child into the family is seen as the means to ensure group viability. Others pamper and cater to pregnant women. Work is adjusted to ensure optimal pregnancy health, and supportive female family members often take over housework, especially toward the end of the pregnancy.

**Prenatal Care.** Mexican-American women generally seek prenatal care early in the pregnancy (first trimester) when social and economic barriers, such as lack of medical insurance or documentation (illegal status), do not exist. Because pregnancy is seen as a healthy state, some women (especially less-educated and more recent arrivals) feel comfortable seeking prenatal care later in the pregnancy. Still others will present to the hospital in active labor without prenatal care. This is more common among undocumented immigrants who generally cannot afford insurance and fear deportation.

Overall, Mexican-American women prefer to receive their care from medical doctors in private clinics, as this is considered to be superior care; however, certified nurse midwives are accepted. Nurse practitioners are often seen as assistants to the obstetrician and, therefore, are less preferable because they do not actually perform deliveries.

---

**NOTE TO THE HEALTH CARE PROVIDER**

Avoid asking about the client's immigration or marital status. Evaluate the availability of family support systems for immigrant women. Consistency of care (same provider) is very important for these clients.

---

## Birthing Process

**Home Versus Hospital Delivery.** Hospital deliveries are preferred over home births, related to the belief that medical care is needed for this final vulnerable stage of the pregnancy. The father of the baby and female members of the maternal family (extended family) are usually present and stay with the woman through the labor and delivery process. The pregnant woman's mother, however, plays the most active role in labor support. Other female relatives fill this role as needed, especially if the immigrant woman is separated from her mother, who may still be living in Mexico. Involvement and support from members of the extended family is crucial. More acculturated or second-generation women are likely to actively involve their male partners in the birthing process.

**Cesarean Section Versus Vaginal Delivery.** Natural childbirth is preferred. Women who cannot tolerate pain may be seen as weak; hence, there may be an inclination to refuse pain medication, even when it is indicated. Fear of cesarean birth is one reason many women choose to arrive at the hospital during the later stages of labor. More acculturated women, however, follow standard medical recommendations to arrive at the hospital in early active labor for fetal assessment and labor management.

**Labor Management.** Warm foods, herbal teas, and massage are offered to women in early labor, and walking is encouraged. When deliveries occur at home, warm baths are believed to help prepare women for birth. There is no special management of ruptured membranes other than their serving as a clue that labor is progressing and delivery is imminent. During contractions the woman is likely to be very vocal and is assisted with emotional and verbal support from family members. Fearing that her uterus will "rise up," family members will discourage the laboring woman from inhaling through her mouth. The baby's father, although in the room, is not likely to be actively involved in labor support. Men who have attended childbirth preparation classes, however, will usually take a more active role. Male extended family members are usually excluded from this event.

**Placenta.**   No special cultural significance or practice surrounds the placenta or its disposal. Individual women may have their own preferences.

### Postpartum

Although the physiologic postpartum period lasts about six weeks, the traditional practice, *la cuarentena,* is a 40-day period of rest and social sequestering. During this time one or more supportive women care for the new mother, usually her mother. The new mother, however, is expected to care for the infant.

The woman is discouraged from getting out of bed for the first few hours after delivery to avoid fainting and, more traditionally, to avoid chilling or exposure to drafts. Women are allowed out of bed only to use the bathroom, and some are encouraged to void in bed on removable linens. To prevent air from entering the uterus, many women wear a girdle or some type of abdominal binder. Likewise, the woman is expected to keep her feet, head, and shoulders covered to prevent chilling or drafts, which may lead to such health complications as arthritis, blindness, or sterility. Light foods, including *caldo de pollo* or chicken broth, herbal teas, and tortillas, are consumed during this period. Showering is also discouraged for several days following delivery because pregnancy is considered a "cold" state and must be balanced by "warm" influences. Drafts from open windows and cold drinks are avoided. For many women employed outside the home, the full observance of la cuarentena is not possible; however, many women still believe that lack of adequate postpartum recuperation leads to poor health integrity later in life.

### Newborn and Infant Care

**Breastfeeding Versus Bottle-Feeding.**   Traditionally, breastfeeding is preferred because it is easier for the mother and less expensive. Statistically, however, Mexican-American women have been shown to be less likely to breastfeed if the father of the baby is Hispanic, indicating that the decision to breastfeed does not rest solely with the mother. This is consistent with the dominant decision-making role that men generally play. Even when deciding to breastfeed, many women believe that they must supplement the infant's feedings with formula. Also, herbal tea is often given to infants. For example, chamomile tea is given for colic; mint tea is a general tonic; and jasmine tea is given as a cleanser to facilitate passage of meconium, the newborn's stool.

**Infant Protection.**   Infants are thought to be especially susceptible to *mal ojo* (evil eye), caused by admiration or envy. Symptoms are sudden unexplained illness, which may include colic and fussy, irritable behavior. To protect against mal ojo, infants may wear a special charm or a religious medal pinned to the clothing. This traditional belief has led to a cultural norm that discourages holding and touching others' children. Also, during the first three months of life, the mother may resist cutting the infant's fingernails, fearing that doing so will cause blindness and deafness in the child. Children are well cared for, and parents are eager to follow medical advice if they have developed a trusting relationship with the provider. Geographic relocation and lack of access to health care may sometimes interrupt follow-up immunization schedules.

**Primary Caregiver.**   While the mother is primarily responsible for the new infant, the entire family plays an active role in caring for the child. This includes the maternal grandmother, aunts, sisters, and cousins. Older siblings also assist in caring for and entertaining baby brothers or sisters. The use of non-familial caregivers is often a source of anxiety and guilt and is usually avoided at all cost. Today, the more acculturated father may also assist with childcare, if required.

---

**NOTE TO THE HEALTH CARE PROVIDER**
Practitioners should recognize and acknowledge the importance of the extended family. Including members of the extended family when providing patient education increases the likelihood of patient compliance.

---

## Middle Age

### Cultural Attitudes and Expectations

Women are considered middle-aged at around 45 to 55 years of age. Modesty and conservative dress and behavior are the norm.

### Psychological Response

The "empty nest syndrome" is not pronounced among Mexican Americans, whose family structure is much larger and includes individuals outside the immediate family. Also, many of these women expand their childbearing years well into their 40s.

### Menopause

**Onset and Duration.**   Menopause, also referred to as *cambio de vida* (change of life), generally occurs during the 40s and 50s, when women report the onset of symptoms. The early onset of menopause may sometimes be blamed on poor diet in North America. During this period, some women report depression and feelings of being "less of a woman" because of their lost fertility. Less acculturated women, on the other hand, may view this period more positively.

**Sexual Activity.**   The onset of menopause is generally not viewed as a deterrent to the maintenance of an active sex life. Older women who care for their appearance and figures are seen as being attractive and may be the objects of flirting behavior. Respect for older women in Mexican culture, however, usually leads to conservative behavior in men.

**Coping.**   The symptoms of menopause, including hot flashes and emotional changes, are seen by many as being "natural." Coping with symptoms ranges from trying to ignore them to such medicinal approaches as herbal teas and, in some instances, the use of hormone replacement therapy (HRT). In general, women do not use HRT unless symptoms of menopause interfere with functioning. Menopause is seen as a natural process with which a woman must cope. More acculturated women do tend to use HRT, however.

---

**NOTE TO THE HEALTH CARE PROVIDER**

Extended responsibilities as caregiver for grandchildren may lead middle-aged women to ignore their own health care needs, such as obtaining routine Papanicolaou's tests and mammograms. Ask the woman about her family responsibilities and remind her about the importance of preventative care.

---

## Old Age

Mexican-American women live into their late 70s. This is younger than the average life span in Mexico, due to a more sedentary lifestyle in North America. Women are considered old after menopause; as elders, however, they are respected and considered sources of wisdom in the family and community. It is common for elder women to live with their adult children and grandchildren or with other members of the extended family.

**Abuela** (grandmother) is a term used broadly for respected elderly women. This respect is accorded women who have lived good lives within expected cultural norms. In addition to being well respected, many elderly women are believed to have special knowledge of folk healing or **curandismo,** which incorporates elements of religion/Catholicism, herbalism, and massages to treat a variety of folk illnesses.

## Death and Dying

### Cultural Attitudes and Beliefs

Death in the elderly is an anticipated event and accepted with the belief that the person's life has been lived. The younger a person is, the more difficult it is to accept the death, and the greater the sense of tragedy. The Catholic and Protestant faiths support the belief in life after death "in heaven," which provides consolation to many during this period of grief.

### Rites and Rituals

For the dying who are Catholic, a priest administers last rites. Following the death of an individual, the family prays at a Rosary service, to ensure the entrance of the departed soul into heaven. There are no gender differences in death rites and rituals.

### Mourning

**Cultural Expectations.** There are cultural expectations for family members to mourn the deceased. During the period of mourning, survivors may adhere to behavior, sometimes called **luto,** in which they dress in black clothing with little or no makeup and avoid dancing or listening to music. The closer the relationship to the deceased, the longer this period is expected to last. Extended periods of mourning that are considered normal among Mexican-Americans may be perceived as being pathologically excessive by non-Hispanics. People observe a holiday called **El Dia de Los Muertos** (the "Day of the Dead"), which occurs on November 1. On this day, family members take food, drinks, and flowers to the gravesites of loved ancestors as offerings to their visiting souls.

**Coping.** Coping is often difficult for women if they have been very dependent on their spouses. An extended mourning period facilitates recovery. Many women are forced to seek employment for the first time. The extended family often assists women through this transitional period.

In the event of an untimely death of a woman, minor children of the deceased woman go to live with female relatives rather than with their father. This practice is related to gender roles for women as caregivers. Godparents (padrinos), usually family members, also assume responsibility for overseeing the child's well being.

---

**NOTE TO THE HEALTH CARE PROVIDER**
Extended periods of mourning are customary; do not diagnose them as pathologic. Referral to group therapy or grief counseling is in order, if acceptable to the client.

---

## IMPORTANT POINTS FOR PROVIDERS CARING FOR MEXICAN-AMERICAN WOMEN

### The Medical Intake

#### Literacy and English Proficiency

Literacy rates vary greatly. Recent arrivals from rural Mexico have lower rates of literacy than urban residents and may require assistance with registration and filling out forms. It should not be assumed that spoken language skills equal written or reading language skills in either English or Spanish. All consent forms and written material should be provided in Spanish. When a language barrier exists, efforts must be made to locate a confidential interpreter. Using friends, relatives, or children as interpreters violates not only patient confidentiality but also cultural rules of modesty, privacy, and respect for elders. Family members often accompany the woman for care, however; and they should be welcomed.

#### Status of the Provider

Health care providers are highly esteemed as educated people: "They are as close to God as you can get." As a result, expecting active participation in care planning and treatment decisions can be culturally confusing, especially for recent arrivals. If the provider presents choices, family consultation is usually required. More acculturated women are far more accustomed to active participation in health-care planning.

#### Communicating Illness and Symptoms

Perceptions of health and illness usually involve viewing health as an absence of illness and pain. Generally perceived as the will of God, pain is handled stoically, care is often sought late, and clients are hesitant to acknowledge pain or request medication. Also, given the social power attributed to health care providers, women are often afraid of offending them or of being judged. An open attitude toward traditional therapies and family caregiving will help to create an atmosphere of respect and trust and thus to secure a more thorough history.

Mexican culture is based on developing close relationships. It is a cultural norm to precede any serious business with a brief period of small talk **(platica)**, which includes inquiring about the patient's family. Women may give detailed descriptions of the illness experience; such story telling is part of establishing rapport and relationship building. Thus, more time may need to be scheduled for visits with traditional women. As many health care providers do not know their clients well, the abruptness of the health-care visit can appear rude or uncaring.

---

**NOTE TO THE HEALTH CARE PROVIDER**
Be tolerant of large numbers of family members accompanying the client to the clinic. Avoid using family members and accompanying friends as interpreters. Be discreet when asking questions pertaining to infertility and reproduction or sexuality.

---

## The Physical Examination

### Modesty and Touching

Mexican women are extremely modest. While they prefer female providers, male providers are acceptable as long these practitioners display sensitivity to the client's modesty needs. Body parts should be covered during the examination, and the presence of a female member of the family or health-care team is recommended during pelvic and other sensitive examinations. Touch by a health care provider is embarrassing, but it is accepted if it is seen as being necessary in the provision of care.

### Expressing Pain

Although stoicism is common (complaining is perceived as a sign of weakness), if the procedure has been poorly explained, the woman may express pain loudly as a way of indicating that an examination is unpleasant.

## Prescribing Medications

### Drug Interactions

Because herbal medicines are commonly used, the practitioner should ask about such use before prescribing medications. Some herbs may actually worsen the patient's condition, which requires that the practitioner have a working knowledge of common herbal medications.

### Medication Sharing

It is common for family members and friends to share prescription medications as a way of facilitating home care or self-medication for those lacking health insurance.

## Compliance

Clients commonly stop taking medication once symptoms disappear. Simplified protocols and clearly written instructions will facilitate completion of the treatment plan. Follow-up phone calls are well received. The importance of and rationale for treatment plan completion must be stressed, including the rationale for taking medications for the recommended time.

## Follow-up Appointments

Follow-up phone calls to remind the client of an upcoming appointment or inquire about a missed appointment are well received, being perceived as a sign of caring, as long as they are respectful. Research shows that women do come in for follow-up treatment, but it may be timed later than recommended or received through a different provider. Barriers to timely follow-up care are largely institutional in nature: inflexible scheduling, transportation problems related to location of the care facility, communication problems with the staff, and discomfort with male providers.

### Orientation to Time

Punctuality is variable among Mexican Americans, depending on level of acculturation to North American societies. As a group, Mexicans are culturally flexible with time constraints and make choices between demands on their time. Family and friend relationships generally take priority over business or health care demands. Humor is often used to apologize for lateness.

## Prevalent Diseases

According to *Healthy People* 2010, Mexican Americans are generally healthier than some other minority groups; however, they have a fairly high incidence of certain diseases. Acculturation appears to increase some diseases or poor health outcomes, with second-generation women faring worse than immigrants. More prevalent health problems in second-generation Mexican-American women are cardiovascular diseases, substance use, and low-birth-weight babies.

Other prevalent women's conditions are obesity (35% compared with 23% of non-Hispanic white women, co-morbid with diabetes and cardiovascular disease) and diabetes (62 per 1000 aged 20 years or older; 23% to 25% incidence in those 60 years or older, which is more than twice that of non-Hispanic whites in that age group). Elderly people are slightly more likely to have hypertension and uncontrolled hypertension than non-Hispanic whites. While less likely to receive regular cholesterol screening, they tend to have a lower incidence of high cholesterol than non-Hispanic whites (18% vs. 21%). There is some tendency toward depression and affective disorders (e.g., Mexican-American women who report feeling **triste,** or sad, especially upon separation from female relatives, demonstrate evidence of major depression), and Hispanic teens are more likely to attempt suicide than are non-Hispanic white teens (2.8% vs. 2%).

# Health-Seeking Behaviors

Generally, women first treat illness with home remedies. Many, especially recently arrived immigrants, seek consultation with a ***curandero*** or ***curandera*** (traditional healer) before using biomedical treatment. Curandero(a)s use a combination of herbal cures, elements of religion/Catholicism, and massage as treatment.

Many women seek health care only when symptoms begin to interfere with role function and often at an advanced stage of the disease process. For a variety of reasons, women generally do not practice preventative self-care, for example, regular exercise or diet. However, educational interventions that promote self-care activities have been shown to be effective in women. Fewer women obtain mammograms and Pap tests than in the general population, although the rate improves with level of acculturation or among women with strong traditional family values.

## BIBLIOGRAPHY

Bell, M. (1995). Attitudes toward menopause among Mexican-American women. *Health Care for Women International*, 16(5), 425–435.

Brittingham, A. (2000). The foreign-born population in the United States. Current Population Reports, March 1999, P20–519. Washington, DC: U.S. Department of Commerce.

Davila, Y. & Brackley, M. (1999). Mexican and Mexican-American women in a battered women's shelter: Barriers to condom negotiation for HIV/AIDS. *Issues in Mental Health Nursing*, 20(4), 333–355.

Ramirez, R. (2000). The Hispanic population in the United States. Current Population Reports, March 1999, 520–527. Washington, DC: U.S. Department of Commerce.

U.S. Department of Health and Human Services (2000). *Healthy People* 2010 (Conference Edition, Two Volumes). Washington, DC: Author.

# Puerto Ricans

## MARIA ROSA, DRPH, RN

### INTRODUCTION

### Who are the Puerto Rican People?

Puerto Rico is the lesser of the larger Antilles in the Caribbean. Measuring 100 by 35 miles, it is located 1400 miles southeast of New York and 1800 miles northeast of Caracas, Venezuela. Ceded from Spain to the United States by the treaty of Paris in 1899, Puerto Rico became a U.S. territory in 1917, and its citizens were awarded U.S. citizenship. In 1952 it became a Commonwealth of the United States.

Puerto Rico has a population of almost 4 million and has undergone a dramatic transformation in the past 50 years. The island has changed from an agrarian economy to an industrial and service economy. These changes have profoundly affected the way Puerto Ricans view education and skills development. The language native to Puerto Ricans is Spanish, spoken very rapidly and often mixed with English words, since English is the second language spoken on the island.

### Puerto Ricans in North America

Over the years, the number of Puerto Ricans migrating to the United States has increased dramatically. During the four-year period from 1991 through 1995, an estimated 168,475 Puerto Ricans migrated to the United States. This compares with 116,571 in the 1980s and 34,703 in 1950.

As a group, most Puerto Ricans have had the experience of moving back and forth to the mainland. In fact, some writers have spoken of Puerto Rico as the "moveable country," referring to the massive population movement during the last 50 years when almost 40% of the Puerto Rican population moved to the United States. Establishment of the hometown island associations on the mainland, particularly in New York City, and the annual Puerto Rican day parades attest to the Puerto Rican presence on the mainland. Puerto Ricans born or reared in the United States who speak English better than Spanish are often referred to as **Neorican** or **Nuyorican.**

An estimated 3,406,417 Puerto Ricans, comprising 9.6% of the Hispanic population, are reportedly residing in the United States, according to Census 2000 figures.

This number is up from the previous 3.1 million reported for the last decade (1990). Additionally, some 130,000 Puerto Ricans are said to have returned to Puerto Rico after living for some time in North America.

Puerto Ricans in the United States reside primarily in the large northeast cities where there are developed ethnic enclaves, such as New York, New Haven, Philadelphia, Boston, and Providence. For example, 66% of Puerto Ricans in the United States were residing in the Northeast in 1990, according to census data.

## 🌐 BEING FEMALE IN PUERTO RICAN CULTURE

The female role is one of nurturing and organizing the family. Early in life the young girl is taught the importance of communicating assertively with boys, keeping a clean and neat home environment, and attending school. Getting a good education and a career is emphasized to "prevent having to depend on a man if you end up alone in life." Finding a good husband and starting a family, with emphasis on maintaining equal rights with her husband, is another goal that is emphasized to the young girl. Female assertiveness is often difficult to accept by men in a culture that promotes "machismo."

## At Birth

### Preference for Sons

Puerto Rican men openly declare the preference for sons, especially the first-born. When a child is born there is a celebration, regardless of gender. When the child is a boy, however, the father can be seen openly celebrating about the birth of a "macho." **Chancletero** is used in a humorous way to refer to a father who has only girls. The ideal family is one consisting of both boys and girls.

### Birth Rituals

Although there are no culturally recognized birth rituals, per se, in this society, during the first months following an infant's birth many Puerto Ricans who are Catholics have what is called a **Bautismo,** baptism of the baby by a Catholic priest; the adults celebrate with a feast.

## Childhood and Youth

### Stages

Individuals up to the mid-teen years are considered children **(los nenes),** and they are expected to be respectful of adults. Sexual activity and childbearing at this stage are considered wrong and shameful, especially for young people coming from so-called "good" families.

### Family Expectations

High behavioral standards are set for young people. All children are expected to attend school as a preparation for their futures. Both parents assume the responsibility for disciplining their children. The mother, however, tends to provide more of a nurturing and less punitive role than the father, who is often called upon as the last resort when the child requires a higher level of punishment.

### Social Expectations

The idea of projecting a "clean" image is very important to the family. Girls and boys are taught to dress neatly and to conduct themselves properly in public so that they do not bring shame to the family.

### Importance of Education

Education is mandatory, and girls, in particular, are expected to attend school to prepare for a career and their financial independence. The importance of a good education is generally emphasized in most Puerto Rican homes, and children are taught from a young age to be competitive in school; sometimes they are even pressured to excel so as to qualify for federal minority scholarships. Academically, girls are expected to compete equally with boys.

## Pubescence

### Psychosexual Development

Generally girls tend to reach pubescence a little earlier than do boys. On average, girls reach puberty between the ages of 10 and 13.

### Rituals and Rites of Passage

There is generally a celebration (**quinceañero**) at age 15 to mark a girl's transition into womanhood. The celebration of this occasion varies depending on the family's religious beliefs. Typically, however, the parents provide a feast, and the girl invites all her relatives and friends. The celebration is initiated with a ceremony in which all the girls' favorite friends participate and dress in a manner similar to that for a wedding. This ritual is more common among more traditional families.

### Teen Sexuality

**Social Restrictions and Pressures.**  During puberty, family members, especially the father, closely monitor a young girl's behavior and dress. Although dress codes largely depend on the family's religious beliefs, most families strive to keep their daughters from dressing in what may be perceived as a provocative or "shameful" manner. Also, all young women are expected to live with their parents until they marry. If they move to a different geographic area to attend school, they are expected to return home on weekends.

**Teen Pregnancy.**  Teen dating, sexuality, and use of contraception are considered taboo and a sign of poor parenting. Teenage pregnancies, although not sanctioned in this culture, are reportedly on the rise. For example, from 1994 to 1997, the percentage of live births involving adolescent mothers rose from 19.6% (out of a total of 12,335) to 20.7% (out of a total of 13,305).

### Menstruation

**Relationship to Health.**   Family members use the phrase *"le cantó el gallo"* when referring to the day a girl has her first menstrual period. This is usually embarrassing to the girl, since menstruation is considered a private matter. Menstruation is seen as a natural process symbolic of reaching womanhood and being healthy. Painful menstruation is viewed as being normal, and women usually carry pain medication for this time of the month. Some women use herbal teas such as **ruda** to ease the menstrual cramps.

**Relationship to Fertility.**   Menstruation signifies that a girl is fertile and can now become pregnant, a very important issue in this culture. A woman who is incapable of menstruating because of a hysterectomy, congenital anomalies, or a medical problem is often viewed as being less of a woman or somehow incomplete.

**Taboos and Restrictions During Menstruation.**   During her menstrual period, a young woman generally continues with her routine activities. More traditional Puerto Ricans, however, tend to restrict the consumption of sour drinks, such as lemonade, during the period, believing that such consumption will reduce the menstrual flow and cause increased cramping.

**Dysmenorrhea.**   Dysmenorrhea is considered a sign of something "not being right," and the young woman is expected to see a doctor. Many women, however, use herbal teas such as **ruda, yerba buena,** and **manzanilla** (chamomile) for treatment of this disorder.

### Female Modesty and Touching

This culture observes female modesty. Expressions of affection, including hugging and kissing, are very normal among family members. It is considered improper, however, for a woman to allow a man who is not her husband to closely embrace her or to touch her sexually.

**Relationship to Health Care.**   Although it is accepted for a female to be assigned to a male practitioner, a female provider is much more preferred. Also, modesty may cause some women to avoid obtaining annual pelvic and breast examinations.

# Adulthood

### Transition Rites and Rituals

A young woman is considered an adult when she marries or, if single, when she becomes self-supporting by finding a job. In this culture it is customary for young women to live with their parents until they get married. The exception is if they pursue out-of-town university studies.

### Social Expectations

Becoming engaged, getting married, and completing her studies are among the expectations shared by both society and her family for a young woman. If parents are elderly or there are younger siblings, it is also expected that the young woman will take care of them.

### Union Formation

**Union Types.**   Polygamy is not a common practice in Puerto Rico. The most usual types of union formation are civil marriages and common-law unions. Several research studies have shown that migrant Puerto Rican women are more likely than non-Latino whites to enter into unions, especially loose, consensual unions, at an early age.

**Social Sanctions for Failing to Enter into Union.**   The derogatory term *jamona* is used to refer to a woman 30 years or older who has failed to marry or enter into a consensual union. The unmarried male of this age, on the other hand, is considered a "playboy."

### Domestic Violence

Although the precise degree to which domestic violence affects Puerto Rican families may never be known because of the unwillingness of many families to report this crime to the authorities, it is nonetheless believed that family violence is quite high among Puerto Rican families. Recent data for 2000 suggest that one out of every three women will be a victim of domestic violence in Puerto Rico at some time in their lives, and 52% of women murdered in Puerto Rico were killed by their husbands or significant others.

### Rape

Because of the shame and guilt attached to rape, Puerto Rican women are often unwilling to report this crime to the authorities. Those living in the United States for an extended period, however, may feel more empowered to seek help from the proper authorities because of the support systems in place to help rape victims.

---

**NOTE TO THE HEALTH CARE PROVIDER**
Women may refuse rape counseling initially because of the stigma attached to this crime. Providers should not coerce the client; gentle persuasion techniques and support are more likely to succeed.

---

### Divorce

**Sociocultural Views.**   The Catholic Church and its teachings maintain a strong influence over the Puerto Rican way of life. For many Puerto Ricans, divorce nonetheless remains the primary solution to marital problems.

**Women and Divorce.**   Following divorce, remarriage of the woman is acceptable in Puerto Rican culture. Many divorced women choose, however, to move to the mainland, hoping to "start their lives all over," far from where the problems originated.

**Child Custody Practices.**   Following a divorce, the male partner is generally expected to maintain ties with the children, including financial support and helping with upbringing. Many divorced women are abandoned by their partners, however, and the women care for the children themselves. The extended family generally provides a good source of support for a divorced woman and her children.

## Fertility and Childbearing

**Family Size.**   Large families were customary among Puerto Ricans. More recently, however, family size has been decreasing for those living in Puerto Rico as well as on the mainland. Today, a total of four children comprise the average Puerto Rican family.

**Contraceptive Practices.**   Puerto Rican women widely accept the use of modern contraception. Today, the birth control pill and intrauterine device (IUD) are the methods most frequently used. Among practicing Catholics, however, the rhythm method remains the method of choice.

**Role of the Male in the Couple's Fertility Decision-Making.**   The choice of a contraceptive method ultimately depends on the woman. Puerto Rican males do not favor condom use, and it is often not an option because it is widely believed to interfere with the sensation and natural enjoyment of sex.

## Abortion

**Cultural Attitudes.**   Although abortion is legalized in Puerto Rico, it not a culturally accepted practice among most Puerto Ricans. Influenced by religious teachings that label abortion a sin, few women will openly discuss abortion or admit to having had one. Because of the secrecy and shame associated with abortion, statistics and other information on the procedure are not readily available.

**Complications.**   Women who seek abortion in medical clinics still face the emotional and spiritual consequences of challenging their cultural beliefs. Others wishing to keep their abortion a secret take a large dose of ruda tea to provoke a hemorrhage and, ultimately, an abortion.

### Miscarriage

A miscarriage is widely believed to be caused by the woman having not been careful and not taken proper care of herself during pregnancy. When pregnancy occurs, the woman is expected to get her rest, eat a well-balanced diet, and take care of herself to preserve the growing fetus inside her. A woman who habitually miscarries is thought to have something wrong with her.

### Infertility

An infertile woman, although not publicly ostracized, is perceived as being incapable of making her husband happy. Consequently, she risks his having children outside the marriage. Adoption, although an option for most infertile couples, is not readily sought because, for many Puerto Rican couples, the child has to be of "their blood."

---

**NOTE TO THE HEALTH CARE PROVIDER**
Couples are likely to be open and receptive to fertility treatments, if affordable, because having their own natural child is most important to most Puerto Rican couples.

---

### Pregnancy

**Activity Restrictions and Taboos.** A pregnant woman, if not ill, is expected to remain active until delivery. In this culture, pregnancy is considered to be a special event, and the pregnant woman is treated with a great deal of respect and consideration. Some people in certain segments of the culture believe that a pregnant woman can be adversely affected by encounters with deformed or disabled people.

**Dietary Practices and Observances.** What a woman eats during pregnancy is believed to be crucial to fetal development. Many pregnant women develop **mala barriga,** morning sickness, for which everyone offers help with different types of remedies. Pregnant women also develop **antojitos,** which are urges for particular foods. For example, some women develop a craving for sour foods and may spend the entire pregnancy sucking lemons. This behavior is generally accepted as a normal part of pregnancy.

**Prenatal Care.** Although not always the case, prenatal care is generally sought during the first trimester. In the days prior to delivery, it is believed that if the pregnant woman keeps very busy, this heightened activity will help the baby "come down" and make for an easier delivery.

Educating clients about their dietary needs, not smoking, and the importance of early and continued prenatal care are particularly important when caring for clients who have recently relocated to the mainland. In Puerto Rico, it is still quite common for women to receive only late prenatal care. Fifty percent of adolescents reportedly have their first visit during the second trimester of pregnancy. Also, low infant birth weight ($<2500$ gm) is listed as the leading factor contributing to infant mortality in Puerto Rico.

### Birthing Process

**Home Versus Hospital Delivery.**   Today, most deliveries in Puerto Rico occur in hospitals and clinics as on the mainland. Women generally prefer anesthesia unless they have made plans for a natural childbirth.

**Cesarean Section Versus Vaginal Delivery.**   Traditionally, vaginal deliveries have been the method of choice for most Puerto Ricans. In the past two decades, however, Puerto Rico has witnessed a dramatic increase in the number of cesarean sections performed, similar to the mainland.

**Labor Management.**   Family members typically stay with and provide support to the woman during the laboring process. Increased contractions and rupture of membranes signal imminent delivery, at which point families will generally seek medical help.

**Placenta.**   The placenta holds no special cultural significance for most Puerto Ricans. It is generally disposed of at the hospital following delivery.

### Postpartum

Following delivery, the postpartum period generally lasts for approximately 40 days. During this period, known as **cuarentena,** family members help with caring for the baby and permit the new mother to get adequate rest. To help the woman regain her strength, family members will typically prepare and serve her chicken broth and other types of soups. The use of herbal teas is also quite common at this time.

### Newborn and Infant Care

**Breastfeeding Versus Bottle-Feeding.** The preferred method of infant feeding is the bottle because of its perceived convenience. Today, however, more women are breastfeeding. For the colicky baby, home remedies are still widely used, including abdominal massages.

**Infant Protection.** Some more traditional families believe in *mal de ojo* (evil eye) and will have the baby wear a neck chain with an *amuleto* for protection. Most families do not believe in mal de ojo but will take their newborn to church for a blessing and protection.

---

**NOTE TO THE HEALTH CARE PROVIDER**
The newborn is generally held and closely examined by many family members who will come to visit and insist on touching and holding the baby.

---

**Primary Caregiver.** The primary caregivers for infants and toddlers are the mother and grandmother. Members of the extended family are also available to assist when needed. Customarily, the male partner does not play a major role in childcare, but he will assist when necessary.

## Middle Age

### Cultural Attitudes and Expectations

Typically, a woman in her late 30s, approaching 40, is considered middle-aged. Few, if any, dress restrictions are imposed on a middle-aged woman; she is encouraged to look good and take care of herself.

### Psychological Response

The "empty-nest" syndrome, associated with midlife, is not as dramatic an event in Puerto Rican culture as it is in some other cultures because of the closeness of the extended family. Even when a woman's children grow up and leave home, the extended family remains very much a part of her life.

### Menopause

**Onset and Duration.** Menopause, often referred to as *cambio de vida* (change of life), signifies the end of the childbearing years for the Puerto Rican woman. Because most Puerto Rican women have already completed their childbearing by this time, they accept the onset of menopause as "normal." The age of onset for menopause varies among Puerto Rican women, based on family history.

**Sexual Activity.** No cultural expectations or limitations are placed on a woman's sexual activity at menopause. In addition to hormone replacement therapy (HRT), many women use over-the-counter vaginal lubricants to overcome vaginal dryness, a side effect of menopause.

**Coping.** Hot flashes and emotional lability are two menopausal discomforts that women find difficulty coping with. Many women use herbal teas, such as *manzanilla, limoncillo,* and *naranja,* to calm the nerves.

# Old Age

## Cultural Attitudes

People older than 65 years of age are considered old and presently comprise the fastest growing segment of society in Puerto Rico. Elderly women are treated with a great deal of respect and viewed as a source of wisdom. Usually, elderly women live with one of their children and their family or some other family member. Although rest homes are now becoming more common, many Puerto Ricans do not view them as an acceptable choice since they believe that these places are for elderly who are not loved and have been abandoned.

# Death and Dying

## Cultural Attitudes and Beliefs

Many in this culture view the concept of death as a natural transition; nonetheless, most Puerto Ricans strive to live a long and healthy life. Over the years the number of Puerto Ricans living well into their 90s and even to age 100 has steadily increased. Improved access to biomedical advances and treatment is implicated.

## Rites and Rituals

Funerals are marked by sadness. Family members will often openly display their grief and sadness by crying out loud, especially when viewing the body. For some families it is still very important to have the body of the deceased returned to the home for viewing and a wake a few days prior to the burial. For Puerto Ricans living on the mainland, inability to observe this cultural practice may present an added burden and stress to the grieving family.

### Mourning

**Cultural Expectations.** The mourning period observed by most Puerto Ricans continues for up to one year. During this time, the surviving spouse and close family members are expected to wear black or dark clothing and to refrain from outward displays of joviality, such as partying.

If the parents of minor children die, custody of the children is decided by the extended family. Most often the maternal grandparents will adopt and raise the children.

**Coping.** Family members provide a very important source of support in helping a widowed woman cope with the loss of her spouse or a child. The death of a child is often more challenging to those left behind than the death of an old person, because of the seemingly untimely nature of the death and feelings that the child "has not yet lived."

## IMPORTANT POINTS FOR PROVIDERS CARING FOR PUERTO RICAN WOMEN

### The Medical Intake

#### Literacy and English Proficiency

English is the second language spoken in Puerto Rico. Hence, some women who have recently migrated to the mainland will not be adequately proficient in English and will require the assistance of an interpreter to explain medical procedures and fill out forms not printed in Spanish.

#### Status of the Provider

The health provider is viewed with a great deal of respect and trust. Unlike some other cultural groups, however, Puerto Rican women are not typically shy and will maintain eye contact with the provider.

#### Communicating Illness and Symptoms

Women will generally be open about their symptoms when speaking with the health care provider. They are more inclined, however, to withhold information about home remedies they may be taking unless they are directly asked about them, fearing disapproval. If, on the other hand, they perceive an honest interest on the part of the health care provider, they are likely to engage in a detailed discussion about their herbal use.

### The Physical Examination

#### Modesty and Touching

Having a female health provider is preferred, but it is culturally acceptable for a male provider to examine the woman with a female nurse or relative present. The woman's privacy should be observed at all times. It is important to cover the body, leaving uncovered only the part being examined.

### Expressing Pain

Women in this culture tend to be very open and expressive about pain. They will cry out loud and request pain medication for what they perceive as severe pain.

## Prescribing Medications

### Drug Interactions

The practitioner should ask detailed questions about other prescription medications and home remedies being taken. Women tend to use many herbs alone or in combination with prescription medications. Often this information will not be volunteered unless questions are directed specifically to it.

### Medication Sharing

Sharing leftover prescription medications with family members and friends is a customary practice. It may be beneficial to have clients bring with them all medications being taken, including self-medications and home remedies.

### Compliance

Often not understanding the importance of completing all doses of the prescribed medication, especially antibiotics, clients will tend to stop the medication or treatments once they feel better.

## Follow-up Appointments

Follow-up medical appointments can be missed if symptoms improve. Many times there is conflict with multiple responsibilities. A telephone call reminding of the appointment is very effective. Also, exploring potential obstacles and planning ahead to avoid them can help ensure that follow-up appointments will be kept.

### Orientation to Time

This group tends to be present oriented and subscribes more to social time than to business time; hence, arriving late for appointments tends to be a problem. Scheduling the client's appointment for at least a half an hour to one hour earlier than the actual time will allow the client to arrive in a more timely fashion without feeling pressured.

## Prevalent Diseases

As a commonwealth of the United States and guided by Puerto Rico's Department of Health, Puerto Rico has adopted the objectives stated in *Healthy People* 2000/2010 to implement new ways of health care delivery. The 10 leading causes of death in

Puerto Rico reported in 1994 by the Health Department were (1) heart disease, (2) malignant tumors, (3) diabetes mellitus, (4) AIDS, (5) cerebrovascular disease, (6) accidents, (7) pneumonia, (8) chronic obstructive pulmonary disease, (9) homicide, and (10) hypertension.

Reductions in such major risk factors as high blood pressure, high blood cholesterol levels, and smoking are having a significant impact in cardiovascular mortality and lung cancer. Diabetes has been identified as one of the most prevalent chronic conditions among Puerto Ricans.

Puerto Rico now has the fifth highest per capita incidence of AIDS in the United States, after Washington, DC. A total of 24,334 cases of AIDS (394 of them children) have been reported in adults and children. Women, especially those of childbearing age, constitute a growing proportion of people with HIV (human immunodeficiency virus)/AIDS infection. Since pediatric HIV infection continues to rise, this illness also will affect many families with children.

As a result of recent improvement in medical care and the availability of antiretroviral therapy, recently reported surveillance data indicate an overall decline in the number of deaths from AIDS. The rate of infection, however, has not declined. An estimate of HIV infection prevalence, using the Centers of Disease Control and Prevention (CDC) formula for projections, suggests that from 32,000 to 55,016 persons are infected with the virus in Puerto Rico.

## Health-Seeking Behaviors

It is customary for individuals to seek medical attention only after they have tried various home remedies and herbal teas. It is often late in the disease process before they seek biomedical treatment. Additionally, if they feel that the biomedical treatments are not effective, it is not uncommon for Puerto Ricans to consult alternative medicine workers (folk healers). Usually, they consult folk healers for a special type of abdominal massage for *empache*. They treat minor illnesses with over-the-counter medications.

### 🌐 BIBLIOGRAPHY

Apontes, I. (2000). La salud de las mujeres: Victimas de violencia domestica. *Boletin Mujer y Salud*, 4(19), 7–10.

Hernandez, D., & Scheff, J. (1996). Puerto Rican geographic mobility: the making of a deterritorialized nationality. *The Puerto Rican Migration Experiences, March* 5,6, 1–20.

Morales, Z. (1996). Los imigrantes residiendo en Puerto Rico: su perfil socioeconomico en el 1990. *Centro de investigacion demografico, Dic*, 1–32.

Oliver, M. (1999). La promocion de la salud de la mujer de edad mayor. *Boletin Mujer y Salud*, 3(2), 11–12.

Rodriguez, C. (1991). *Puerto Ricans in the United States*. Boulder, CO: Westview Press.

*17*

# Russians (Former Soviets)

KAREN J. AROIAN, PhD, RN, CS, FAAN

## INTRODUCTION

### Who are the Russian People?

"Ethnic Russians" are of Slavic background and have roots in Czarist Russia or the Republic of Russia. In the United States, however, the label "Russian" has come to be applied to anyone from the former Soviet Union (FSU), including ethnic minorities that do not have Russian Slavic roots (e.g., Soviet Jews, Armenians, Ukrainians, and Moldavians). In this chapter the terms Russian, Soviet, and former Soviet are used interchangeably to include ethnic Russians as well as the various ethnic minorities in the FSU.

The Soviet Union was formed in 1917 when the Russian Revolution overturned Czarist rule and replaced it with communism. The Soviet Union consisted of 15 republics of ethnically and culturally diverse people from two continents: Europe and Asia. The Asian republics were and continue to be primarily agrarian, rural, and traditional societies; whereas the European republics are mostly industrial, urban, and more contemporary. In 1991 communism collapsed, and the republics were transformed into independent nation states.

During communist rule, there was considerable internal migration with ethnic Russians and ethnic minorities moving from their original to other republics. With the collapse of communism, there has been some return migration to the republic of one's ethnic heritage. Presently, however, people in the FSU are shaped by the republic where they lived most of their lives.

### Russians or Former Soviets in North America

There were four contemporary (post 1917 or post-revolutionary Russia) waves of migration from the FSU to the United States. The first three waves (1917 to 1993) were comprised primarily of national or religious ethnic minorities. Soviet Jews are the largest ethnic minority group of immigrants, followed by Soviet Armenians,

**ACKNOWLEDGMENT**
The author would like to acknowledge the assistance of Galina Khatutsky and Gulnara Ogarkova for their expertise on the culture of Russian women.

Pentecostals, and Evangelicals. Emigration among ethnic minorities was facilitated by their refugee status, which was awarded on the basis of their ethnic or religious persecution in the Soviet Union. The fourth wave (1993 to present) of migration from the FSU was spawned by the transformation of the Soviet Union into independent nation states in 1991. This development resulted in freedom to emigrate, sociopolitical turmoil, economic hardship, and in many areas, increased ethnic conflict and strife. The shift from communism to a market economy also widened the gap between rich and poor. Emigration was no longer restricted to minority groups with refugee status. Only a small number of ethnic Russians, however, have been able to emigrate to North Amerca. Unlike former Soviet minorities with refugee status, ethnic Russians are subject to U. S. immigration quotas, job requirements, or family sponsorship.

As of 1998, about 30,000 immigrants from the FSU are in the United States. Slightly more than half of these immigrants are women. Of the total U.S. former Soviet immigrant population, just over one-third is from the Republic of Russia and just under one-third is from the Ukraine. The remaining republics of origin are mostly European. Regardless of republic of origin, most former Soviet immigrants are from urban areas and, similarly, have settled in major American cities such as New York, Boston, Baltimore, Philadelphia, Chicago, and San Francisco. They are highly educated and were mostly professionals in their homeland. For example, in 1990, 1 in 6 Soviet immigrants was a scientist, engineer, or former medical doctor. Unlike many other immigrant groups, a number of immigrants came as older adults, in part because Russian immigrants often immigrate as extended, multigenerational families.

The 1996 Census enumerates 272,335 people of Russian heritage in Canada, 51% of whom are women. They live predominantly in Toronto, Vancouver, and Montreal. People of Ukrainian heritage number 1,026,475 and live mainly in Edmonton, Winnipeg, and Toronto.

## 🌐 BEING FEMALE IN RUSSIAN SOCIETY

Women have been a part of the work force, including the professional sector, since the early 1900s, when communism was established. Similarly, most former Soviet women were and continue to be highly educated. However, the Russian culture has always valued traditional feminine behavior and the roles of mother, spouse, and homemaker. Many Russian women and men view North American women's emphasis on equal rights as militant and a disavowal of femininity. Russian women pursue their education and occupational goals while assuming full domestic responsibility for their families. Fulfilling multiple roles is possible for Russian women because they often live in multigenerational households and have assistance from their mothers and grandmothers.

## At Birth

### Preference for Sons

Children, regardless of gender, are highly valued. Female children are not neglected or abandoned. With the exception of more traditional subgroups (e.g., Russian Orthodox Jews, Russians in rural areas), sons are not preferred over daughters.

### Birth Rituals

No rituals are associated with birth except that girls are dressed in pink and boys are dressed in blue.

# Childhood and Youth

## Stages

Childhood is not demarcated into stages. At age 16, children in the FSU are awarded passports or identity cards even though they are not generally recognized as adults until age 21. The literal translation for the Russian term for an adolescent, **podros-toka,** means growing but not fully grown. In more rural and/or non-European former Soviet republics, age 16 (rather than 18) is the legal age for marriage. Nonetheless, a recent trend throughout the FSU is to delay marriage and childbearing until at least age 18 to 20.

## Family Expectations

Youth are expected to assist with household chores. Chores are assigned according to traditional gender expectations with one exception—both boys and girls assist with food shopping. Girls help with cooking and cleaning and are never expected to engage in physically demanding work. Boys help with household repairs and physical labor, such as digging and harvesting family vegetable gardens. Girls spend more time at home with their families, but both genders are expected to be good students.

## Importance of Education

Regardless of gender, education is highly valued in the FSU. Even in more traditional and rural areas (e.g., the Caucasus), men desire as brides women who are more highly educated. Beginning with the post World War II era and continuing today, almost all former Soviets have at least a high school degree. Before the collapse of communism, the state provided vocational or college education to everyone in the FSU who demonstrated ability. However, the educational level of the population may decrease now with the privatization of higher education.

# Pubescence

## Psychosexual Development

Girls mature faster than do boys, both emotionally and physically. The average age of onset of puberty for girls is age 12 or 13, compared with ages 14 or 15 for boys. There are no physical, genetic, or nutritional reasons that delay or accelerate the onset of puberty (e.g., breast development, onset of the menstrual cycle).

## Rituals and Rites of Passage

No special rituals or observances celebrate a young girl's transition into womanhood.

## Teen Sexuality

**Social Restrictions and Pressures.**   Just one generation ago, teenage girls were expected to downplay their sexuality by braiding their hair, wearing uniforms, and not using make-up or nail polish. These behavioral norms no longer apply. Teenage girls are not expected to marry once they enter pubescence, although marriage at age 16 was the norm in southern or Asian regions of the FSU. As already noted, the current trend is to delay marriage until at least age 18. For those who have migrated to the United States, many of these behaviors and norms are retained, due in large part to socialization within the ethnic enclave.

**Teen Pregnancy.** Contraception and sex education are not provided for teens, mostly because public discussion of sexual topics is considered inappropriate, and teens are not expected to engage in sexual activity out of wedlock. Also, contraception, when available, is financially prohibitive for teens. Pregnancy out of wedlock is considered shameful and is usually handled by abortion. Parental consent is required for unmarried girls younger than age 18 seeking an abortion at a gynecologic clinic.

### Menstruation

Menstruation, like sexuality, is considered a topic that is inappropriate for public discussion. Much of what the girl learns about menstruation is learned from her mother.

**Relationship to Health.** Beliefs about the relationship of menstruation to health are based on biomedical knowledge, not on cultural beliefs.

**Relationship to Fertility.** The general population clearly understands the significance of menstruation for fertility. The cultural value of fertility is higher among some subgroups and in some regions, such as in the Caucasus. Generally, however, infertility is considered a personal disappointment and is ascribed to a health problem rather than being viewed as a punishment for transgression or a failure of femininity.

**Taboos and Restrictions During Menstruation.** There is a general perception that it is unhealthy to engage in physical activity, including swimming, during one's period. Thus, schoolgirls are routinely excused from physical education when menstruating. Some restrictions may have resulted from the former unavailability of tampons.

**Dysmenorrhea.** Attributions for dysmenorrhea, like beliefs about menstruation, are based on biomedical knowledge. Russian women use painkillers similar to Tylenol (when available) for relief of menstrual cramps.

### Female Modesty and Touching

Female modesty is not pronounced in the Russian culture, but older generations of women are more modest than younger generations.

Female physicians were and continue to be common in the FSU. Most Russian women have no preference regarding the gender of their health care practitioners. There are no taboos against touching or exposing women's bodies. In fact, crowded housing and health-care facilities afford little privacy. Modesty does not limit Russian women's readiness to obtain annual pelvic examinations. However, pelvic examinations are customary only for married women and women with gynecologic problems. Mammography is not offered routinely.

## Adulthood

### Transition Rights and Rituals

Marriage and starting a family signify the transition into adulthood. Typically, Russian women marry and start their families at a younger age than North American women (as early as age 16 in rural republics and age 18 to 25 in urban areas). Most Russian women are married by age 25 and begin their childbearing while completing secondary education. No formal ceremonies, other than marriage, mark the young woman's transition into adulthood.

### Social Expectations

Young Russian women are expected to be married and to begin having children (at least one child) by age 25. Living with a man before marriage or having a child out of wedlock is not acceptable. Young Russian women are also expected to finish secondary education and establish their careers while starting a family. Although education and work are very important in this culture, having a good husband carries more social pressure.

### Union Formation

**Union Types.** A civil ceremony was the most common way to be married in the FSU, but Russians are increasingly choosing religious ceremonies. Although there is some matchmaking, most marriages occur through personal choice

**Social Sanctions for Failing to Enter into Union.** There is social pressure for Russian women to marry and begin having children by age 25. Men are expected to begin their families around age 30.

Women who value their careers over marriage and remain unmarried are labeled "*blue stockings*." This term has negative connotations and describes an overly intellectual, cold woman who is more interested in her career than in having a family life. The term for an unmarried woman, regardless of her career aspirations, is *staraya deva,* which literally means "old maid," a pejorative label.

### Domestic Violence

Domestic violence is common and related mostly to men's high incidence of alcohol abuse. Women usually deal with this problem themselves or seek refuge with friends or relatives. There are no hotlines or shelters in the FSU for this type of problem.

---

**NOTE TO THE HEALTH CARE PROVIDER**
Unaccustomed to the availability of support services in the FSU, Russian clients in North America are unlikely to report domestic violence/battery to the authorities. Also, since psychiatry has been a tool of repression in the Soviet Union, these women may also be disinclined to seek out counseling.

---

### Rape

Rape is not publicized in the FSU; thus, it is very difficult to get information or statistics on its occurrence or prevalence. There are no rape crisis or counseling services. The concept of date rape is not recognized, and the state is not expected to pursue personal crimes of this nature. Russian women in North America are very unlikely to pursue legal action or seek out counseling in the event of rape, given the casual nature with which this crime is viewed by the authorities in their homeland.

## Divorce

**Sociocultural Views.**   There are no taboos against divorce. Most former Soviet citizens are not religious, in part because communism did not approve of religion. Thus, most Russians do not embrace religious sanctions against divorce.

Divorce rates are high in the FSU, and they are even higher among immigrants to North America. Theories about the rise in divorce after immigration are that (1) Russian immigrant women become more independent as they acculturate, which causes more family disharmony; (2) the general stress of immigration causes divorce; and (3) women in unhappy marriages are more apt to choose divorce after immigration.

**Women and Divorce.**   Divorced women in the FSU are not viewed negatively. Remarriage is common and there is no proper or improper time for one to remarry.

**Child Custody Practices.**   In the FSU, male partners pay a fixed amount (e.g., 25% of their salary) for child support. This amount is automatically deducted from their paychecks. Child custody is never awarded to men. Although there are exceptions, divorced men usually do not remain active in their children's lives; rather, they tend to move on and establish new families.

## Fertility and Childbearing

**Family Size.**   Family size has decreased over the years. Small families are typical, mostly as a result of economic hardship. The average family size is one child in urban areas and not more than two children in rural areas.

**Contraceptive Practices.**   There are no taboos, including religious sanctions, against female contraception. However, quality contraception was not readily available until recently in the FSU. For example, condoms were made of thick rubber. Oral contraceptives, when available, were of poor quality and caused side effects (e.g., non-menstrual bleeding). Presently, because of past experiences with poor quality, Russians are generally suspicious of hormonal preparations and tend to avoid birth control pills. Men often refuse to use condoms because they interfere with their pleasure. Men avoid vasectomy because it is seen as a threat to masculinity. Consequently, rhythm, douche, intrauterine devices, and abortion were and continue to be popular methods of contraception.

---

**NOTE TO THE HEALTH CARE PROVIDER**
Discussing vasectomy as a family planning option is likely to alienate male partners. Extra education is needed about the side effects of birth control pills.

---

**Role of the Male in the Couple's Fertility Decision-Making.**   Contraception is the woman's responsibility. She often makes her choice without asking her partner's opinion. Both men and women are knowledgeable about contraception, but couples typically do not discuss the topic.

With the exception of vasectomy and, to some extent, birth control pills, choices about contraception are made according to cost and availability. Cost is also an issue for new immigrants since they are usually living on limited finances. Thus, health professionals should include cost considerations when recommending a method of contraception.

## Abortion

**Cultural Attitudes.**   Abortion is not encouraged, and repeated abortions are recognized as a health risk. Nonetheless, abortion as a method of family planning is still highly prevalent and is considered a painful necessity. Russia has the world's highest abortion rate. According to official figures, two out of three pregnancies end in abortion. Abortions are likely to be sought early in the pregnancy.

**Teen Abortions.**   Teenage out-of-wedlock pregnancy is not common. When it does occur, abortion is the usual response regardless of social class.

**Sources of Abortions.**   Abortion is legal in the FSU as long as it is preformed by a health care professional. Abortions are often performed without anesthesia. Anesthesia, when available, is costly, and the patient bears the expense.

Megadoses of vitamin C and hot baths are used as abortificents in the FSU. These abortificents are less likely to be used in North America since professionally performed abortions are preferred when anesthesia is available.

---

**NOTE TO THE HEALTH CARE PROVIDER**

Do not be surprised if married Russian women seek abortion. Practitioners should refrain from a judgmental attitude toward using abortion as a method of family planning.

---

## Miscarriage

The rate of miscarriage in this population is not unusually high, perhaps because parity is low and because the cervix is not compromised from multiple abortions until after women have borne their desired number of children.

Miscarriage is perceived as an unfortunate accident or the consequence of a health problem. No specific procedures are taken to prevent a woman from miscarrying. However, bed rest is commonly prescribed in the FSU for many complications of pregnancy, including threat of miscarriage.

## Infertility

Although statistics are only recently available, incidence of infertility in the FSU is high, with estimates ranging from 10% to 25% of all couples. Ascribed causes for infertility are based on biomedical knowledge. For example, Russian citizens acknowledge that multiple abortions are a likely cause for the high rate of infertility. Infertile women are not ostracized. However, women with known fertility problems are less desirable as potential spouses. Women who voluntarily choose to remain childless are rare. Although choosing to not have children is considered selfish, no blame is attributed to involuntary childlessness.

Infertility may lead to divorce if the partner highly values having a child. However, individuals vary greatly in this regard.

---

**NOTE TO THE HEALTH CARE PROVIDER**

Russian immigrant women and their partners are highly receptive to fertility treatment if the treatment is covered by their medical insurance or if they can afford it.

---

### Pregnancy

**Activity Restrictions and Taboos.**   Pregnant women are advised to refrain from heavy lifting and physically demanding activity. Bed rest is commonly prescribed. Maternity leave in the FSU is generous and has recently been lengthened from seven months to three years postpartum. Women are paid their full salary for three months and then one-third of their salary for the remainder of their maternity leave.

Women are not expected to stay indoors when pregnant. There are no beliefs that the developing fetus might be harmed by contact with deformed or disabled people or specific animals that may frighten the woman during pregnancy.

Russian women are accorded more respect and given special consideration when they are pregnant.

**Dietary Practices and Observances.**   No cultural norms surround diet during pregnancy other than eating healthy foods (e.g., foods high in iron, calcium, and other vitamins) and avoiding foods that can cause infant allergies (e.g., strawberries, citrus, chocolate). Eating nonfood items (e.g., pica) during pregnancy is not common.

**Prenatal Care.**   Russian women seek prenatal care from health professionals early and throughout their pregnancies. Frequency of prenatal visits in the FSU is greater than in North America.

No special procedures, rituals, or preparations are used in the weeks or days prior to delivery to enhance the delivery.

### Birthing Process

**Home Versus Hospital Delivery.**   By far, hospitals are the most common site for delivery in the FSU. Physicians and midwives perform deliveries. Home deliveries are rare and are not preferred by most individuals, and the choices are similar in North America.

**Cesarean Section Versus Vaginal Delivery.**   Most deliveries are vaginal. Cesarean sections are used only as a last resort and are considered a complication in the delivery process. There is often no choice regarding natural childbirth or anesthesia because anesthesia is not routinely available; it is used only when there are complications or if the couple agrees to bear the extra cost. For average citizens, the cost of anesthesia is prohibitive.

**Involvement of the Male Partner.**   Traditionally, husbands and female relatives are not only excluded from the delivery but also are not allowed to make postpartum visits to the hospital. However, some contemporary birthing centers have recently opened that offer many Western features, including husbands' active participation in the delivery process. The cost of these contemporary birthing centers is high and borne by the couple.

**Labor Management.**   Labor management is the same as it is in Western biomedical practice. However, many couples will typically offer extra money to ensure that health practitioners will be attentive during labor.

**Placenta.**   No special significance is accorded to the placenta or "afterbirth."

---

**NOTE TO THE HEALTH CARE PROVIDER**
Some families may not be responsive to practitioners' efforts to involve husbands or significant others in the birthing process. Russian women may interpret having a cesarean delivery in North America as indicative of a very serious birth complication. They may also resist the trend toward early hospital discharge.

---

## Postpartum

Typically, women remain in the hospital for five days postpartum. At home, women recuperate for one or two weeks unless the delivery was complicated. There are no postpartum restrictions nor are specific cultural practices observed during this period. However, postpartum women are encouraged to improve their breast milk by eating nuts and drinking special herbal teas and black tea with milk.

### Newborn and Infant Care

**Breastfeeding Versus Bottle-Feeding.** Breastfeeding is the typical method of infant feeding, in part because infant formula was often not available or of poor quality. Although the availability and quality of infant formula has recently improved, it is costly. Women who breastfeed are encouraged to pump "extra" breast milk to share or donate to others. Government-run "milk kitchens" offset the lack of quality infant formula and milk products by providing this donated breast milk as well as coupons for milk products. If the neonate is assessed as "weak," which is a common neonatal assessment in the FSU, the mother is discouraged from breastfeeding. Instead, a nurse will bottle-feed the infant with the mother's pumped breast milk. Homemade compresses of various sorts (e.g., honey, onion, and flour, or vodka and honey) are used to relieve mastitis. Dill water, a preparation that is available in pharmacies in the FSU, is used for colicky infants.

**Infant Protection.** Health personnel monitor infant and toddler growth and development regularly. Immunizations are required but are of poor quality. Thus, parents try to avoid the risk of immunization, fearing that it will harm their children. Russians do not believe in the effects of evil eye and discredit the notion that malevolent wishes, such as another woman's jealousy, can harm infants.

**Primary Caregiver.** Mothers and grandmothers are the primary caregivers for infants and toddlers. Joint care giving is facilitated because multiple generations often live together. However, grandmothers may be burdened by caring for their own mothers in addition to having responsibility for their grandchildren. Although there are exceptions, male partners seldom contribute significantly to childcare.

---

**NOTE TO THE HEALTH CARE PROVIDER**

Grandmothers' advice is highly regarded. Be sure to include grandmothers in decision-making and education on infant care. However, living arrangements often change after immigration, and grandmothers may be less available. Given that fathers do not typically help with childcare, new immigrant mothers may be overburdened with multiple role responsibilities if their mothers are not available to help them.

---

# Middle Age

## Cultural Attitudes and Expectations

Women are considered "mid-life" once they begin having children, which is usually by age 25. Middle-aged women are expected to dress more maturely than young girls do. For example, very short skirts are inappropriate for women once they enter motherhood.

### Psychological Response

The "empty-nest" syndrome is not relevant in this culture. Multiple generations live together, and women become grandmothers and primary caretakers for their grandchildren at a fairly young age.

"Mid-life crisis" occurs in Russian culture, but it is generally ascribed only to men. The typical manifestation is for men to become interested in younger women, perhaps even divorcing their wives to pursue this interest.

### Menopause

**Onset and Duration.**   The term for menopause is *climax,* drawing from the Latin word climacteric. The average age range for the onset of menopause is 45 to 50 years.

There is little to no information about the typical course of menopause in Russian women, in part because the topic is not discussed publicly or considered important.

**Sexual Activity.**   Menopause does not signify the loss of womanhood or have any implications for a woman's sexuality. However, many women are not sexually active at menopause because of a shortage of men (the average life expectancy for men is 12 years younger than that of women).

**Coping.**   Women do not complain about or seek help for symptoms of menopause. Given the hardships of daily living and the preponderance of other, more serious health problems in the FSU, menopause is not considered an important or difficult transition.

Women usually ignore hot flashes and emotional changes. If women do acknowledge hot flashes and attribute them to menopause, they may treat them by drinking herbal teas. Hormone replacement therapy (HRT) is not used in the FSU. Russian immigrant women may also be reluctant to use HRT in the United States because of their general distrust of hormonal preparations.

---

**NOTE TO THE HEALTH CARE PROVIDER**
If HRT is indicated, be sure to provide extensive education about its risks and benefits.

---

## Old Age

### Cultural Attitudes

The average life expectancy in the FSU is 57 to 58 years for men and 69 to 70 years for women. The death rate in the FSU is staggeringly high because of lifestyle, environmental hazards, health problems, and health-care shortages. For example, alcoholism, diets high in fat and salt, poor air quality and work conditions, cardiac disease, and a lack of preventative health care are common in the FSU.

Women are considered old by age 60. Elderly women are not accorded more respect than their younger counterparts. However, elderly women are valued as an important source of financial support and childcare for their offspring.

Households in the FSU are typically multigenerational, with elderly and widowed women living with their adult children and grandchildren. Multigenerational households, however, are less common among the new Russian elite (i.e., people who have prospered in private businesses since the collapse of communism) and among Russian immigrants. In the United States, many elderly Russians choose to live in elderly housing, in part because such housing is less isolating than living with adult children who are working all day. If elderly women are not living with their adult children, they often live alone, mostly because they are widowed or divorced.

Family members typically care for elderly women if they cannot care for themselves. Rest homes are used as a last resort and are often perceived as an abdication of family responsibility. Rest homes are scarce in the FSU and are of poor quality.

## Death and Dying

### Cultural Attitudes and Beliefs

Untimely death is considered tragic, but death in the late 50- to early 60-year-old age range is expected and accepted as a part of life.

Although there is a recent resurgence of religion in the FSU, most former Soviets are not religious. Thus, few people believe in an afterlife.

### Rites and Rituals

Funerals and wakes are adorned with flowers. Caskets are often open, even among Russian Jews. Observant Russian Jews may sit shivah at home, at which time visitors pay their respects for seven days following the death. More typically, Russians observe a pre-Revolutionary tradition: family and friends gather with food and drink (usually vodka) on the 9th, 40th, and 365th days following the death to remember and celebrate the deceased. They also pour a glass of vodka for the deceased. It is considered respectful to properly bury the dead. However, burial sites are at a premium, expensive, and available mainly to important and wealthy people; they are a status symbol in the FSU.

There are no gender differences in the burial practices or the amount of respect accorded the deceased.

#### Mourning

**Cultural Expectations.**   The typical mourning period is one year.

Mourning is expressed by crying openly at funerals, wearing black, and keeping a picture of the deceased in a black picture frame. Leaving flowers at the grave on holidays is a way of showing devotion to the deceased. It is acceptable for spouses to remarry after one year.

When a mother dies, a family member, usually a grandmother, cares for the children.

**Coping.**   Grief is openly expressed in the FSU. Women often respond to widowhood by busying themselves with their grandchildren. For women, the death of a spouse usually signifies the loss of a breadwinner. Support is usually forthcoming from extended family.

---

**NOTE TO THE HEALTH CARE PROVIDER**

Treat grandparents as the primary caregivers rather than trying to involve fathers in the care of children who have lost their mothers.

---

## 🌐 IMPORTANT POINTS FOR HEALTH PROVIDERS CARING FOR RUSSIAN WOMEN

## The Medical Intake

### Literacy and English Proficiency

Russians, including the elderly, have a high rate of literacy. There are no gender differences in literacy and, for immigrants, proficiency in English. Most Russian immigrants, with the exception of the elderly, become proficient in time with English. When language is a problem and medical translators are unavailable, family members or friends are likely to assist with translating the health-care encounter.

### Status of the Provider

Health providers, particularly physicians, are accorded high status in the FSU. The status of "American medicine" is even higher. Consequently, Russian immigrants may have unrealistic expectations for medical cures. Russians, regardless of gender, expect and prefer health providers to be authoritative and to make health care decisions for them. Nonetheless, they are not passive in voicing their needs.

### Communicating Illness and Symptoms

Women openly offer information about their health and illness, including medical history and current symptoms. However, they may not offer information about using home remedies or being treated simultaneously by more than one health practitioner.

Russian women are quite verbal, discussing their somatic symptoms in detail. Emotional symptoms are also typically communicated as bodily complaints. Practitioners who take the time to listen are perceived as being caring and responsible.

Disease is attributed to biomedical beliefs as well as the belief that psychosocial stress and trauma can cause various illnesses. Cancer, for example, is often attributed to stressful life events such as divorce.

Women are considered capable of seeking and using health care without family assistance. However, family members will often accompany one another to medical appointments to provide support and help with making health-care decisions.

---

**NOTE TO THE HEALTH CARE PROVIDER**

Women may not be open and forthcoming with their answers because they do not expect health care providers to inquire about sexual activity or psychosocial issues that they consider highly personal, such as quality of their marital relationship.

---

## The Physical Examination

### Modesty and Touching

Female modesty and gender of the health provider are not issues when conducting physical examinations.

Russians are used to less personal or body space than are North Americans. Touching female clients is appropriate. Women are not considered unclean or untouchable when menstruating.

### Expressing Pain

Life in the FSU is full of hardships and, as previously stated, anesthesia is not routinely available. Thus, most women have a high threshold for pain. Nonetheless, they express pain openly and without restraint. Women may also exaggerate pain, complaining loudly and demanding relief as a way to secure scarce health-care resources.

## Prescribing Medications

### Drug Interaction

Former Soviets use a variety of herbal preparations and home remedies. They are unlikely to share information about herbal preparations and home remedies with health care providers unless explicitly asked. Some of these herbal preparations are dangerous when combined with other medications.

### Medication Sharing

Friends and family members often share leftover prescribed medications.

Clients are likely to seek medications simultaneously from more than one health practitioner, operating on the principle that greater professional input and more medication are better. Practitioners may be unaware of the full complement of their clients' medication regimens. Thus, problems stemming from polypharmacy, including interactions with herbal and home preparations, are common.

### Compliance

Medication compliance is generally not a problem with former Soviets. They are not only used to biomedical solutions but also idealize them. Nonetheless, clients may discontinue antibiotics and save prescriptions for later use if they begin to feel better. For financial reasons, former Soviets will continue to use medications that have expired.

Taking a thorough medication history about use of herbal and home remedies and prescribed medications, as well as providing education about potential untoward drug interactions, will increase compliance. Compliance, specifically not sharing prescriptions or using outdated prescriptions, will also be greater if cost is not a problem.

## Follow-up Appointments

Generally, missing appointments is not a problem for this group. They tend to keep follow-up appointments even when they are feeling better.

### Orientation to Time

Orientation to time is a combination of present and future. The future orientation is necessitated by the common shortage of consumer goods in the FSU and the need to stockpile goods that might not be available in the future. People are usually punctual for medical and other business appointments.

Follow-up visits and care are not a problem for this group, in part because they highly value health care.

## Prevalent Diseases

Health in the FSU is worsening because of economic hardships. Alcoholism, depression, heart disease, hypertension, diabetes, gastrointestinal disorders, arthritis, lung disease, and asthma are prevalent. Alcoholism is less prevalent among women and Jews.

Many of the prevalent diseases in the FSU are related to lifestyle. For example, smoking and diets high in fat and salt are common. Other contributory factors include environmental hazards, food shortages, and a lack of medical equipment and health services.

## Health-Seeking Behaviors

People seek medical attention at the first sign of illness. Although they consult health professionals at the earliest opportunity, they will seek lay persons' advice and self-treat while they are waiting for medical attention. Many Russians will also seek treatment from healers who heal with "extra senses" and employ such techniques as energy fields and therapeutic touch.

Herbal and home remedies are commonly used to treat minor illnesses. Compresses of various sorts, as well as tea and vodka preparations, are especially popular. If they have time, some newer immigrants and refugees engage in health promotion activities, such as walking or swimming, and attention to diet, especially adding more fruits and vegetables. However, others simply add more meat because of its higher quality and availability in North America.

Home remedies are not the treatment of choice for major illnesses. Rather, surgery or more radical forms of treatment are preferred.

## 🌐 BIBLIOGRAPHY

Aroian, K. J., & Norris, A. E. (1999). Somatization and depression among former Soviet immigrants. *Journal of Cultural Diversity*, 6(3), 93–101.

Aroian, K. J., Khatutsky, G., Tran, T. V., & Balsam, A. L. (2001). Health and service utilization among elderly Russian immigrants from the former Soviet Union. *Journal of Nursing Scholarship*. 33, 265–271.

Lassey, M. L., Lassey, W. R., & Jinks, M. J. (1997). *Health care systems around the world*. Upper Saddle River, NJ: Prentice Hall.

Remennick, L. I. (1999). Preventive behavior among recent immigrants: Russian-speaking women and cancer screening in Israel. *Social Science & Medicine*, 48(11), 1669–1684.

Remennick, L. I., Amir, D., Elimelech, Y., & Novikov, Y. (1995). Family planning practices and attitudes among former Soviet new immigrant women in Israel. *Social Science and Medicine*, 41(4), 569–577.

# CHAPTER 18

# South Asians

## RACHEL ZACHARIAH, DNSc, RN

🌐 INTRODUCTION

### Who are the South Asian People?

"South Asia" refers to the Indian subcontinent and surrounding nations, including India, Pakistan, Bangladesh, Bhutan, Nepal, Sri Lanka, and the Maldives. In addition to a person from any of these nations, "South Asian" also refers to anyone of South Asian ancestry who settled in England, Fiji, Kenya, Tanzania, South Africa, Malaysia, Canada, the United States, Trinidad, or Guyana. For example, one billion people reside in India, but there are more than 15 million Indians around the world. Most settled in the former British colonies as indentured servants and have lived there for many generations. In Trinidad and Guyana, Indians are one of the major ethnic groups.

Because of enormous national and ethnic diversity as well as influences from the country of resettlement, the information in this chapter cannot be generalized to all segments of the South Asian population. Indians are emphasized based on the author's knowledge and because Indians comprise the largest South Asian population in North America. However, India itself is second only to the United States in ethnic diversity. South Asians in North America speak more than 20 languages, and most identify themselves by the region of their village and language; for example, Indians from the region of Gujarat speak the Gujarati language. Other languages include Bengali, Malayalam, Tamil, Telugu, Kannada, Marathi, Punjabi, Urdu, Hindi, Kashmiri, Assamese, Oriya, Sindhi, and Sanskrit.

The Indian subcontinent is religiously diverse. Eighty-three percent of Indians are Hindus, but there are more than 120 million Muslims in India. Pakistan, Bangladesh, and the Maldives are Islamic countries. South Asians also include Christians, Sikhs, Jains, Buddhists, and Parsis. There is also social structure diversity within groups, that is, the caste system. In the context of the global South Asian diaspora, however, not all South Asians can identify their roots.

---

**ACKNOWLEDGMENT**
Rahel Mathews MPH, Boston Department of Public Health, provided valuable research assistance relating to introduction, domestic violence, and chronic disease sections and personal communication regarding the experiences of adolescents as second generation South Asian-Americans.

## South Asians in North America

The first wave of Indian immigrants to North America came as laborers in the 19th century. Most early immigrants were Punjabi Sikhs who settled in the United States and Canadian Northwest and worked in lumberyards, steamship companies, farming, and railroad construction. Organized labor, however, lobbied to ban Asian immigration in 1917; the ban was lifted in 1946. Between 1946 and 1965 approximately 6000 Indians entered the United States as wives or minor dependents of Indians already in the country. In 1965, immigration laws abolished the quota regulation and nullified laws that discriminated against those of Asian descent. As a result, 15,000 South Asians entered the United States annually between 1970 and 1980, more per year than the total number of South Asians who resided in the United States during the entire period from 1904 to 1947. With increased numbers came increased diversity of social background and geographical areas from which people originated. Later immigrants were more urban and educated compared with the earlier group. Currently, Indians are the fourth largest (12%) Asian group in the United States.

For the last 30 years, immigrants have lived with the myth that all South Asians are well-educated professionals who prosper in North America. In reality, there is economic stratification, and studies contradict the "model minority" image of South Asians. Although the mean income level is relatively high because of numerous health care professionals, information technology specialists, engineers, and business owners, many South Asians drive taxis or work in assembly lines, restaurants, and personal caregiving. The level of poverty in this population is rising, particularly among female-headed households and the elderly. For example, recent legal changes have allowed poor immigrants from Bangladesh to seek refugee status based on economic and environmental disasters.

The 2000 U.S. Census counted more than 1.6 million Indians. As of 1998, there were about 585,000 Pakistanis in the United States. Some 44,000 Bangladeshis immigrated in the years 1991 to 1997. Most Indians live in the states of California, New York, New Jersey, Illinois, and Texas and the cities of New York, Chicago, Los Angeles, San Francisco, and Washington, D.C. The 1996 Canadian Census listed 723,345 South Asians, 548,080 East Indians, and 38,655 Pakistanis, of whom the great majority live in Toronto, followed by Vancouver.

### Demographics of South Asian Women in North America

South Asian women are diverse in education, language skills, occupation, and income levels. They differ in their access to education, resources, and control within families. They earn a fraction of what their male counterparts earn, and they may have little control over financial decisions. A large percentage of women engage in semi-skilled, unskilled, or homemaking labor. The levels of education and English skills are considerably lower for females than for males, and female poverty rates are higher.

There are generational differences within families and in South Asian communities. For example, those who have lived in North America for 30 years have acculturated to the dominant culture, although they still retain many of their customs and values. This generation organized social, cultural, and religious activities that connect South Asians from the same background. Second-generation children have grown up with the mix of North American ideals and South Asian values. First- and second-generation people may clash on economic, religious, social, and health issues. A third group consists of young couples who are recent arrivals from South Asia, are just starting families, and have not yet experienced years of culture shock or the North American educational systems.

> **NOTE TO THE HEALTH CARE PROVIDER**
> Providers must be aware of the ethnic, language, religious, and generational diversity of South Asians. They should begin assessment by asking where the patient grew up; when she immigrated; whether she is Hindu, Muslim, Christian, or of another faith; and her mother tongue. Providers should listen for variations in food habits, values, customs, and lifestyle patterns.

## 🌐 BEING FEMALE IN SOUTH ASIAN SOCIETY

In parts of South India, Hindus had a matriarchal system and, thus, daughters held important roles and responsibilities within the extended family. Because their history did not include gender segregation **(purdah)**, the women were relatively more independent and relaxed than other South Asians. Muslim communities, in which some degree of purdah is the norm, are strongly patriarchal, and unmarried adolescents and women are usually restricted from socializing with unrelated males. They must demonstrate extreme modesty in dress and behavior.

The female role is first and foremost that of wife and mother. The extent to which a good education and career is emphasized depends on whether the subculture is more traditional or cosmopolitan. Girls are married to well-to-do husbands in their early 20s when parents can afford it. South Asian women have held prominent political and professional positions throughout history and have demonstrated leadership roles in both the home and host societies. Examples include Rani of Jhansi (1835–1857), an Indian nationalist heroine and a symbol of Indian patriotism who fought valiantly against the British soldiers in 1857; Indira Gandhi (1917–1984), Prime Minister of India (1966–1977, 1980–1984); Benazir Bhutto, ex-Prime Minister of Pakistan (1988–1990, 1993–1996); and Chandrika Bandaranaike Kumaratanga, President of Sri Lanka (1994 to present). Despite the stereotype of women's subordination, the women's movement is very strong in India.

Indian women wear many kinds of draped clothing, as well as different kinds of pants, trousers, blouses, jackets, and long skirts in fabrics that are woven and embroidered. Their style of dress reveals geographic region, religion, and caste of origin. Modern young women wear a mix of ethnic styles: shalwar kameez, saris, mundu, western style dresses, and long pants.

South Asian women have formed organizations related to nationality, religion, domestic violence, legal needs, economic needs, and professional interests. There are referral lines providing support and advice. Immigrants came for different reasons and faced different barriers on arrival. Some women came to marry men they hardly knew, lacked a support system, and faced fear and uncertainty in new relationships. Others came as elderly widows, completely dependent on their children. Still others came as caregivers for extended family members and had to work outside the home. Another group sent their children home for their parents to look after so that they could concentrate on higher education and employment to help support immediate and extended families in North America or in their home countries. Finally, some women come to North America to work for a time to support their husbands and children in the home country.

## At Birth

### Preference for Sons

People in some castes believe in a particular type of hell, called **put,** from which only a son, **putra,** can save his parents. Almost all families wish for a male heir to continue their lineage, provide support in old age, and perform the last rites at the funeral to ensure that the parent's soul makes the journey to the home of the ancestors without difficulty. There is greater jubilation at the birth of a son than of a daughter, especially in poorer families in which boys grow up to earn money and will take responsibility for the parents until their death. Daughters are provided with a dowry and marry out of the family.

### Response to the Birth of a Female

Birth of a daughter is often met with mixed emotions. While there is excitement over the first child, after several girls, parents worry about whether they will have a son. Reservations are reflected in such statements as, "Well, we will try again, hopefully for a boy next time." The dowry system may also be a factor. Parents who have girls need to save a large sum of money and jewelry for the girls' marriages; whereas boys' marriages bring dowry into the family. Since grandparents want to see a grandson carry on the name of the family, the in-laws of a woman who fails to produce a son may respond to the woman with anger and frustration. In some communities, the husband may leave the woman and marry another to have a male child.

In some Indian villages, there have been reports of termination of pregnancies when ultrasound revealed that the woman was carrying a female fetus. While sons are especially well cared for to ensure normal growth, poverty and stress may sometimes cause neglect of female children. Infanticide or neglect or abandonment of female infants is rare, but it has been reported in one Indian state.

### Birth Rituals

South Asian Indian families openly celebrate the birth of a son, especially when the baby is born after one or more girls. Several religious rituals celebrate birth. In South India, a closely related woman who is held in high esteem gives a drop of honey mixed with gold to the baby on its tongue. In some Hindu communities, a special type of loud cry by women called **kurava** follows the birth of the baby. Beating on the ground with long poles is heard throughout the neighborhood. On the 28th day after birth, there are family celebrations to tie the waistband of gold, silver, or cotton thread on the baby. In certain castes, the child's hair is not cut until it is two or three years old, at which point the hair is cut in a temple and offered to a god. Other communities celebrate the girl's ear piercing like a wedding. Wealthy Hindus at times give their gods and goddesses gold or silver equal to the weight of the baby soon after the hair shaving or ear piercing ceremony. Some events and rituals of Jains, Buddhists, and Sikhs are similar to those of Hindus. Muslims, Christians, and Parsis have their own celebrations.

Female circumcision is not practiced. Male circumcision is mainly practiced among Muslims.

# Childhood and Youth

## Stages

Childhood is a prolonged process with no clearly delineated stages. Individuals up to their mid-teen years (13 to 15) are considered children and are expected to conduct themselves accordingly. Emphasis is on obedience to parents; respect of elders; and being courteous, caring, and polite in social and family situations. Although various languages and dialects use different words, they have separate words for children and youths. For example, in Malayalam, a child is **kutty,** and male and female adolescents are **kumari** and **kumaran**, respectively. Tamil adolescents are called **selvi** and **selvan**.

South Asians love children, as do people in most cultures. Parents often are willing to sacrifice all their comforts to provide the best education and life experiences for their children. Infants are breastfed on demand until they are 2 or 3, or even older. Children have unlimited freedom up to the age of 5 or 6, and they lead a carefree life. Babies and small children are indulged, not allowed to cry, and play without clothes, urinating wherever they like. In the context of the tradition of extended families, families in large cities without a supportive network find it difficult to allow children to grow up with the traditional comforts. The ideal of indulging children remains, however, and if economic conditions allow, small children continue to have someone—if not a grandmother, an older sibling or a servant—to take care of them.

There is no social activity from which children are excluded, and they attend even classical dances and music performances. After the age of 6, boys are still allowed considerable freedom, but girls are increasingly expected to comply with the standard of behavior considered appropriate for girls. Children in extended families have almost constant attention from the women of the household. Children are encouraged to play in groups with cousins and children from the neighborhood.

## Family Expectations

Children are not expected to become independent. They are fed, dressed, bathed, and carried by others even when they are old enough to handle these tasks by themselves. From birth until preschool, children sleep with their parents, and afterward, with their siblings, so they are rarely, if ever, alone. They learn to walk, talk, and use the toilet from watching others, quickly coming to understand and fit into the expectations and norms of the family.

Children are expected to obey and respect adults. Indian children tend to address all grown-ups as "aunty" or "uncle" because using the person's surname is considered too formal and using the first name shows lack of respect. Restricted contact between the genders in Indian groups may be very frustrating to second-generation immigrants, but it has little effect on young children. Families expect children to bring honor to the family and maintain its name and status.

## Social Expectations

Girls are brought up to follow and become the keepers of the customs and traditions. Religious traditions are very important in each community, and children are expected to participate in cultural activities and celebrations. The factors that distinguish South Asian young people are religion, race, and class, and families follow "people specific" and "region specific" codes, even in North America. Young people's socializing with each other across religious, racial, and class lines often causes family conflicts.

Girls are expected to help actively with household chores, cooking, and entertaining, among other responsibilities. Indian parents expect them to become self-supporting and independent before they get married. Muslim girls and women from Pakistan and Bangladesh are subject to stricter rules and may remain in the family until they marry. They may wear the **Burkah** to cover their head and/or body at puberty and are expected to dress modestly and not to socialize with unrelated boys. Young girls are protected, chaperoned, and not allowed to be out by themselves in the evening or night.

Girls are not prepared to cope adequately with cross-cultural issues in dating, courting, and marriage. Whether she has grown up in North America or elsewhere, a young girl is expected to be obedient and respectful to the family. She can have a successful academic, athletic, or extracurricular career, but she is also expected to help the family as needed at home. She is usually not allowed to date, although some teens date behind their parents' backs. Hiding their dating may be embarrassing because they may think that their friends view their parents as "horrible" and they may feel guilty. A young woman often plans to marry the person she dates; but if she has a sexual relationship that failed, this may cause tremendous stress and distress. Among very strict Muslims, a young woman might even be killed for bringing shame to the family through a premarital sexual relationship.

### Importance of Education

Families emphasize children's education as an investment in the future. This investment should be repaid by fulfilling obligations such as obedience and respect and making large contributions to the family economy. Parents consider education more important for boys than girls. However, the literacy rate in some states, such as Kerala in India, is almost 100%.

## Pubescence

### Psychosexual Development

Most South Asian girls reach pubescence between 12 and 15 years of age, with an average onset of menses at 13. Boys reach pubescence between 13 and 18 years of age. These averages apply even among undernourished boys and girls.

### Rituals and Rites of Passage

In several castes, there are special rituals to celebrate a girl's transition into womanhood and a boy into manhood. For example, in some areas, a girl is dressed in sari, and the family holds a celebration when she starts menstruating.

### Teenage Sexuality

There are considerable restrictions on a girl's behavior, activities, and dress once she enters pubescence. She is instructed and assisted to dress appropriately and to assume additional responsibilities at home. Although she may be expected to marry during adolescence, dating, sexual activity, and childbearing at this stage are usually considered taboo, especially for young people in upper-class families.

**Teen Pregnancy.** There are strong cultural sanctions on teen dating, sexuality, use of contraception or family planning, pregnancy, and abortion. None of these activities is approved by most South Asian families. Indeed, use of contraception before marriage, teen pregnancy, and abortion are all considered sources of shame for the family and guilt for the girl. Adoption of an unwed teenage mother's baby is unacceptable.

### Menstruation

**Relationship to Health.** The amount, type, regularity, and color of her menstrual flow are believed to demonstrate the state of a woman's health, and a change in these variables indicates a change in health. It is generally agreed that rest and relaxation are important during menstruation. Otherwise, there are different attitudes and practices among South Asians. For example, some women fear that losing a lot of blood through menstruation may adversely affect their health or strength. It is important to provide information about the anatomy and physiology of menstruation, and about proper personal hygiene during the period.

**Relationship to Fertility.** Menstruation is considered a sign of fertility. However, a woman incapable of menstruating because of a hysterectomy or other congenital medical problems is not valued less for that reason.

**Taboos and Restrictions During Menstruation.** A girl's mother or an older female in her family may teach her the folk practices when she starts menstruation, although many families do not speak freely about menstruation and sexuality. Immigrant girls usually receive information regarding menstruation in school and from their friends.

Taboos and restrictions vary with religion and the position of women in the family, or within the specific South Asian subculture. Hindus believe that menstrual blood is a source of ritual pollution, as is blood associated with childbirth. In the past, menstruating women had to retire to an outhouse **(veliku marri,** meaning "she stays outside") and three days of seclusion. Even now, in many orthodox families, a menstruating woman should not enter the kitchen, touch the salt, go to the temple, or participate in any religious ceremony. Nobody is allowed to touch her, and she sleeps outside the regular sleeping areas. Women may leave the cooking to the servant, an older daughter, or even the husband if no one else can do it. Orthodox Hindu Brahmin women who are menstruating are not even allowed to touch their family members on the first day of the cycle.

Some orthodox Hindu women take birth control pills to regulate their periods so they can take part in important ceremonies. In some communities, Hindu adolescent girls sit in a tent in the backyard for the first week. On the seventh day they are given a special ceremonial bath and taken into their homes.

Syrian Christian women from South India are discouraged from participating in church worship and religious ceremonies during menses. Muslim women follow strict cultural and religious practices during and after menstruation. According to Islamic law, blood is unclean and renders the female impure. Menstruating women are forbidden from entering a mosque, praying, or participating in the feast following Ramadan. Sexual relations are forbidden during one's period. When the flow stops, the woman performs a special ritual washing to purify herself, after which she can again participate fully in religious activities.

**Dysmenorrhea.** Missed periods, light or shortened periods, or the passage of clots are all causes for concern. Herbal and Ayurvedic treatments are used to deal with such problems. Herbal teas, tonics, oils, exercises, and hot applications are used to ease discomfort.

### Female Modesty and Touching

Female modesty is strongly emphasized. It has a basis in Islam, Hinduism, and Christianity. Women in general consider modesty, simplicity, and chastity important virtues. Touching each other in public is unusual among adults, between the sexes, and in churches and other public gatherings. Men and women are seated separately in churches and public places. Hugging and kissing takes place only between members of the immediate family. People are greeted with folded hands.

**Relationship to Health Care.** In North America, a female can be assigned to or treated by a male practitioner, although it is not appropriate in the home country. Annual pelvic examinations are not customary, and modesty may adversely affect a woman's willingness to obtain them.

---

**NOTE TO THE HEALTH CARE PROVIDER**

Cultural issues may inhibit physical contact with or touching a girl's or woman's body, even during physical, breast, and gynecologic examinations. Explain what is to occur and provide a choice of a female practitioner.

---

# Adulthood

### Transition Rites and Rituals

A young woman is considered an adult at 21 years of age. Different subcultures and castes hold different celebrations to herald adulthood. In the past, young women were married long before the age of 21, but many women now marry during their early and late 20s. Young women are often expected to seek education and employment before getting married.

### Social Expectations

Parents prefer to arrange the marriage of a daughter to a young man from a similar background. Young women, caught between the values of older family members and those of their age peers, may struggle to balance the traditional South Asian cultural practices of socializing within one's own cultural group and the North American practice of socializing freely across class, religious, and ethnic boundaries.

Young women may also be caught between the more egalitarian models of marriage in North America and the roles of women as mothers and wives who are subordinate to their husbands in traditional South Asian families. Young women have close and loyal relationships with parents and siblings and are more likely to assume responsibility for elderly or sick parents or younger siblings than other members of the family. Extended family interdependence is a strong value and young women may feel the pressures of family obligations and responsibilities for caring for family members.

### Union Formation

**Union Types.**   Parents prefer arranged marriages. Until recently, Southern Hindus favored a cousin or even a maternal uncle as the husband, so that the girl moved into a family she already knew. Her mother-in-law was also her aunt. Even though such practices are considered old-fashioned by the current generation, the relationship between the husband and wife is closer and more intimate in South India. Many young people are encouraged to meet and select suitable partners from North America or the home country through "matrimonials" (advertisements in newspapers published in their language or on the Internet) and other means of introduction.

**Social Sanctions for Failing to Enter into Union.**   Women are encouraged by parents and family to marry during their early to late 20s. They are also encouraged to be employed and financially independent before they get married. A woman who marries at an advanced age is not ridiculed or otherwise adversely affected. There is no particular word designating a woman who is single after the age of 30.

### Domestic Violence

Domestic violence is underreported. A study in Massachusetts showed that 30% of South Asian survey participants reported having experienced physical abuse, and 19% had experienced sexual abuse. Sixty-five percent of the women reporting physical abuse also reported sexual abuse.

Across the United States there are shelters and organizations with multilingual staffs offering services designed specifically for South Asian women, including immigration and legal information as well as job training resources. Most women need information on how to protect their immigrant status, as they rely on their husbands to fill out the papers. Threatening to have his wife deported is an example of the batterer's emotional abuse of his new wife. Isolation from both family and non–South Asian people based on language barriers decreases the chance of finding support and help.

South Asians consider the family the foundation of society and attempt to protect family relationships at all costs. Family members and the church leaders (in the case of Christians) will try to counsel the couple to settle their disputes. In extreme cases the woman will take shelter with her parents, brother, or relatives. Domestic violence is often seen as a disgrace to the family. It is a family secret that is not often shared with others. Therefore, women who are abused are unlikely to report it to the authorities.

### Rape

There are no statistical data on the incidence of rape in South Asian communities, although sexual assault is prevalent among girls and married women. These societies view rape as a crime of anger and retaliation by the man who is responsible. Women are supported and assisted by family members in the crisis, but many do not tell their families until pregnancy is detected. Pregnancy may be terminated through abortion, or adoption may be arranged through agencies. Many South Asian college students experience date rape or rape by boyfriends, involving both Indian and non-Indian young men.

Listen non-judgmentally, and screen all patients for violence in their intimate relationships. Ask the woman directly whether she is safe in her relationship, beginning the interview with, "Because violence is so common, I ask these questions of all my patients." The woman may not disclose a violent relationship during the first visit, but she may do so when she trusts you. Assure her that the violence is not her fault. Talk to her alone, do not ask questions if the husband or boyfriend is present, and do not allow a family member to interpret. Help the woman with plans for immediate safety or refer her to services. Report to the police only with the woman's consent or pursuant to state law. Respect and be sensitive to the preferences and wishes of the woman and family.

### Divorce

**Sociocultural Views.** The word for divorce in Malayalam is **vivaha mochanam,** and it is **vivaharathi** in Tamil. In South Asian subcultures, divorce or separation is strongly stigmatized, particularly for women. Economic difficulties may also discourage women from seeking divorce even though they are in abusive or unhappy relationships. Catholics do not accept divorce, and divorced Catholics cannot remarry in the church.

The rate of divorce has increased among Christians in their home countries, although it used to be unheard of among South Asian Christians. With increasing mobility among South Asians, marriages have weakened. The stabilizing influence of extended family on young families is also lacking. Divorces are also more frequent among South Asians in North America.

**Women and Divorce.** Divorced women are viewed negatively. The individual is not blamed, but the family may be considered dysfunctional. It is much more difficult to arrange remarriage for a divorced woman. The acceptable time for remarrying varies with individuals and families.

**Child Custody Practices.** Since divorce is rare in South Asian countries, some men may be inclined to abandon their families, move on, and establish new families. South Asians in North America abide by court decisions regarding child custody, which is often given to the mother. The father is expected to provide financial support and to participate actively in his children's upbringing.

## Fertility and Childbearing

**Family Size.**   In the past, large families were typical, but family size has decreased with the availability of contraceptive technology. For example, some women plan on being sterilized after three children. Employment of women outside the home and higher education for women also contributed to this change. The goal for India was to reach 2.5 children per family. In many areas this goal has been met. In North America, the family size of South Asians is usually two or three children.

**Contraceptive Practices.**   In the past, some women had to undergo sterilization or accept a specific type of contraceptive technique. Today, contraceptives are available to and used by most married women who want to control the number of pregnancies. However, Catholics may experience restrictions. Muslims are also restricted from using contraceptives because one "should not stop or deny what Allah provides." The use of contraceptives is slowly increasing in Bangladesh, in which use increased from 8% in 1986 to 54% in 2000, and in Pakistan, in which use increased from 5% in 1975 to 18% in 1994. Women generally do not use local or indigenous methods of contraception, preferring the biomedical or other modern contraceptives.

---

**NOTE TO THE HEALTH CARE PROVIDER**
Explore the client's understanding, feelings, and fears regarding the use of contraceptives in a culturally sensitive manner. Provide sufficient explanation and teaching as to the use, advantages, disadvantages, and related precautions of each method to help the woman make an informed decision. Make the services of an interpreter available, if necessary.

---

**Role of the Male in the Couple's Decision-Making.**   Decisions about fertility and type of contraception are most often made by the woman with her health care provider. If there are specific concerns after this decision, the husband may be included. Because of the availability of effective female methods of contraception, males may not be receptive to the use of condoms.

## Abortion

**Cultural Attitudes.**   Abortions are viewed negatively by most South Asians. Abortion was not legalized until the 1970s, so therapeutic abortions were not performed on a regular basis. Many women, especially those who are college educated, believe it is a woman's right to have a safe abortion. Christians do not accept abortions, even when recommended as an alternative.

In North America, women seek abortion in cases of unwanted pregnancies on rare occasions, such as for accidental pregnancy, but abortion is not prevalent. It is highly unlikely that abortion will be used as an additional form of birth control.

**Teen Abortion.**   Teen abortions are infrequently performed in North America. While some pregnant teens use abortion, the community is generally negative about this choice.

**Sources of Abortions.** There are no legal or professionally run abortion clinics in South Asian counties. Therefore, women resort to unskilled practitioners who use herbs and native medicinal leaves to stimulate labor, as well as rods and crude instruments to abort the fetus. South Asian immigrant groups in North America do not use these methods.

**Complications.** There is a high incidence of abortion-related complications and death reported in women after illegal abortions in the home country, because of infection, perforation, shock, and bleeding. Abortion is likely to be sought late in pregnancy because of delay in confirming the pregnancy. In North America, women can test for pregnancy very early, and safe and legal abortion services are available.

## Miscarriage

Miscarriages may be seen as being due to spells, punishment from God, or other unexplainable causes. Women who habitually miscarry are treated with extra care and receive medical consultation. The condition causes a great deal of sorrow for both the couple and the extended family. Pregnancy is an important event, and prevention of miscarriages or other complications is a priority of women and their families. If there is any sign of bleeding, women take such precautions as staying in bed.

## Infertility

Infertility is a cause for concern for the couple and their family. It may be viewed as punishment for sins or a curse on an individual or family. Most communities support an infertile woman, and she will not be publicly ostracized. However, she may be considered an ill omen in the community. The term for an infertile woman in the Malayalam language is **machi,** and it is not a derogatory term. In Tamil, a barren woman is called **maladi.**

The husband usually treats his infertile wife with love and care. However, some husbands or family members may treat the woman with contempt, depending on the individuals concerned and the cultural group. Questions regarding heirs to the family's land and wealth may cause additional tension for the woman and within the family. The wealth will usually be divided among other brothers or sisters who have children.

In North America, South Asians will seek medical intervention for infertility.

## Pregnancy

**Activity Restrictions and Taboos.** Pregnant women are treated with special consideration and respect. South Asians consider pregnancy, birth, and the immediate postpartum period as a time of great vulnerability for women and their newborns. Therefore, women are carefully watched and protected by their mothers or older relatives. They are advised not to lift heavy objects, stand for long periods, or work outside the home; and they are encouraged to get as much rest as possible. They are expected to avoid exposure to uncomfortable events; activities that exhaust them; strong emotions such as fear, anxiety, and anger; and places where evil spirits might be present. Some believe that the developing fetus may be affected by encounters with deformed or disabled people or specific animals that frighten the woman during pregnancy. During the third trimester (seventh month), a pregnant woman usually returns to her mother's residence to be cared for in a special way to prepare for delivery and for special care during labor, delivery, and the postpartum period.

**Dietary Practices and Observances.** Pregnant women receive Ayurvedic medicines **(lehiam)**, tonics, herbal medicines, and health food items. Medicinal oils are used to massage the body to strengthen the body systems for safe delivery. Some women are advised (by older women) that healthy food may increase the size of the baby and cause difficult labor.

Pica (eating non-food items) is uncommon, but there are reports of women eating raw rice, raw flour, and clay during pregnancy. Women may crave and demand food items that are quite uncommon, and they are not prevented from eating anything they desire. In the belief that the woman or baby may be harmed if the cravings are not satisfied, the husband or family members try to satisfy the cravings.

**Prenatal Care.** Women receive prenatal care from health care providers of the Western medical system. Hindus have a special ritual for pregnant women in either the seventh or ninth month of their pregnancies, called **valaikappu.** In other groups, there are no special rituals before delivery, but women rest and relax in preparation for delivery. They take oil baths and have massages during the few weeks before delivery. These practices do not conflict with the practices of mainstream health care in North America.

---

**NOTE TO THE HEALTH CARE PROVIDER**

Some women and their partners regard prenatal classes and exercises as being unfamiliar and unnecessary. Be prepared to provide detailed information regarding the benefits of health supervision and participation in prenatal classes, if needed.

---

## Birthing Process

**Home Versus Hospital Delivery.** Traditionally, South Asian women delivered at home under the supervision of lay midwives and family members. Currently, in both home countries and North America, women deliver in hospitals.

**Cesarean Section Versus Vaginal Delivery.** In the past, vaginal deliveries were most common, assisted by midwives or untrained individuals, except in very difficult labors, during which women were taken to the hospital and delivery was assisted with instruments or surgery. However, there is a trend toward hospital and cesarean delivery over the past few years encouraged by the increase in the number of hospitals and adequately prepared health care professionals. Women usually prefer to be relieved of pain and discomfort during labor, so they are willing to resort to pain medications and anesthesia, if necessary. However, they are very particular about the safety of the baby, and if the baby's health may be affected by anesthesia, they are apt to forgo it.

**Involvement of the Male Partner.** Traditionally, fathers were not involved in the labor and delivery process. The woman's mother and female relatives assisted with labor and delivery. More recently, in both North America and the home country, husbands have become more actively involved in assisting and supporting their wives during the delivery.

**Labor Management.** Women are encouraged to walk about during early labor. They are usually cared for and deliver in bed after rupture of the membrane. In case of postmature pregnancies, labor is stimulated.

**Placenta.**   Traditionally, the placenta or "afterbirth" is carefully examined for intact delivery and is then buried. In hospitals, the placenta is buried in a designated area or is incinerated with other waste. It is believed that harm will come to the mother and baby if the placenta is left outside for animals or birds to touch. The blood and all associated products of the birth are disposed of similarly. It is also believed by some that the placenta will protect the mother and baby from evil spirits. South Asians in North America do not believe in or follow these practices.

### Postpartum

The postpartum period is 56 days among Syrian Christians of South India. After delivery, the woman is put on a special schedule of ceremonial oil baths every morning: The water is boiled and cooled with special medicinal leaves **(vedu).** Women eat special diets prepared at home with Ayurvedic medicines, herbs, and ghee (clarified butter). Special spices are used as ingredients to cool the body and shrink the stomach. The woman's mother is responsible for supervising and providing care for the 56 days.

Women believe that their future health and strength depend on strict compliance with all the prescribed routines. There are times during the postpartum period when the woman is not allowed to drink water because of the types of medicines ingested. She is not allowed to go out of the room or visit with too many people during postpartum. The baby is brought out of the room by the grandmother for visitors to view for a few minutes, and it is then returned to the mother. The husband and his family pay ceremonial visits to see the mother and baby during this time. There are expectations as to what each family should bring for the mother and baby; examples are sweets, gold or silver items, and clothes.

At the conclusion of the postpartum period, the woman is given a strong laxative to rid her body of the baby's hair and nails left inside and also to cleanse her body of all impurities. After 56 days the mother and baby return to the husband's home, with attendant rituals and ceremonies associated with the return. These practices vary among different groups of South Asians.

### Newborn and Infant Care

**Breastfeeding Versus Bottle-Feeding.**   Breastfeeding, the only method for centuries, is still the preferred method of infant feeding. More recently, however, women are selecting bottle-feeding for convenience, especially when they work outside the home, and some women believe that bottle-fed babies are healthier than breastfed babies. Some women avoid certain foods that they believe will cause the baby to be colicky. Traditional and folk remedies for colic include herbal medicines and homeopathic medicines such as *senna* to ease the discomfort.

**Infant Protection.**   In the past, risky practices for newborns included covering the umbilical cord with cow dung to dry it, which could cause infection and death. Modern women in South Asia and North America are aware of the importance of immunizations for children. They have their baby's growth and development monitored on a regular basis by health care personnel.

Many South Asian women believe in the evil eye **(kannu vachu),** which causes sudden sickness in the infant, such as fever, vomiting, or diarrhea, or the infant's sudden fall that causes injury or even death. The belief that someone can project harm by gazing or staring at another person or his or her property persists among newer immigrants in North America and those who maintain a strong ethnic heritage. Traditional preventive practices include protective objects or substances worn, carried, or hung in the home; religious rituals such as burning candles and offering prayers; and amulets (charms) worn on a string or chain around the neck, wrist, or waist to protect the wearer. Amulets may be worn for luck or to prevent evil or the evil eye. One method of removing the effects of the evil eye is massaging the whole body of the infant with leaves of a certain plant **(panal),** during which the person doing the massage should not talk to anyone.

---

**NOTE TO THE HEALTH CARE PROVIDER**
Provide information and reminders about scheduled immunizations. Do not remove amulets or other substances placed on the infant to prevent the evil eye.

---

**Primary Caregiver.**   The mother is the primary caregiver for infants and toddlers. Fathers usually do not contribute significantly to childcare, although extended family members, if available, will assist with it. South Asian women in North America usually bring the parents of the husband or wife from the home country to assist with childcare. They are very reluctant to leave children with babysitters. The baby may sleep with the parents, be picked up anytime it cries, and be fed on demand, all of which are usual practices.

---

**NOTE TO THE HEALTH CARE PROVIDER**
When giving care to a newborn, be very familiar with the cultural practices and preferences regarding newborn care. For example, babies may be given additional food at stages that may conflict with the recommendations of Western health care providers. Verify the parents' understanding of dietary needs of infants and newborn care to prevent conflicts.

---

# Middle Age

## Cultural Attitudes and Expectations

Women are considered middle-aged or at mid-life between 45 and 65 years of age. There are no socially sanctioned behavioral or clothing restrictions. However, middle-aged women are expected to demonstrate a high level of maturity and modesty and efficiency in management and leadership in whatever they are responsible for. Their clothing will conform to the religious and social traditions of the community. They are expected to set an example for the younger generation with their behavior.

## Psychological Response

The "empty-nest" syndrome is not relevant in South Asian cultures because of the extended family system. Mid-life women may live with their married son, daughter-in-law, and grandchildren without any difficulty. On the whole, they are not lonely because they maintain close connections with relatives and immediate family. The concept of "mid-life crisis" is also uncommon and is not significant in this culture. Middle-aged women are respected, and they share responsibilities of the family. They usually feel important and needed.

Menopause

**Onset and Duration.**   There is no specific word for menopause, other than its description. The age range for onset is 45 to 55 years of age. Early or late menopause is atypical unless there are associated pathologic conditions.

**Sexual Activity.**   Menopause does not affect a woman's sexuality. Sexual relations continue during and after menopause. Hormone replacement therapy (HRT) may be used to keep hormones in balance and prevent problems in sexual activity.

**Coping.**   Most women generally cope with this life transition without difficulty. The extended family is of assistance in dealing with any problems. Hot flashes and emotional changes are usually not serious issues among South Asian women. The symptoms are usually ignored if they are not very serious. Herbal remedies and Ayurvedic treatments are available. HRT is also used by some women to deal with the problem.

---

**NOTE TO THE HEALTH CARE PROVIDER**
South Asian women are not familiar with HRT. Thoroughly explain its advantages and disadvantages to help the client make an informed decision. Potential drug interactions of HRT with herbs taken for menopause are also not clearly understood.

---

# Old Age

## Cultural Attitudes

Genetic factors, poor nutrition and health habits, chronic illnesses, and stress influence life expectancy, which in India is 63.4 years for men, 64.3 years for women. A woman is usually considered old at 80 years of age, although 70 is considered old by some women.

Elderly women are revered and respected and viewed as a source of wisdom in the community. Elderly and widowed women usually live with adult children and grandchildren or other members of the extended family. Family members care for them if they are unable to care for themselves. This tradition has changed in recent years as sons and daughters have moved to urban areas or to other countries. As a result, many elderly in the home country are being looked after by personnel in rest homes or other institutions managed by churches or private organizations. In North America, first-generation South Asians are reaching old age and are faced with the challenges of obtaining assistance from appropriate sources. In addition, some elderly have difficulty obtaining services because of decreased mobility, limited English, and economic constraints. Most of the elderly are looked after by children and families.

# Death and Dying

## Cultural Attitudes and Beliefs

Beliefs regarding death and dying are based on religion. For example, Buddhists believe that illness is inevitable and a consequence of actions taken during both this life and previous lives. Death is accepted as a peaceful movement into the next existence in the presence of loving family and friends. Some South Asians believe that such omens as a crow bathing in water or a message in a dream warn of approaching death. Breaking a taboo may also be believed to cause death. For example, entering a Hindu temple area and spitting on the grounds may anger the spirit and cause an individual's death. Muslims from Bangladesh and Pakistan rely on daily prayers, including reciting verses from the *Quran*, when illness strikes. A religious authority or older relative may write selected Quranic verses on a small piece of paper that is placed in a small cloth or metallic necklace **(taweez)** worn around the neck or upper arm. Bengalis may sacrifice a goat, called **chadka,** to thank Allah for helping someone recover from illness or for divine assistance in healing. Divine intervention may also be sought by praying at a **majar** (holy place, usually a burial site).

The type of death also has an impact on its meaning. Suicide shames the individual and the entire family. Christianity prohibits suicide, even to the point of denying a Christian burial in the church cemetery. Suicide is strictly forbidden under Islamic law. Sudden, untimely, or violent death, and death during childbirth, are considered bad deaths that disturb the individual's spiritual balance. Death from cancer is as accepted as death from any other disease. The death of an elderly woman is accepted as natural and expected. However, the death of a mid-life or younger woman who leaves her spouse and young children behind is viewed as a crisis situation.

---

**NOTE TO THE HEALTH CARE PROVIDER**
Family members assist a mortally ill patient, taking turns in keeping vigil. South Asians may try to protect the dying person by not disclosing the seriousness of his or her condition, thus preventing the experience of shock and panic for the individual. They may expect the practitioner to do the same.

---

Rites and Rituals

Funeral homes and mortuaries are unfamiliar to South Asians, and they may need support and explanations about North American customs. A few will accompany the coffin to the homeland to bury the dead relative next to his or her ancestors. Many immigrants adhere to their traditional customs of same-gender family and friends washing and preparing the body for burial.

Different religious groups have different practices. South Indian Christians wash the body, wrap it in the wedding sari with the head covered with the end of the sari, and leave the gold wedding pendant with the cross **(minnu)** tied around the neck as it was tied during the wedding ceremony. The body is faced toward the east, and candles and a cross are put at the head of the bed for viewing the day before the funeral. The family and friends gather for hymns, reading the Bible, meditation, and prayer. A priest conducts the funeral service at home. Family members and friends then join in a procession to the church for another service before the body is buried in a homemade, unadorned coffin, followed by dinner or refreshments in the home.

Among Hindus, there are different caste-related rituals, and various family members and religious officials have special duties in preparing the body for cremation. The son lights the pyre on which the deceased is cremated. One ritual is spreading the ashes over the waters of the holy river Ganges so that the soul can attain Nirvana. The Hindu religion emphasizes Karma, in which the person's life after death takes on other forms of life to finally reach Brahma, the ultimate reality.

### Mourning

In the more relaxed life pace in South Asian countries, the mourning period is extended according to the individual situation. The spouse and family members wear white or other plain-colored clothing, and make-up is not worn for several days. South Indian Orthodox Christians offer prayers in memory of the deceased every year on the anniversary date. On the 40th day after the death, the family invites relatives and friends for a service and dinner in memory of the person.

**Coping.** Extended family members stay with the family to assist in dealing with death and mourning, often filling the family roles and easing the trauma of bereavement and economic pressures for the family. The surviving spouse is encouraged to express anguish and grief openly and is given the time to talk about the experience and reminisce about the couple's life together. He or she is also helped to plan for the future of the family, such as educating the children, finding work if the individual has not been working, or sometimes assisting the individual to move in with parents or other immediate family. Patterns of coping with death, as well as the resources available to the bereaved for coping, depend on the educational and socioeconomic background of the bereaved.

Custody of children, in the case of the mother's death, is decided on by the father, both sets of grandparents, and immediate relatives. The father and the paternal grandparents usually take responsibility for the children, but in some instances the maternal grandparents and uncles assume this responsibility.

---

**NOTE TO THE HEALTH CARE PROVIDER**
Encourage women to express their grief openly, when necessary. They will often seek a family member or clergy for support in times of bereavement. The stress of caring for a sick person and later losing him or her may render the surviving relative or partner vulnerable to illness or psychosomatic symptoms if she does not go through the normal grief process. Be aware of differences in culture-related practices in mourning.

---

## IMPORTANT POINTS FOR HEALTH PROVIDERS CARING FOR SOUTH ASIAN WOMEN

### The Medical Intake

#### Literacy and English Proficiency

In 1990, 75% of the South Asian residents in the United States spoke a language other than English at home, but one study showed that women do not speak less English than do men. Family members are likely to accompany women to a clinic to assist with translation, when necessary, and many women prefer a family member to an interpreter.

---

**NOTE TO THE HEALTH CARE PROVIDER**
Assess how the client speaks English to see if an interpreter is needed, but be aware that clients with strong accents may speak very good English.

---

## Status of the Provider

Health care providers, particularly physicians, are afforded high status and respect in most situations. Women are generally shy, modest, non-verbal, and passive, and they refrain from making direct eye contact with unrelated men, including health care providers. However, the behavior will vary according to the educational, socioeconomic, and religious background of the individual. Some women listen to the provider and follow recommendations based on this respect, while women who are well informed and confident may question recommendations.

## Communicating Illness and Symptoms

Accompanying family members typically participate in providing information. Confidentiality is less prominent in South Asian families because the extended family is expected to share the responsibility for the health care of its members. Due to lack of familiarity with the health-care system, not knowing the significance of the information, shyness, or lack of English or knowledge of anatomic terminology, less acculturated women may not volunteer significant medical history information, current symptoms, or home remedies that they have taken. Some examples are excessive bleeding during or between periods, a lump in the breast, and constipation. However, educated and acculturated women will usually not hesitate to provide the necessary information.

Use open-ended and culturally sensitive questions to obtain information about sexual history, home remedies, and family violence. Questions that women consider offensive are influenced by the woman's religious, educational, and socioeconomic background. Sexual matters are considered private by most women, and they are more comfortable discussing such matters with the provider than with their family members. Giving detailed introduction and having a female provider will be helpful. For example, saying, "I ask this of all my patients, we are concerned about your health, I am going to ask you this about. . .stop me if it is inappropriate."

Women may give elaborate explanations or tell lengthy stories to explain their illness, including, in rare cases, spiritual causes or symptoms (e.g., breaking taboos or a pledge to a religious saint). Healing also may be explained as being due to faith or related to rituals and practices associated with different castes. As routine breast and pelvic examinations are not common in South Asia, the provider needs to inquire sensitively about past examinations.

## The Physical Examination

### Modesty and Touching

Modesty and covering the female body are major issues. Women cover their bodies from neck to foot with long drapes or trousers and blouses. It may take longer than normal for a woman to undress and dress. It is essential that some women (e.g., traditional Muslim women) be seen by a female health care provider. South Asian women are not used to being touched by a non-family member, so do not touch her except during a physical examination or in the course of nursing care. Avoid touching or exposing private parts of the body except during gynecologic or breast examinations. The health care provider needs to explain the procedures and their purposes to the woman very clearly before initiating the examination. Having a female family member present will be helpful; allow the family member to be present during screening.

### Expressing Pain

Complaining may be perceived as a sign of weakness or as eliciting the disapproval of the health care provider. Women are generally quiet when in pain and do not loudly complain or demand relief. Some women will wait until the pain becomes intolerable to ask for help, but others, whose tolerance level is low, will demand relief of pain without waiting.

## Prescribing Medications

### Drug Interactions

Women may use herbal teas and roots for medicinal purposes. They may be unaware of the possibilities of drug interactions or overdosing with prescribed medications. Therefore, the use of herbal medicines may not be relayed to the healthcare provider.

### Medication Sharing

Some women may share leftover medications with family members or friends. They may take medications prescribed by other health care providers without the knowledge of current practitioners and, depending on education level, they may be unwilling to share this information with the current practitioner.

## Compliance

Take a comprehensive health history, including a checklist of medications, to identify potential compliance problems. The problem will vary according to the educational and socioeconomic levels of the individual. There may be a tendency for
clients not to complete the full course of prescribed medications, discontinuing the
medication either when the symptoms disappear or when they do not disappear after a day of two following initiation of the treatment. Health teaching about the importance of medication and treatment compliance may well be needed.

## Follow-up Appointments

It is typical to keep follow-up medical appointments, even when women feel better.
However, appointments are sometimes cancelled if there are problems with transportation, illness in the family, inclement weather, or the like. It is helpful to call the
day before the appointment to remind the patient, and to encourage the woman to
bring her family members.

### Orientation to Time

Time orientation depends on the situation, and it can have a past, present, or future
orientation. Some South Asians tend not to use clock time for social activities, and
they are rarely "punctual" in the North American sense. However, men and women
are generally punctual in work and health care or other appointments. Providing detailed information about follow-up visits, written materials that reinforce the information, and telephone calls to remind the patient will help.

## Prevalent Diseases

South Asians are hospitalized for heart disease more than any other Asian immigrant group, and coronary artery disease is three times the general U.S. rate. Mortality from coronary artery disease is greater in South Asian women compared with
women of other ethnic backgrounds. High blood pressure, high serum total cholesterol level, cigarette smoking, high fat diet, and obesity fail to explain this high
prevalence of heart disease entirely, although low HDL cholesterol and high triglyc-
erides, LDL cholesterol, and lipoprotein (a), along with a genetic predisposition for
insulin resistance and hypertension, may be responsible.

There is a high prevalence of type 2 diabetes, which is related to a genetic propen-
sity to insulin resistance, as well as abdominal obesity, in Asian Indians. Gestational
diabetes is higher in immigrant women, especially Asian Indians. Breast cancer in
Pakistani women in Karachi is more prevalent than in any other Asians; in men, lung
cancer is the most frequent malignancy. Karachi also has the highest incidence of
larynx cancer in males in Asia; mouth, throat, and larynx cancer are high in both men
and women.

Stress-related disorders or mental health problems may be associated with low
self-esteem, lack of support in the new environment, physical isolation, lack of language or job skills, and financial obligations to local and extended family members
in the home country. A patriarchal family system expects women to place low priority on their own needs and focus on the needs of the family, including extended

family members. Multiple caregiving roles, doing all the housework, and employment outside the home can put enormous pressure on immigrant women, leading to depression, anxiety, and stress.

---

**NOTE TO THE HEALTH CARE PROVIDER**

Mental illness, believed to be hereditary, is a source of shame and denial, and may create problems for marriages. Seeking help for psychiatric problems is usually a last resort and is done only when problems are severe. Treatment may be sought from religious gurus, mullahs, or other indigenous healers. Use great care when mentioning diagnoses and making referrals. A patient might agree to treatment by a family physician or psychologist in a primary care setting, but will refuse a referral to a psychiatrist or mental health clinic because of the stigma involved. Involve the woman's family members and friends by providing information and support.

---

## Health-Seeking Behaviors

Health-care-seeking behavior of South Asians depends on their education, language skills, employment, and health insurance coverage. Younger women tend to seek medical attention at the first sign of illness, but some wait until the disease process is advanced. They may consult family members and friends, and they may try known family remedies until the condition worsens. In general, South Asians have great faith in Western biomedicine.

Ethnic and folk healers are not prominent, although people may seek Ayurvedic and homeopathic treatment. Some may visit India to undergo Ayurvedic treatment at a famous center (Kottackal) in South India, which is especially effective for arthritis and other musculoskeletal conditions. The treatments include mud therapy; massage; oils condensed from herbs, leaves, and roots; tonics; powders; teas; and other preparations. These are prescribed for joint and muscle pains, jaundice, swelling of the extremities, tonsillitis, lung conditions, anemia, postpartum period, and heart ailments. There are also Ayurvedic treatments for cancer. In North America, homeopathy is popular for all illnesses, particularly skin conditions and systemic illnesses.

Taking care of one's health is holistic and includes exercise, eating well, reducing stress, and striving for balance in one's life. In a study of Indian immigrants in three counties in California, 27% were vegetarians, 59% experienced a weight increase, and 74% did not exercise regularly. Health teaching is important to promote effective health seeking behaviors for South Asian women.

## ⊕ BIBLIOGRAPHY

Ahmed, S. M., & Lemkau, J. P. (2000). Cutural issues in the primary care of South Asians. *Journal of Immigrant Health*, 2(2), 89–96.

Emerging Communities. (1996, January). A health needs assessment of South Asian women in three California counties: Alameda, Santa Clara, Sutter. National Asian Women's Health Organization.

Koland, G. (1994). *Culture shock! India. A guide to customs and etiquette.* Portland, OR: Graphic Arts Center Publishing.

Massachusetts Department of Public Health. (2000, June). *Refugees and Immigrants in Massachusetts 2000: An Overview of Selected Communities*. Boston: Office of Refugee and Immigrant Health Bureau of Family and Community Health.

Spector, R. E. (2000). *Cultural diversity in health and illness*, 4th ed. Norfolk, CT/San Mateo, CA: Appleton & Lange.

# CHAPTER 19

# Vietnamese

## THU T. NOWAK, MS, RN

### INTRODUCTION

## Who are the Vietnamese People?

Vietnam, a country of 127,330 square miles with a population of more than 75 million people, is located at the southeastern corner of the Asian mainland along the South China Sea. It has rugged mountains, coastal and lowland plains, and tropical forests. Its recorded history is more than 2000 years. In 1954, the Geneva Accords divided the country into the Communist north and the non-Communist south.

Vietnamese are a Mongolian racial group closely related to the Chinese. Their skin varies from pale ivory to dark brown, and they are typically of small size (adult women average 5 feet and weigh 80 to 100 pounds), with almond-shaped eyes, sparse body hair, and dry earwax. Not all people from Vietnam are ethnically Vietnamese. Many refugees who came to North America from Vietnam after 1975 are Chinese, Hmong, or other highland minorities, having their own languages, cultures, and special needs. Most Vietnamese are Buddhists, and about 5% are Christian, mostly Catholic.

Ethnic Vietnamese speak a single polytonal language, with northern, central, and southern dialects that can be mutually understood. Most words are single syllable, although a hyphen sometimes joins two words to form a new word. Although the grammar is simple, non-Vietnamese find pronunciation difficult because each vowel can be spoken in five or six tones that may completely change the meaning of a word.

Vietnamese is written in the Roman alphabet. Some common terms are *ong* (form of address equivalent to Mr.), *ba* (used to address older and/or married women), *co* (used to address young women), *cam on* (thank you), *xin* (please), *chao* (used in combination with a name or form of address to express greeting), *manh gioi* (how are you), and *khong* (no).

Many Vietnamese learned at least rudimentary English during the American military presence (1960 to 1975), and many are studying it today. Most Vietnamese who came to the United States in the first large refugee wave in 1975, or who had arrived previously, either knew English or learned it soon after arrival in the United States. Most of those in subsequent waves of immigration, which generally represented lower socioeconomic groups, did not know English, and some still have not learned it.

## Vietnamese in North America

Approximately 1,200,000 Vietnamese are now in the United States. The largest populations are in California and Texas, with the highest numbers in Los Angeles, San Francisco, Houston, Dallas, and San Diego. Another 140,000 Vietnamese live in Canada, nearly half of them in Ontario. There are many more men and teens and young adults than women, elderly people, and small children in the population. About 30% of those in North America are Catholic.

Vietnamese came to North America in four waves of immigration. At the end of the Vietnam War in 1975, people closely associated with the American-supported South Vietnamese or who otherwise feared retribution from the winning Communist side were admitted as refugees. A second refugee wave began a few years later, as people became disenchanted with Communism and falling standards of living. That period also saw deteriorating relations between Vietnam and China and consequent antagonism toward the Chinese minority, who joined the exodus. A third wave of immigration started in 1979 with creation of the Orderly Departure Program, which provided safe and legal exit for Vietnamese seeking to reunite with family members already in North America. The fourth wave was based on programs to bring in former South Vietnamese military officers and other political detainees. Most recently, the Amerasian Homecoming Act of 1987 provided for the entry of the children of American servicemen and Vietnamese women and their close relatives. Since arrival in North America, there has been some secondary migration, especially a tendency to move to the West coast.

Vietnamese immigrants experienced dissimilarity of culture, absence of local family or relatives to offer initial support, and a negative identification with the unpopular Vietnam War. Many Vietnamese are involuntary immigrants. Their expatriation was unexpected and unplanned, and their departure precipitous and often tragic. Escape attempts, especially during the second wave of immigration, were typically long, harrowing, and, for up to half of those involved, fatal. Survivors often were placed in squalid refugee camps for periods of up to seven years.

Some refugees considered their journey to the West as only temporary and planned to return when conditions improved. Few have actually done so. Despite some problems of adjustment, most see the opportunity for a better life in North America than in their home country. Although arranged marriages are now rare, many young men have made temporary visits to Vietnam to find a wife of their own choosing. Some people still visualize spending their old age back in Vietnam, or at least plan to have their ashes returned there.

## ⊕ BEING FEMALE IN VIETNAMESE SOCIETY

The traditional Vietnamese family is strictly patriarchal. A woman's primary traditional role is to continue the family by giving birth and rearing young. The trauma of dislocation and drastic lifestyle changes in North America, however, have challenged that role. A father may no longer be the undisputed head of the household, and the parents' authority may be undermined. Immigrant families frequently experience role reversals, with women or children adapting more easily than men do to the Western workplace and becoming the primary providers, thus gaining increased authority. In established families, a woman still is expected to be a wife and mother, but she is often expected to have a career outside the home as well.

These challenges, together with centuries of war, migration, and frequent loss of male family members, may have resulted in a tendency for Vietnamese women to be more self-reliant and independent of men than are women of other Asian cultures.

Vietnamese have joined wholeheartedly in pursuit of the North American dream, with recognition of the importance of good education and jobs. Many women have seized the opportunity to attain equal rights and a major role in controlling family decisions.

## At Birth

### Preference for Sons

Traditionally, and even now in Vietnam itself, there is a preference for male children, at least the first born. If a woman has only daughters, she may consider herself a failure. Families in North America are placing less and less emphasis on birth sequence, though there remains a desire to try to have at least one son.

### Response to the Birth of a Female

A family with only female children may be viewed socially as less meritorious than others. The father is unlikely to totally abandon his family, but he may seek another woman with whom he can have sons. Infanticide or total abandonment of a female child is unknown. Severe disregard or neglect of daughters is rare and does not normally occur among Vietnamese in North America.

### Birth Rituals

There sometimes may be prayers of gratitude following a birth and, at times, prayers for a boy the next time. Traditionally, neither sex is circumcised, but male children now may be circumcised if recommended by a doctor for health reasons.

## Childhood and Youth

### Stages

Childhood is long, with no definite stages. The general word for child is **con.** Small children are **con nit** or **tre con.** Parents, however, may use the word **con,** as well as other terms indicating a parent-child relationship, well into their children's adulthood. Teenagers are **vi thanh nien,** and passage into maturity (at 18 to 21 years of age) is **truong thanh.**

### Family Expectations.

Vietnamese children are prized and valued because they carry the family lineage. For the first two years, they are primarily cared for by their mothers; thereafter, their grandmothers and others take on much of the responsibility. Traditionally, children are expected to be obedient and devoted to their parents, their identity being an extension of the parents. Children are obliged to do everything possible to please their parents while they are alive and to worship their memory after death. The eldest son is usually responsible for rituals honoring the departed.

### Social Expectations

Young people are expected to continue to respect their elders and to avoid behavior that might dishonor the family. For boys, emphasis is on achieving success in education and career development. For girls, traditional emphasis is on avoiding premarital sex and pregnancy and learning to serve the family. American Vietnamese are beginning to make less of a distinction of those roles.

### Importance of Education

A good education always has been important in Vietnam, even for girls. Illiteracy is not common in either sex. Parents now expect their children to achieve a higher education than they did. In North America, especially, parents place great pressure on children of both genders to advance in education.

## Pubescence

### Psychosexual Development

The term for a pubescent girl is *day thi,* and that for an adolescent is *thieu nien.* There is little gender difference in age of pubescence. The average age of puberty in girls was 14 to 16 in Vietnam, with breast development at around 13 to 14 years of age and menstruation shortly thereafter. Mainly because of nutritional differences, however, Vietnamese girls born in North America are now developing breasts as early as 9 to 10 years of age and starting menstruation at 13 to 14.

### Rituals and Rites of Passage

No special traditional rituals are associated with passage of either sex into adulthood.

### Teen Sexuality

**Social Restrictions and Pressures.** Traditionally, a young girl is expected to be modest in behavior and conservative in dress, assuring that most of her body is covered. To this day in Vietnam, the standard garment for a girl, the *ao dai,* exposes only the head, hands, and feet. Contact with boys is highly limited, though an annual village celebration, the *cung dinh,* allows formal interaction between the sexes. Such traditions are changing in North America, the extent depending largely on the will of the parents.

Social pressure is considerable for a young girl to marry. Indeed, it was normal in Vietnam for marriages to be arranged well before pubescence. Arranged marriages are now declining and are very rare in North America.

**Teen Pregnancy.** In general, the Vietnamese culture opposes teenage dating, any display of sexuality, and contraception. Pregnancy in an unmarried teenager and abortion are loathed. In Vietnam, however, acceptance of family planning is growing. In North America it has become normal, if not fully acceptable, for teenage girls to date and to wear clothing exposing much of the body.

### Menstruation

**Relationship to Health.**   A clean, regular, and abundant menstrual flow is considered a favorable omen and good for the health.

**Relationship to Fertility.**   A good menstrual flow signifies fertility and improves a woman's status. If she undergoes a hysterectomy or otherwise becomes incapable of menstruating, she may be viewed as less of a woman and not be afforded the same respect as one who still can produce children.

**Taboos and Restrictions During Menstruation.**   Many traditions are associated with menstruation. During the period a woman is considered unclean and should not go into a temple or prepare certain foods. She also should not even look at a newborn child, as doing so is thought to adversely affect its health.

**Dysmenorrhea.**   Disruption or abnormal menstrual flow is considered a bad omen. Problems with menstruation are traditionally treated by a special herbal concoction known as *o kim.*

### Female Modesty and Touching

Female modesty is critical in the Vietnamese culture. It is ingrained so strongly into a girl's upbringing that she becomes extremely reluctant to be touched by a male or any stranger, even in the context of health care. Shaking hands as a greeting is unusual for a woman in Vietnam, but it is becoming more acceptable in North America.. Both Catholicism and Buddhism favor modest behavior, though traditional social standards probably have a more dominant influence than religion. The term *nam nu tho tho bat than* refers to the need to restrict contact between the sexes, thereby preventing problems and maintaining harmony within the community.

**Relationship to Health Care.**   Treatment of a female by a male practitioner in Vietnam would generally be unexpected and may cause difficulty. It has become acceptable in North America, though only among well-educated and liberal-minded women. It is not customary to have an annual pelvic examination, and women may wait until severe problems develop.

Touching or exposing a young girl's or woman's body, including physical, breast, and gynecologic examinations, is accompanied by great reluctance and embarrassment, even when done by a female practitioner. In addition to the basic traditions of modesty, a girl may fear that having a cervical examination will reveal that she has become sexually active.

---

**NOTE TO THE HEALTH CARE PROVIDER**
Health care providers can alleviate problems associated with the physical examination of a young girl by using female practitioners and persistent education. Allowing the presence of the girl's mother, sister, or some other trusted female acquaintance is helpful. A teenager may be more comfortable if an unrelated friend accompanies her, especially one who has already undergone the experience.

---

# Adulthood

## Transition Rites and Rituals

A young woman commonly is considered an adult at ages 18 to 21. The term for this stage is **truong thanh.** No special rites mark the transition.

## Social Expectations

A young woman is expected to be married by age 21. She is trained all her life for this role, particularly in caring for the needs of her husband, parents-in-law, and children. There is considerable pressure in traditional Vietnamese society to keep the children close by, partly to facilitate their eventual service to the elderly. In North America, acceptance of the need for good education and employment is increasing, and families place pressure on young women accordingly.

## Union Formation

**Union Types.** Arranged marriages had a long tradition in Vietnam but are now declining, and they are very rare in Vietnamese American society. Most marriages now result from typical one-to-one acquaintanceships.

**Social Sanctions for Failing to Enter into Union.** Traditionally, young women were strongly pressured into formal marriage by age 21. Fear is great that a daughter may lose her virginity before that time and thus become unable to enter a good marriage. These views have declined somewhat in North America. Young men generally have no such constraints.

Women who do not marry when young are subject to some ridicule, though the acceptable age limit has now been pushed back to about 30. **Lo thoi** is the equivalent of "old maid" in Vietnamese.

## Domestic Violence

Domestic violence is common, mainly because men traditionally have a controlling role and wish to continue to demonstrate their power. The prevalence of alcoholism among Vietnamese men also is growing, a factor that contributes to more violence. Women often accept this situation, although in Vietnam they are now speaking up more because the new government has become more sympathetic to the problem.

Women are reluctant to report domestic violence because of shame and embarrassment, and they do not wish to call attention to the situation. They also fear reporting the problem because they realize that they must continue to live with their husbands and do not wish to anger them further. They also may be concerned that a husband in prison will be unable to support the family. There is a long-standing mistrust of the police and government interference, although younger women are becoming more ready to go to the authorities. These patterns are common both in Vietnam and in Vietnamese communities in North America.

No resources or safe houses for battered women are found in Vietnam. They are potentially available to Vietnamese women in North America, but to date there has been little use of such resources.

### Rape

The incidence of rape in Vietnam is high and increasing. It often involves adult male abuse of young girls. Extensive breakup and rearrangement of traditional family structures are partly responsible. Stepfathers and uncles frequently molest female children. Increasing alcoholism also contributes to the problem. It also is common for men to rape females employed as domestic workers. There is a growing practice of luring young women and girls with the promise of honorable employment, then raping them and forcing them to serve as prostitutes. Many girls are sold into prostitution, sometimes by their own families, and then transported to work in other countries, particularly Cambodia.

Traditionally, rape is considered a serious crime and is unacceptable. Although rape victims are not usually held responsible, the government offers little support, especially if the rape occurs among family members or involves a well-to-do man and his employees. Women tend not to report rape. It is kept quiet to avoid associated embarrassment and other problems. The same problems have been carried over to Vietnamese communities in North America.

### Divorce

**Sociocultural Views.** Traditionally some stigma is associated with divorce, though perhaps less in Vietnamese society than among some other groups. Centuries of war, revolution, break-up of families, and demographic disruption have all tended to make Vietnamese women more self-reliant, while contributing to opportunities for unfaithfulness by men. Many women seek and receive a divorce because of a husband's philandering. Men generally are more reluctant to divorce than are women. Buddhism sanctions divorce if both parties agree, although Catholicism does not officially allow it. The word for divorce is **ly di.**

The new revolutionary government has made divorce relatively easy, and the procedure has become common in Vietnam, although exact statistics are not available. It also has increased among Vietnamese who have migrated to North America.

Divorced women in Vietnam are treated reasonably well. Remarriage is acceptable and often comes quickly. There was a traditional wait of 3 years before remarrying, but now 1 year is socially acceptable. In North America, young Vietnamese women may quickly and easily remarry.

**Child Custody Practices.** If divorce occurs, the father may become upset, remarry, and establish a new family. He is often inclined to give up responsibility for his former wife's children and provide care only for his new family. Traditionally, there is less fear of losing a father than a mother because the woman is mainly responsible for maintaining the family.

> **NOTE TO THE HEALTH CARE PROVIDER**
> A divorced woman commonly does not want to talk about what happened and is interested only in moving on with her and her children's lives. Providers should not pry further if she says she is divorced.

## Fertility and Childbearing

**Family Size.**    Traditionally, a large family was typical and desirable. That situation now is changing both in Vietnam and in Vietnamese society in North America. As recently as the 1970s, the average woman of childbearing age in Vietnam underwent six pregnancies and four live births. Now, the average number of children there is 2.53. The government has been encouraging restriction to two children per couple. Education and increasing work outside the home by women have been factors. Contraceptive procedures also have contributed to the decline, but they are not yet fully developed in Vietnam.

**Contraceptive Practices.**    There is a traditional dislike of contraception, the term for which is *ke hoach gia dinh.* Parents generally oppose it, and young people conceal their use of it. Buddhism has no problem with contraception, though Catholicism officially opposes all unnatural forms of contraception (both religions proscribe abortion).

Various traditional contraceptive methods are available, but they are seldom used now, especially in North America. Oral contraceptives and the intrauterine device (IUD) are commonly employed. Some women are reluctant to use oral contraceptives because of a fear of cancer. Men may not like their wives to use the IUD, though women often do so surreptitiously.

> **NOTE TO THE HEALTH CARE PROVIDER**
> Misinformation in the Vietnamese community is extensive regarding use of oral contraceptives, particularly the belief that the pill causes cancer. Providing educational information in that regard is important, as is emphasizing that any dangers may be more than balanced by the risks of too many births.

**Role of the Male in the Couple's Fertility Decision-Making.**    The male is traditionally dominant with respect to fertility decision-making. Surveys indicate that women are often glad to try contraception but may be overruled. They then may try to conceal use of contraceptive devices. Males are reluctant to use condoms because of alleged reduced sensation. Education and encouragement are needed, especially in sessions bringing the husband and wife together, to improve family planning.

## Abortion

**Cultural Attitudes.**    Abortion is traditionally abhorred by Vietnamese society and is strongly opposed both by Buddhism, which considers the soul to enter the being at the time of conception, and Catholicism. Acceptance of abortion is increasing in Vietnam, however, even up to 6 months into pregnancy. While formerly acceptable only in cases of medical necessity, it now has become common, partly through encouragement by the new revolutionary government.

Abortion is becoming accepted as a form of birth control in both Vietnam and North America, although it is less common than other methods.

**Teen Abortion.**   Teen abortions are becoming common in Vietnam, often to protect family reputations. Young women of higher social class are more likely to seek abortions. There is much advertising by clinics that serve such clientele. Young women from lower social classes are less able to obtain abortions, and they are more reluctant to do so because of religious proscriptions and feelings of guilt.

**Sources of Abortions.**   Prior to 1975, abortions generally were available only through traditional midwifery, but the new revolutionary government has established modern clinics. In the United States and Canada, clinics are readily available and well known to circles of young people.

The concoction known as *o kim* is believed to be effective as an abortificent during the first 6 weeks of pregnancy, but it is not generally available in the United States and Canada.

**Complications.**   Prior to 1975, complications, particularly infections, occurred in 80% to 90% of abortions, frequently leading to serious illness and sometimes death. These complications resulted mainly from the primitive facilities then available. The situation subsequently has improved.

---

**NOTE TO THE HEALTH CARE PROVIDER**
Vietnamese society and family tradition do not accept abortion, and both major religions of Vietnam strongly oppose it. If abortion becomes advisable to protect the mother or prevent birth of an abnormal child, providers must approach the subject cautiously and provide education.

---

Miscarriage

Miscarriage is very common in Vietnam, probably because of a lack of prenatal education and care, as well as a tendency by women to continue heavy lifting and other routine work in the fields through late pregnancy.

Tradition holds that evil spirits and spells cause miscarriage. They may be overcome through ritual prayers known as **tam the tu.** A woman who habitually miscarries may be viewed as weak and, in accordance with Buddhist doctrine, as one who is being punished for misdeeds (particularly for having abortions) in a previous life.

---

**NOTE TO THE HEALTH CARE PROVIDER**
The typical immigrant woman may be especially subject to miscarriage because of a lack of knowledge regarding prenatal care and a tendency to do heavy work during pregnancy. Miscarriages tend to occur early, during the first trimester, because proper education regarding prenatal care has not been provided.

---

## Infertility

Infertility is viewed as a curse or punishment for misdeeds in a previous life. An infertile woman may be treated badly and designated a *gai doc khong con,* "the poison woman without children." People may openly encourage her husband to seek another wife. Depending on the husband's character, he might ignore his wife and find another woman with whom to begin a family, or he may continue to support his wife but quietly have a relationship with another woman.

---

**NOTE TO THE HEALTH CARE PROVIDER**

Women are likely to be receptive to modern infertility treatments, though they may also wish to continue with traditional ritual prayers known as *cau tu.* Husbands will support their wives in this regard.

---

## Pregnancy

**Activity Restrictions and Taboos.**   Few restrictions are placed on a woman until late in the pregnancy. A typical country woman may continue to work in the fields, carry heavy loads, and not seek professional advice unless a severe problem develops. An upper-class or better-educated woman may avoid strenuous work and even lifting her arms above her head. The new revolutionary government has helped disseminate educational information and provide prenatal care.

Vietnamese women believe that encounters with certain people and animals may adversely affect the developing fetus. Conversely, a pregnant woman may frequently look at pictures of happy families, healthy children, or religious figures to ensure a successful birth. Pregnant women are respected and assisted, but they are considered bad luck at weddings, funerals, and the New Year celebrations. Older women are ready to help and advise a young pregnant woman. "Home-based" prenatal care includes ritual prayers, commonly said at an altar in the family home.

**Dietary Practices and Observances.**   An extensive regimen of foods is prescribed for women at various points of pregnancy, in accordance with the balance known as *yin* and *yang* in Chinese. The corresponding terms in Vietnamese are *am* (cold) and *duong* (hot). These terms have nothing to do with temperature and are only partly associated with seasoning. In addition, foods are classified as "tonic" and "wind."

During the first trimester, a woman is considered to be in a weak, cold, and antitonic state. She should correct the imbalance by eating hot foods, such as soups with chili peppers, salty meat and fish, and wine steeped with herbs. To provide energy to the fetus, she should also follow a basic diet of tonic foods, such as steamed rice and pork. In the second trimester, the woman is considered to be in a neutral state; cold foods are introduced, and the tonic diet is continued. During the third trimester, cold foods are prescribed, hot foods are avoided, and tonic foods, which are believed to increase fetal weight and thus make birthing difficult, are also avoided. Wind foods, including leafy vegetables, beef, mutton, and glutinous rice, are avoided throughout pregnancy. In practice, most women use this regimen only as a general guide, commonly restricting, rather than totally abstaining from, the proscribed foods.

Eating of nonfood items is uncommon.

**Prenatal Care.**   Prior to 1975, it was normal for a woman to wait until late in her pregnancy or until a severe problem developed before seeking care. With subsequent increases in education and availability of assistance, women begin to seek care at a modern clinic after about 3 months of pregnancy.

---

**NOTE TO THE HEALTH CARE PROVIDER**

The language barrier, the sight of unfamiliar medical equipment, and, especially, the presence of men among clinic personnel may intimidate the immigrant woman. Providers should welcome female relatives who may accompany her and try to have women providers see her as much as possible.

---

### Birthing Process

**Home Versus Hospital Delivery.**   In the Vietnamese countryside, children are commonly delivered by certified midwives in a screened-off portion of the family home or in a special birth house. In large cities, most births occur in hospitals or obstetric clinics, and a midwife usually handles the procedure. In North America, most Vietnamese women deliver in hospitals.

**Cesarean Section Versus Vaginal Delivery.**   Most deliveries are vaginal. Cesarean sections are accepted in a life-threatening situation. Midwives generally handle the delivery and determine whether a cesarean section is necessary and if a physician should be called. Natural childbirth is preferred, though Vietnamese women tend to request anesthesia more frequently than do women in some other ethnic groups.

**Involvement of the Male Partner.**   The mother and sisters of the pregnant woman are regularly present during birth and will try to provide comfort and advice. The father is traditionally kept out and may be chased away if he persists.

**Labor Management.**   Pain medication is not usually prescribed during contractions unless severe complications develop. This practice is often related to a scarcity of medicine in Vietnam. During labor, women attempt to stay in control, and they may even smile continuously. After rupture of the membranes, delivery tends to be more rapid than is generally observed in North America.

---

**NOTE TO THE HEALTH CARE PROVIDER**

Refrain from strongly encouraging the father to be present during the birth. The mother and the other women present might be adamantly opposed to his involvement. Discussing the matter beforehand with all concerned is best.

---

**Placenta.**   The placenta is usually buried, in accordance with the tradition of returning to the soil. In some cases, if the placenta looks especially healthy, family members may cook it into a dish and eat it. Among those in North America, there is likely little or no interest in obtaining the placenta or burying it.

## Postpartum

Typical recuperation time is 3 months. In Vietnam, women who work are commonly given paid leave for that length of time. The word for baby is *be* and for mother, *ma*.

Because body heat is lost during delivery, Vietnamese women avoid "cold" foods and beverages and increase consumption of "hot" foods to replace and strengthen their blood. Ice water and other cold drinks are usually unwelcome. Women will take most raw vegetables, fruits, and sour items in lesser amounts. Because water is "cold," women traditionally do not fully bathe, shower, or wash their hair for 1 to 3 months after delivery. Postpartum women also avoid drafts and strenuous activity, wear warm clothing, and stay in bed or indoors for about a month. Traditional practices include sleeping on a bed raised above hot coals or applying a hot, salty towel to the vaginal area.

---

**NOTE TO THE HEALTH CARE PROVIDER**

Do not encourage the woman to bathe after birth. Make sure that hot (or at least room-temperature) fluids are provided at the bedside. Talk with her about what she prefers regarding traditional practices. Some women have welcomed the opportunity to shower or bathe and to give up certain other traditional practices. Many, however, are reluctant to do so. Pericare with a warm cleansing solution is usually agreeable and should be suggested.

---

## Newborn and Infant Care

**Breastfeeding Versus Bottle-Feeding.** Breastfeeding is traditional in Vietnam, although there has been a trend toward using formula or bottled milk in the mistaken belief that it is better for the child. With careful education on the natural health benefits of breastfeeding, women tend to return to that approach. Immigrant, working women might not realize that, in selected workplaces, they can continue to breastfeed through pumping and refrigerating breast milk.

**Infant Protection.** The Vietnamese government now provides free immunizations. Regular monitoring of growth and development, however, is minimal. Although less attention is paid to the beliefs in spells and curses than previously, there still is a widespread tradition of avoiding praising the child, lest he or she be stolen by jealous spirits. The infant may also be given an unattractive name and dressed in old clothes to protect it from such spirits. In North America, these practices are still found to some extent. In particular, a happy, attractive, well-behaved baby may be dressed in old clothes and given an unattractive nickname to protect it from evil spirits.

---

**NOTE TO THE HEALTH CARE PROVIDER**

Health care professionals in the vicinity of the baby should not compliment the baby on appearance or good behavior, as that may create the opposite spiritual effect, causing the child to cry all night. It is best to avoid touching the head of a baby to the extent possible.

---

**Primary Caregiver.** Although the mother remains the primary caregiver, aunts and the grandmother on the mother's side take much responsibility. Extended family members are also commonly available. Males traditionally are not involved but, with both spouses now often working outside the home, fathers are starting to participate in basic care of young children.

---

**NOTE TO THE HEALTH CARE PROVIDER**

Do not incorrectly interpret the tendency of a Vietnamese mother to depend on other women to care for the newborn, and her own state of inactivity, as apathy or depression. In this culture, other women normally take such a role. Also, do not encourage men to handle and care for the baby without first discussing the matter with all concerned.

---

## Middle Age

### Cultural Attitudes and Expectations

Women are generally considered middle-aged at about 45 to 50 years. Middle-aged Vietnamese women traditionally wear less bright colors and more conservative clothing. As women age, roles commonly change. In particular, by middle age (after 40) women tend to have increased authority in the family and to be treated with growing respect. Among the Southern Vietnamese, especially, elderly women (after 60) may come to dominate the family.

### Psychological Response

The "empty-nest" syndrome can be especially severe in a culture that traditionally depends on extended family units and keeping children close to the elders. With the increasing disruption of families and mobility of children, crises may develop. In such cases parents can do little except seek acceptance of children's departure through religion or meditation.

The extended family system in Vietnam traditionally has alleviated mid-life problems. Such emotional support is often lacking in North America, and increasing rates of separation and divorce may aggravate the situation. Some women seek help through religious organizations, while others may gain support through renewed social and even romantic activity.

### Menopause

**Onset and Duration.** The Vietnamese term for menopause is **tat kinh,** which specifically means completion of the job of the woman. Menopause begins at age 45 to 50 years. In Vietnamese culture, a relatively early onset is considered favorable. Late onset indicates bad karma reflecting misdeeds in an earlier life. It is not unusual, however, for onset to occur after 50 years. Genetic factors are probably involved.

**Sexual Activity.** Some women consider their sexual role to terminate with menopause, but this view reflects cultural and religious influence rather than physical inclination. The husband of a woman who makes this choice may object and perhaps seek another sexual partner. Vietnamese women in North America are more likely to want to extend their sex lives, sometimes with the help of hormone therapy or various stimuli.

**Coping.** Some Vietnamese women cope with menopause by becoming more religiously active. Others, particularly in North America, try to compensate through increased socialization and partying.

Hot flashes and emotional changes are common, and a woman may anger easily. Often such symptoms are ignored, and most women do not believe in hormone treatments. Many women try herbal teas and other traditional remedies, however.

---

**NOTE TO THE HEALTH CARE PROVIDER**
Many Vietnamese women actually welcome menopause and feel satisfaction at no longer being sexually active. They may be reluctant to take hormonal therapy, which may lead to continued sex that culturally they would view as unfavorable and for which they are too old. Some women also fear such therapy because of a presumed association with cancer. An understanding attitude in broaching the topic of such therapy may be helpful in explaining its usefulness.

---

# Old Age

## Cultural Attitudes

The average life expectancy of a female in Vietnam is about 72 years, which is shorter than that for North American counterparts. The difference largely relates to maternal demise during childbirth, reluctance and inability to seek good health care, more disease and trauma, and inadequate treatment of infections in Vietnam. A woman may be considered old at age 50. At age 60 there is a happy celebration, known as **mung luc thuan,** to mark the achievement of old age. Elderly women generally are respected, even venerated. The expression **kinh lao dac tho** suggests that the more one respects the elderly, the greater the chance he or she has to reach old age.

Older women and widows traditionally remain a part of the Vietnamese extended family system, which cares for them. Such an arrangement is ingrained into Vietnamese society. Society will view anyone who places an elderly relative in a nursing home unfavorably.

# Death and Dying

## Cultural Attitudes and Beliefs

Death is given much attention in Vietnamese culture, perhaps even more than marriage. It is accepted as a normal part of the life cycle, and preparation for the time that one will become a venerated ancestor is considerable. This practice, however, is more prevalent among the elderly. Premature death (e.g., a woman dying in childbirth) is traumatic to the family. A dying person is encouraged to release life easily, without fear or anger.

Buddhism holds that desire causes suffering and that life is a cycle of ordeals: to be born, grow old, fall ill, and die. A soul is reincarnated through several cycles. People's present lives predetermine their own and their dependents' future lives. Karma is accumulated through misdeeds during one life cycle and must be paid for in the next one. Proper prayers and deeds lead to reincarnation into a better life.

### Rites and Rituals

Vietnamese families may wish to gather around the body of a recently deceased relative and express great emotion. They use various traditional prayers and rituals to help accept the situation. Men handle the traditional preparation of deceased males, while women handle that of deceased females. The body is dressed in good clothing, usually red if the person is old. Buttons and metal objects are not used. Rice is sometimes placed within the mouth. To prevent shifting of the body, the coffin may be filled with tea leaves, if the family can afford it, or crumpled paper, if not. There is a traditional importance of being buried in an area where descendants may maintain the grave, although decades of war and demographic disruption may have overwhelmed that tradition. In North America, some Vietnamese immigrants have tended to favor cremation, so as to allow remains of the departed (ashes) to be kept in the home.

### Mourning

**Cultural Expectations.** Traditional mourning practices include wearing white clothes for 14 days. After that period, men wear black armbands, which indicate membership in certain associations, and women wear headbands or cloths, which are usually white in the south and black in the north. Prayers are said every day for 45 days following death, after which it is believed that the soul is reincarnated. There is a yearly celebration of the anniversary of a person's death.

A surviving spouse and other close female relatives are expected to dress conservatively, avoid jewelry and makeup, and restrict social activity. Traditionally, a woman was not supposed to remarry for 3 years, though the generally accepted period now is 1 year.

If a mother dies, responsibility for the children passes to the aunts or grandparents on the mother's side.

Women attempt to cope with spousal loss through prayers and support from the extended family. Loss of a father is considered less significant than loss of a mother.

---

**NOTE TO THE HEALTH CARE PROVIDER**
A woman in mourning requires some quiet time. Practitioners should support her beliefs and assist her to reach a temple or church. It is especially important to allow the family, and appropriate monks or clergymen, to come in to pray together and support the woman.

---

# IMPORTANT POINTS FOR PROVIDERS CARING FOR VIETNAMESE WOMEN

## The Medical Intake

### Literacy and English Proficiency

The literacy rate for women in Vietnam is about 91%. Because men traditionally are responsible for business matters and paperwork, however, many Vietnamese women cannot fill out forms, even if they are literate and the forms are printed in Vietnamese. It is best to have a well-qualified interpreter available, preferably not a child. An adult female relative who is fluent in English is the ideal interpreter both for forms and when asking about female health issues. Indeed, since the presence of a man may intimidate a woman and she may be reluctant to mention certain things, health care providers should be certain that the female client receives correct information on female health issues through a female relative. Lack of organized language services is a critical obstacle to dissemination of information needed by Vietnamese women relative to the early detection of cervical cancer.

### Status of the Provider

Women are traditionally shy, modest, and passive. Eye contact is commonly considered rude. These factors apply especially in the case of health care practitioners, who women view as authority figures. These women may be extremely reluctant to discuss personal matters with a male provider; women may express such feelings not by direct negativity but by giggling, shrugging the shoulders, or averting the eyes.

### Communicating Illness and Symptoms

Vietnamese women may be unlikely to volunteer significant medical information openly. There is a strong tradition, influenced by the Confucian code of ethics, to maintain self-control and avoid complaints. A woman may smile and say she is fine, even if she is in pain. The practitioner should use a quiet, unhurried manner and watch for behavioral cues. Building the trust and good relationship that will yield the necessary information and compliance requires time.

Once a woman does open up, she may voice elaborate explanations and tell lengthy stories to explain her illness. It is then best for the practitioner to allow some leeway, but set limits.

Belief in spiritual causes of sickness is common, even among immigrants and Vietnamese Americans. Many spiritual healers are in the United States and Canada. The term **mac dang duoi** refers to a spirit taking over the body. Women will typically share such beliefs with friends and relatives, but not with Western health care practitioners.

Family members sometimes accompany the woman client and participate in providing information. Through judicious use of such relatives, particularly adult women who are fluent in English, a practitioner may obtain valuable information. A male relative may attempt to explain a change in the client, but such information is best obtained from another female.

## The Physical Examination

### Modesty and Touching

Modesty is extremely important, and difficulty in obtaining information or doing a physical examination can be overcome only through a quiet and understanding approach, detailed but easily understood explanations, and taking time to build trust. The Vietnamese concept **nam nu tho tho bat than** indicates that males and females are allowed to communicate but not to have bodily contact, and this restriction is instilled in girls from early childhood. A female health care provider is always best, although not essential, particularly if appropriate female friends or relatives can accompany the client.

Touching should be kept to a minimum. Male practitioners should avoid touching females except when absolutely necessary and in the presence of another female, preferably a friend or relative. Practitioners should not do a pelvic examination on an unmarried woman during the first visit or without careful advanced explanation and preparation. The head is considered a sacred part of the body; providers should not touch it. They should avoid contact to the extent possible during menstruation.

### Expressing Pain

Vietnamese are traditionally stoic and consider complaining about pain to be a sign of weakness. Once a relationship is established with a practitioner, however, especially by an older client, the client may voice extensive complaints and demands for relief.

## Prescribing Medications

### Drug Interactions

Vietnamese frequently use traditional Oriental medicines and have little understanding of side effects or interactions with Western drugs. The practitioner should provide education on such matters and specifically ask about the use of traditional remedies.

### Medication Sharing

Sharing prescribed medications is common. Clients are likely to take medications from several different traditional and Western practitioners. They also are quite reluctant to advise their current practitioners that they are doing so. Health care providers must explain the potential for severe health problems when taking some medications together and encourage clients to list all the medications they are taking. They should also strongly assure clients that they will not tell former or other health care providers that a client divulged what medications they were prescribed. Some clients may fear that such providers may be "insulted."

### Compliance

Medication and treatment compliance is a severe problem among immigrants. There is a strong tendency to stop taking medication if the immediate symptoms are alleviated. This is especially true of tuberculosis medication. Much checking, home visits, observation by trusted relatives, repetition of instructions, and persistent education may all be necessary to ensure medication and treatment compliance.

## Follow-up Appointments

It generally is advisable to call to remind the client the day before the appointment. Vietnamese Americans have a tendency to miss follow-up appointments, especially if they feel better or if they hear that acquaintances with similar symptoms had no consequent difficulties.

Vietnamese generally have a more fluid concept of time than do Westerners, and they may be less concerned about the present and about precise schedules. They frequently arrive late for appointments. Established families in North America, however, generally are fully aware of the importance of punctuality.

To increase adherence to follow-up visits and care, it may be necessary to carefully explain the problems that may result (e.g., the effect of inaction if nothing is done about abnormal Papanicolaou's test result). Women should be made to understand that lack of symptoms or pain may be only temporary and that experiences of acquaintances may not apply to them. Persistent reminding, as part of an overall effort to improve communication and dissemination of information, is the best way to encourage women to undergo regular cancer screening and follow-up treatment. To encourage cervical cancer monitoring and prevention, it is useful to remind women that the disease, even if survived, could lead to hysterectomy.

## Prevalent Diseases

Vietnamese are especially susceptible to tuberculosis, hepatitis B, diabetes, hypertension, lung cancer, and depression and other psychiatric conditions associated with the trauma of war and social disruption. Lung cancer is associated with a high rate of smoking among Vietnamese men (56% vs. 32% among the general population), whereas smoking is less common in Vietnamese women (9% vs. 27% for women in general). Vietnamese women, however, have the highest rate of cervical cancer of any female population that has been surveyed. Yeast infection is another persistent urogenital problem among Vietnamese women.

The prevalence of cervical cancer in Vietnamese women may be linked to a lack of education, a great reluctance to seek early treatment, a fear that nothing can be done, low use of annual Papanicolaou's tests, and failure to follow-up on abnormal Papanicolaou's test results. Some evidence also implicates human papillomavirus (HPV), a sexually transmitted etiologic factor in the pathogenesis of cervical cancer. The enormous and lengthy military activity and social disruption in Vietnam may have led to extensive sexual relations with multiple partners by males and spread of sexually transmitted problems, including HPV, to women. Cancer and other problems common to Vietnamese may also be associated with widespread use of chemical agents during the Vietnam War.

## Health-Seeking Behaviors

Vietnamese commonly wait until medical problems are in an advanced stage before seeking care from modern practitioners. They may first consult friends, relatives, and traditional healers. Many practitioners of traditional Oriental medicine, as well as untrained folk and spiritual healers and sorcerers, are in the Vietnamese community. Vietnamese women may seek their services for any physical or psychological problem. The following are some of the common treatments practiced in Vietnam and to some extent in North America.

**Cao gio,** literally meaning "rubbing out the wind," is used for treating colds, sore throats, influenza, sinusitis, and similar ailments. An ointment or hot balm oil is spread across the back, chest, or shoulders and rubbed with the edge of a coin (preferably silver) in short, firm strokes. This technique brings blood under the skin, resulting in dark striped bruises so the offending wind can escape.

**Be bao** (skin pinching) is a treatment for headache or sore throat. The skin of the affected area is repeatedly squeezed between the thumb and forefinger of both hands, as the hands converge toward the center of the face. The objective is to produce ecchymoses or petechiae.

**Giac** (cup suctioning), another dermabrasive procedure, is used to relieve stress, headaches, and joint and muscle pain. A small cup is heated and placed on the skin with the open side down. As the cup cools, it contracts the skin and draws unwanted "hot" energy into the cup.

**Xong** is an herbal preparation relieving motion sickness or cold related problems. Herbs (or an agent such as Vicks Vaporub) are put into boiling water and the vapor is inhaled.

Acupuncture, acupressure, and acumassage relieve symptomatic stress and pain.

Moxibustion is used to counter conditions associated with excess cold, including labor and delivery. Pulverized wormwood or incense is heated and placed directly on the skin at certain meridians. Balms and oils, such as Red Tiger Balm (available in Asian shops), are applied to certain areas for relief of bone and muscle ailments. Herbal teas, soups, and other concoctions are taken for various problems, generally in the sense of using cold measures to overcome hot illnesses.

These treatments may be tried in the initial stages of major illness. Vietnamese commonly attribute illness to the yin/yang or am/duong imbalance. It is typical to try traditional and supposedly natural remedies before consulting a modern doctor. Such inclination, unfortunately, makes Vietnamese reluctant to seek early screening and treatment for problems such as cervical cancer.

With regard to health promotion, upper-class Vietnamese in North America use such preventive measures as regular examinations, exercise, and careful diets. Lower-class people and recent arrivals are usually too concerned with securing the immediate basic needs of life for themselves and their children to worry about long-term prevention programs. Prayer and meditation are common, though attendance at temple is rare except when there is serious illness or a threat of death.

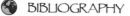 **BIBLIOGRAPHY**

Bong, J. (2000). 2000 Assembly on cervical cancer among Vietnamese-American women. Annandale, VA: Health Awareness Program for Immigrants and National Asian Women's Health Organization.

Calhoun, M. A. (1985). The Vietnamese woman: Health/illness attitudes and behaviors. *Health Care for Women International*, 6, 61–72.

D'Avanzo, C. E. (1992). Barriers to health care for Vietnamese refugees. *Journal of Professional Nursing*, 8(4), 245–253.

Nowak, T. T. (1998). Vietnamese-Americans. In L. Purnell & B. Paulanka (Eds.). *Transcultural health care: a culturally competent approach*. Philadelphia: F. A. Davis, pp. 449–477.

Stauffer, R. Y. (1991). Vietnamese Americans. In J. N. Giger & R. E. Davidhizar (Eds.). *Transcultural nursing: Assessment and intervention*. St. Louis: Mosby–Year Book, pp. 402–434.

# CHAPTER 20

# West Indians

## PATRICIA F. ST. HILL, PhD, RN, MPH

### 🌐 INTRODUCTION

### Who are the West Indian People?

West Indians, often distinguished as Jamaicans, Trinidadians, Tobagonians, Barbadians, Grenadians (depending on the island of origin), are predominantly an Afro-Caribbean people. Individuals of East Indian, Chinese, and European ancestry (most often Spanish and British) are also found in large numbers on these islands, making West Indian society truly multicultural and multiracial. Additionally, interracial marriages are very common among the varying ethnic groups, accounting for the many skin tones, facial features, and hair textures commonly seen in the West Indies.

The language native to most West Indians is English, spoken with a distinct West Indian accent. West Indian groups from islands previously colonized by the Dutch, Spanish, or French speak primarily Dutch, Spanish, or French, many with little or no proficiency in English. For this group of West Indians, communications may be a problem.

### West Indians in North America

Pushed primarily by economic pressures, West Indians, from as early as the 1800s, have fought their way to the United States in search of work and a better life for themselves and their families. By the 1960s, West Indian immigration to the United States reached an all-time high. The Immigration Act of 1965, which did away with the old quota system and expanded immigration opportunities for people of color, largely contributed to this development. Between 1965 and 1974, 18% of all immigrants admitted to the United States came from the Caribbean. More recent immigration statistics suggest that the number of legal Caribbean immigrants reaching the United States has stabilized.

**ACKNOWLEDGMENT**
The author would like to acknowledge Michele Salmon, RN, BSN, who contributed valuable cultural information to the chapter.

The greater New York and New Jersey area along with several large cities in Central and South Florida (especially Miami) serve as home to the largest numbers of West Indian immigrants in the United States. Over the years, the supportive ethnic niches have allowed West Indian immigrants to enjoy life similar to that experienced "back home," by providing ethnic foods, music, and other pleasures reminiscent of the Caribbean.

Canada has also been the recipient of large numbers of West Indian Immigrants. According to Canada's 1996 census, the number of West Indians is 305,209, almost 6% of Canada's immigrant population. They reside mainly in Toronto and Montreal.

## 🌐 BEING FEMALE IN WEST INDIAN CULTURE

In Caribbean society, the woman's role is first and foremost that of wife and mother. Although a good education and career are recognized as desirable for girls, finding a "well-to-do" husband and starting a family is the dream of almost all parents for their daughters. Likewise, equal rights for women are verbally espoused; nonetheless, the leadership role played by men, both at home and in the community, goes without question.

## At Birth

### Preference for Sons

Preference for sons, especially with the firstborn child, is openly declared by West Indians of East Indian ancestry. Other groups are much more receptive to the birth of a daughter, even when she is the firstborn. Nevertheless, when the child is a boy, a father may be seen openly celebrating and even boasting about the birth of "his son." The mother, too, appears to get special recognition from her husband and family and is especially proud of her male offspring.

### Response to the Birth of a Female

This society has never practiced infanticide or abandonment of female children. Instead, following the birth of a daughter, parents will often "try again" for a son. A family consisting of both boys and girls is most ideal and sought-after. The woman who bears only female children may be at risk for abandonment by her spouse, or, more likely, he may seek an outside woman with whom he starts a second family. This development is more likely among rural and lower-class residents.

### Birth Rituals

This culture never practices female circumcision; only rarely are male children circumcised.

## Childhood and Youth

### Stages

In West Indian culture, childhood is a prolonged process with no clearly delineated stages. Individuals up to their mid-teen years (13 to 15 years of age) are considered children or **pickney** and are expected to conduct themselves in that manner. Dating, sexual activity, and childbearing at this stage are considered taboo, especially for young people from middle-class and upper-class families.

### Family Expectations

Extremely high behavioral standards and expectations are set for young people, especially girls. The idea that "children should be seen and not heard" remains the basis for discipline. Most families assign children perceived age-appropriate and sex-appropriate household chores. Thus, boys are generally assigned more "manly" chores, while girls are assigned more "domestic" or "feminine" chores (e.g., cooking and assisting with the care of younger siblings), intended to prepare them for their future roles of wife and mother. Very masculine women or very feminine men are not well received in this society.

### Social Expectations

The ideas of social respectability and not "bringing shame" to the family's name are impressed upon children, especially young girls. Anything deemed negative that the child does outside the home is believed to reflect badly on the family, especially the parents.

### Importance of Education

Female illiteracy is generally not a problem among West Indian girls and women, although education beyond elementary school is neither mandatory nor free. Most West Indian homes stress the importance of a good education, and children tend to be extremely competitive in school. Many are pressured to excel in order to obtain a scholarship to high school. Academically, girls are encouraged to compete equally with boys. If family resources are limited, however, the tendency is to educate male children to prepare them for their roles as "breadwinner" and provider for their future families. An exception to this general rule is a case in which a young girl is exceptionally bright.

This society has never encouraged or practiced child labor.

## Pubescence

### Psychosexual Development

No discernible gender differences are found at the age at which most youngsters reach pubescence. On average, girls reach puberty between ages 11 and 13 years, with some variations that may be attributed more to familial rather than cultural tendencies or characteristics. Often, emotional or psychological maturation lags behind physical maturation. Thus, although they may appear physically mature, these adolescent girls may act shy and even somewhat childish in social situations.

### Rituals and Rites of Passage

Generally, no recognized rituals or observances celebrate the girl's transition into womanhood. The same is true for the boy's transition into manhood. At or about the age of 12, it is customary for young Catholic or Protestant boys and girls to be "confirmed" by the church.

## Teen Sexuality

**Social Restrictions and Pressures.** Family members, typically older women, closely monitor the pubescent girl's behavior, dress, and sexuality. Families, especially middle-class families, strive to prevent their daughters from growing up "too quickly." Consequently, steady dating and engaging in sexual activity are strongly discouraged. If the teenage girl does date, the young man must meet parental approval (e.g., be of the same social class as the girl's family).

**Teen Pregnancy.** Taboos against teen pregnancy are strong. Although parents seldom, if ever, discuss sex and birth control with the teenage girl, and seldom will a parent readily consent to birth control use by the minor child, a pregnant teenager is a perceived disgrace to her family. If pregnancy does occur, abortion is not a likely solution. Instead, the tendency is for the girl's mother or an aunt to raise the child while the young girl resumes her education.

## Menstruation

**Relationship to Health.** For the West Indian girl, menstruation signals her entry into adulthood. She is now perceived as a young woman capable of childbearing, and hence is subjected to even greater parental scrutiny. The inextricable linkages between menstruation and health and menstruation and fertility resonate in this culture. In fact, menstruation has frequently been reported as a "barometer of one's good health and fertility" for the West Indian woman. It has also been deemed a time of bodily cleansing, and hence is expected to be regular. This means the same duration, amount, and type of flow each month. Any deviations from this pattern signal either pregnancy or poor health, which is likely to be treated with various herbal teas obtained from locally grown plants and shrubs. Severe menstrual cramping, typically viewed as an abnormality, is similarly treated with herbal teas of a different variety.

**Relationship to Fertility.** Because of the close cultural linkages between menstruation and health and menstruation and fertility, the woman who is incapable of menstruating following a total hysterectomy may experience a perceived loss of her "barometer of health." As a consequence, she is likely to experience grief, remorse, and sadness about "fertility lost." This is particularly poignant in a society in which the woman's fertility frequently defines who she is and her worth (as a person) in terms of her ability to bear children.

**Taboos and Restrictions During Menstruation.** No culturally recognized taboos or restrictions are placed on activities during menstrual periods. Many women, however, avoid taking cold showers or baths, fearing exposure of the uterus to "cold." Likewise, many women deem sexual activity as undesirable and curtail it during the menstrual flow.

**Dysmenorrhea.** Menstrual activity that deviates from the perceived norm, including the failure to menstruate a "satisfactory amount" each month, signals a health threat or problem. Studies done with this population point to the ever-present fear expressed by women of accumulating too much blood and developing high blood pressure if menstrual flow is insufficient. Light or short periods as well as the passage of clots or menstrual cramping are equally troublesome to West Indian women, who are likely to treat such problems with herbal teas.

### Female Modesty and Touching

No religious or social mandates dictate the observance of female modesty. Women, however, tend to be very conservative and maybe even embarrassed and reluctant about exposing their unclothed bodies to strangers, including health care professionals. Likewise, they view hugging and touching by people outside the immediate family as inappropriate or "fresh."

If given a choice, the woman will greatly prefer to be treated by a female practitioner. Among those of East Indian ancestry who are practicing Hindus or Muslims, treatment by a female practitioner may be mandatory. Annual pelvic examinations, mammograms, and breast examinations, including self-breast examinations, are seldom observed because of the discomfort and embarrassment associated with touching one's own body as well as having strangers touch one's private parts.

---

**NOTE TO THE HEALTH CARE PROVIDER**

Be extremely careful about preserving the young woman's privacy during a physical or gynecologic examination. At all times, a female staff member or the adolescent's mother should be in the examination room. Also, providers should be expeditious with the procedure.

---

## Adulthood

### Transition Rites and Rituals

No one specific age stands as a point at which a young woman is considered an adult. No rites of passage or ceremonies are observed. Around age 18 to 19 years, however, Caribbean students generally complete their higher education (college), which prepares them for full-time employment. Accordingly, they are permitted more liberties and adult choices at this point in time.

### Social Expectations

Because of society's validation and promotion of education and career achievement, little or no pressure is placed on middle-class and upper-class young women during their teens and early 20s to marry and start a family. By their mid-20s, however, parents may begin to exert some pressures on young women to marry, since failure to enter into union and have children is still highly stigmatized in this culture. A clear double standard exists for women and men. While the unmarried man is viewed as a playboy or **saga boy,** the unmarried woman older than age 30 years is pitied and viewed as a "spinster" or "old maid."

### Union Formation

Monogamy is the prevailing type of union formation. In rural areas and among the lesser educated and poor, polygamy—the result of multiple common-law unions—is still likely to be found.

### Domestic Violence

Consistent with the authority/leadership role afforded to men, domestic violence is frequently a part of many family systems. It is not unusual to hear a Caribbean man refer to his wife as "his" or "belonging to him." Accordingly, this sense of ownership may lead the man to be violent toward or to batter his wife for such minor things as not cooking dinner or leaving the house without his knowing.

Because of the stigma and shame attached to domestic violence, it often remains within the family—the unreported crime. With younger or more liberated women, however, there may be exceptions to this rule, especially those living in North America.

The culture views children as belonging to the parents; consequently, parents will spank their children, seeing it as their responsibility to "train" or discipline their children. They consider such behaviors to be nobody else's business.

---

**NOTE TO THE HEALTH CARE PROVIDER**

Women, especially older women, are unlikely to report or admit to being victims of domestic abuse. In cases of suspected domestic abuse or violence, practitioners should be very tactful and supportive when addressing the subject. If not, the woman is likely to be offended and shut down previously established communication.

---

### Rape

Acts of sexual violence committed against young girls and women are unspeakable crimes surrounded by secrecy and heightened feelings of shame and guilt on the part of both the victim and her family (as if to blame the victim). Because of the stigma and shame attached to rape, many victims are unlikely to report this crime to the proper authorities, especially those who are illegal immigrants or who have recently migrated.

### Divorce

**Sociocultural Views.**  The frequency of divorce among young adults has increased over the years. Accordingly, the stigma and shame once attached to divorce no longer applies. The society is less forgiving, however, of the woman who remarries shortly after divorce, especially if she has in her custody minor children from the previous marriage. Among West Indians living in North America, issues of separation and divorce may be partly attributed to the stressors of migration as well experiences of marginalization or "not belonging" in the dominant society.

**Women and Divorce.**  Neither divorce nor remarriage is stigmatized anymore. The woman who marries multiple times, however, is subject to criticism. At the same time a man with a similar history of multiple marriages is viewed less negatively. Upon dissolution of the marriage, the divorced woman will often move in with family members or friends, at least during the initial period following the divorce, until she "gets back on her feet." If her parents are alive, they are generally the primary source of support for her and the minor children.

**Child Custody Practices.**  The woman generally assumes custody of the minor children with the expectation that her ex-husband will continue to provide financial support for them. Often, however, this does not happen because child support laws in the Caribbean, when observed at all, are very lax. Additionally, the anger and bitterness that often develop between the man and his ex-in-laws further separates him from his family. Furthermore, very commonly the ex-husband will enter into a new relationship soon after the divorce, in which he may start a new family.

---

**NOTE TO THE HEALTH CARE PROVIDER**
West Indians look primarily to family and close friends for support during difficult times. Women going through divorce, illness, financial difficulties, and the like may refuse counseling sessions initially. Providers should not force discussion; gentle persuasion techniques are likely to be more successful.

---

### Fertility and Childbearing

**Family Size.**  Historically, large families typified West Indian households. Although family size has decreased in recent years, the number of offspring in the average family may still range from four to eight (or even more), depending on the family's economic status and residence. Generally, rural residents tend to have more children than do urban residents. Women in urban areas tend to be better educated, work outside the home, and be more receptive to use of contraceptives. Family size for West Indians in North America tends to closely approximate that of middle-class America, partly because of the acculturation of American fertility beliefs and practices.

**Contraceptive Practices.**  Although contraception is used in the Caribbean, several factors limit its influence: cost, positive cultural views and values surrounding fertility and childbearing, and perceptions of modern contraception (especially among lesser educated and rural residents) as unnatural and a possible health hazard. The pill, for example, is feared as a cause of cancer. Lastly, the increasing influence of Rastafarianism in the West Indies must be considered. Rastafarianism is a religion with roots in Ethiopia but a long history in Jamaica. It is based on the premise of living a "natural" or "holistic" life and excludes the use of contraceptives. For the Rastafarians, or **"Rastas"** as they are often referred to, prolonged lactation is the one and only means by which pregnancies are spaced and family size is limited.

**Role of the Male Partner in the Couple's Fertility Decision-Making.**  In this culture, contraceptive use is generally thought of as "the woman's" responsibility. Many men, especially younger men, tend to view the ability to impregnate a woman as a testimonial to their masculinity, and hence they divorce themselves from the contraceptive decision-making process. Patient education, involving both partners, will be most effective in increasing the use of contraceptives.

---

**NOTE TO THE HEALTH CARE PROVIDER**
West Indian men are likely to reject suggestions of condom use. Providers should emphasize the benefits of condom use (especially with single men) in reducing the risk of sexually transmitted diseases (STDs), especially human immunodeficiency virus (HIV), given its extremely high incidence in this region. Also, they should help the client explore and support use of so-called "natural" methods of contraception if other methods are unacceptable.

---

## Abortion

**Cultural Attitudes.** Abortion is not socially sanctioned in this society. Much secrecy and shame surrounds abortion; hence, the extent to which it occurs is unknown. Today, the procedure is generally conducted in a hospital (outpatient clinic setting). Nevertheless, women from some of the smaller Caribbean islands whose financial resources and access to medical care are limited may occasionally resort to using locally grown herbs/abortificients (commonly used in the past) during the early stages of pregnancy despite the many inherent dangers.

**Teen Abortion.** Because of the veil of secrecy surrounding the abortion issue, statistical figures and specific information regarding its incidence and circumstances among teens is unknown.

---

**NOTE TO THE HEALTH CARE PROVIDER**

Be extremely careful to preserve client privacy and reassure her of the confidentiality of the information provided. Take this opportunity to educate client about both STDs and female methods of contraception. Helping her select a method that is appropriate and acceptable to her is important. Providers should try to ask as few direct questions as possible about client's sexual activity/behavior.

---

## Miscarriage

When a woman becomes pregnant, extreme measures are taken to ensure a healthy pregnancy and good outcome. The occurrence of a miscarriage induces feelings of responsibility, guilt, and sometimes shame on the woman's part. If the miscarriage was unexpected or seemingly suspicious, its cause may be attributed to witchcraft/voodoo or **obeah,** especially if the woman who lost the child can readily identify someone (e.g., an envious or childless woman) as the possible source of her difficulties. Similarly, women who habitually miscarry often will view this as a punishment from God for some misdeed perpetrated by her or her husband. To correct this, she generally will seek God's help through prayer.

---

**NOTE TO THE HEALTH CARE PROVIDER**

The stressors of pregnancy, migration, and living conditions in North America may put many of these women at increased risk for miscarriage. Encouraging early prenatal care and monitoring these women closely are important interventions.

---

## Infertility

Fertility is a highly prized asset from both the male and female perspectives. Many women, especially the rural poor, view fertility and childbearing as a means of demonstrating their womanhood and achieving social status in the community. The infertile woman, on the other hand, is made to feel as though she is "less than whole." Such derogatory statements as "she can't breed" or "mule" may often be used to describe the infertile woman. Accordingly, many husbands/male partners feel justified in seeking out an "outside woman"(often a neighbor) with whom they can have children. Often, the infertile woman tolerates such infidelity because she believes that her value as a woman is "depreciated" and fears total abandonment.

Technology related to fertility treatments is still not available in the Caribbean. Cost is also an issue, putting such treatments out of the reach of most.

---

**NOTE TO THE HEALTH CARE PROVIDER**

Feelings of hopelessness, helplessness, and loss of self-esteem may need to be addressed for the infertile woman. Initially, fertility treatments, even if affordable, may not be culturally acceptable to the couple. First, counseling sessions should be suggested.

---

## Pregnancy

**Activity Restrictions and Taboos.** Pregnancy is viewed as a special state. This society treats the "big" or "full" woman (terms used for pregnant women) gently since the woman is considered to be carrying a prized possession. Family and friends will often remind the pregnant woman that she is "eating for two," needs her rest, and should remain as free from stress and comfortable as possible. Often the pregnant woman will retain her job if employed outside the home. Frequent periods of rest with the feet elevated are customary and encouraged. Stretching or reaching above the head is discouraged, because of the fear that the umbilical cord will become tied around the fetus's neck. The pregnant woman's mother and older female relatives are likely to warn against coming into contact with deformed, disfigured, or disabled people and various animals, especially goats (often used during voodoo rituals), for fear of them *salting* (negatively affecting) the fetus.

Family support systems are generally very strong. Commonly, the pregnant woman's mother or an older female relative will assist with household chores (especially strenuous activities) during the final months. Throughout the pregnancy, the woman may drink various herbal teas intended to assist and ensure a healthy pregnancy.

The diet of this culture tends to be high in starchy foods (rice, potatoes, and "ground foods" such as yams and cassava/yuca); nonetheless, a well balanced diet is sought during pregnancy. In addition, many of these women frequently report of "pica" (the consumption of nonfood items), including starch, chalk, clay, and dirt.

**Prenatal Care.** Whether or not the woman receives prenatal care, the point at which care is initiated and from whom the woman seeks the care (i.e., lay or licensed midwife or medical doctor) is determined primarily by socioeconomic status and location of residence. Generally, women from urban areas will seek prenatal care early in the pregnancy and from a medical doctor or licensed midwife.

---

**NOTE TO THE HEALTH CARE PROVIDER**

Be sure to have clients identify all herbal teas and nutritional supplements that they are taking to avoid potential drug interactions or complications. Patient education should include information on the dangers of pica during pregnancy.

---

## Birthing Process

**Home Versus Hospital Delivery.** Today, home deliveries are no longer common. Most deliveries, especially in the urban areas, occur in the hospital under the supervision of a licensed health care professional. In the rural areas, however, where access to medical personnel may be limited, home deliveries under the supervision of a lay or licensed midwife still occur.

During the birthing process, it is customary for the pregnant woman's mother or another older female relative to be in attendance, helping and coaching the woman through labor and delivery. Traditionally, men are not present during the birthing process. This practice has been changing over the years, however, especially with younger couples.

**Cesarean Section Versus Vaginal Delivery.** Natural childbirth is preferred. Most deliveries are vaginal except in the event of an emergency.

**Labor Management.** Labor contractions are managed using breathing techniques and lower back massages. The use of pain medication is minimal, if at all. Following rupture of the membranes, the woman is placed on strict bed rest and monitored closely.

**Placenta.** Because of certain cultural and superstitious beliefs about the placenta, it is customary to dispose of it by burial in the backyard if the delivery occurs at home or outside the hospital setting. After delivery of the placenta, the patient may request to inspect it to make sure that it is intact.

---

**NOTE TO THE HEALTH CARE PROVIDER**

Offer pain medication to the client if she appears to be experiencing discomfort. Client will likely not request medication. Also, providers should expect female members of the family to be present throughout the entire labor and delivery process. Women may want to see the placenta and possibly inspect the cord after delivery, since some supernatural beliefs are associated with the placenta.

---

## Postpartum

The postpartum period can last up to 10 days. During this time, the woman remains on bed rest and is "binded." This means that a white flat sheet is wrapped tightly around her waist and abdomen to promote the return of the uterus to its pre-pregnancy size. Also, she is advised to stay indoors, away from "drafts" (cold breezes), and to avoid walking without shoes on the cold floor. To promote the production of breast milk, she is provided large amounts of herbal teas and soups.

---

**NOTE TO THE HEALTH CARE PROVIDER**

Avoid serving cold drinks or foods to the postpartum woman. Also, avoid turning on air conditioning systems and maintain an ambient temperature that is comfortable for the woman.

---

Newborn and Infant Care

**Breastfeeding Versus Bottle-Feeding.** Breastfeeding is the preferred method of feeding. It is considered a "natural" process. The breastfeeding period may extend for as long as 9 months to 1 year. Breastfeeding may also serve as a form of birth control for pregnancy spacing. If the mother works outside the home, she will be receptive to pumping her breasts and saving the milk for feeding the baby while she is away from home. Colicky infants are frequently fed herbal teas (chamomile and anise) as well as "gripe water" (a mixture of sodium bicarbonate and ginger) by bottle.

**Infant Protection.** It is generally believed that the young infant is highly vulnerable to cold ambient temperatures and cold breezes; hence, extra efforts are made to keep the infant well wrapped and warm. Evil forces from the outside world, such as evil spirits, envy, and the evil eye or *mal ojo* are also perceived as threats to the infant. For their children's protection, mothers will often avoid taking their newborns outdoors (unless absolutely necessary), fearing their children's exposure to jealous women capable of casting the evil eye. Symptoms associated with the evil eye include vomiting, diarrhea, irritability, and colic. For added protection against evil spirits or the evil eye, a bible, cross, or other religious artifact may be placed in or near the child's crib. A religious relic or blue ribbon may be pinned on the inner aspects of the child's clothing.

---

**NOTE TO THE HEALTH CARE PROVIDER**
Limiting the number of people/staff who hold and touch the child to those directly involved with the child's care is helpful. Staff members should avoid paying excessive compliments to the child about his or her appearance.

---

**Primary Caregiver.** The mother is usually the primary care provider to the children. Traditionally, men have not played an active role in childcare. This, however, is gradually changing, and the modern man may provide some assistance with the care of his children especially if his wife is ill. The role of the extended family, especially the maternal grandmother, is one of support and nurturing.

## Middle Age

### Cultural Attitudes and Expectations

At or about age 50, women are considered middle-aged. Accordingly, they are expected to dress and conduct themselves conservatively. If single and dating, the woman is expected to date a man in her age range or older. Society frowns on the older woman dating or marrying a younger man but is more forgiving if an older man marries a much younger woman.

### Psychological Response

The concept of the "empty nest" syndrome, typically occurring at midlife when the children grow up and move away from home, is generally a nonevent for Caribbean people because of both the physical and emotional closeness that the extended family maintains. Likewise, "midlife" crisis is generally not a recognized phenomenon in this culture. Most women take great pride in their roles as mother and later grandmother, anticipating their role in helping to raise the grandchildren.

### Menopause

**Onset and Duration.**   Menopause, referred to as "change-of-life" or "the change," demarcates the end of a woman's fertile years. Although fertility provides a source of pride, self-worth, and identity for many of these women, at the time of menopause few express regret at its onset, because they see menopause as a " naturally occurring" phenomenon. Early or late onset of menopause can be attributed to genetics, as can the intensity of the associated discomforts of menopause. The costs of hormone replacement therapy (HRT) coupled with the fear of breast cancer, long associated with the use of HRT, account for the limited demand and use of these drugs among West Indian women.

**Sexual Activity.**   The menopausal woman remains sexually active. Hot flashes, vaginal dryness, and emotional lability are all recognized as "real" and an expected part or the body's response to menopause.

**Coping.**   Menopause marks the beginning of another phase of life for women in this culture. They may be concerned about hot flashes and unexpected bleeding and will consult with their friends or older women who have already gone through "the change." Herbal teas or "cooling," such as **serasy** and **mauby,** are often used to control the discomfort of hot flashes. Only if the various prescribed herbal remedies do not work will women generally seek biomedical treatments.

---

**NOTE TO THE HEALTH CARE PROVIDER**
Educate and reassure women of the improvements in and increased safety of HRT. Be aware of possible drug interactions or potentiation with HRT and herbal remedies. Clients often will not volunteer this information unless directly questioned.

---

# Old Age

Many West Indians live well into their late 80s or 90s. It is believed that the simplicity and decreased stressors that accompany life in the Caribbean contribute to the extended life span. At the same time, the diet includes many fried foods; highly seasoned foods; and the use of high-cholesterol products in cooking, including coconut cream, lard, and large amounts of cooking oil. The use of these products can contribute to the high incidence of hypertension, stroke, and cardiac disease that kill a significant number of individuals in their 40s or early 50s.

## Cultural Attitudes

This culture greatly respects the elderly. Women in their late 60s or early 70s are considered old and afforded respect from both their family and community. Most elderly women tend to live with their adult children and their families. Those who live alone remain in close contact with their adult children and grandchildren, who are readily available to assist with errands and chores that the elderly woman cannot perform. For most West Indians, placing an elderly relative in a nursing home is unacceptable.

## Death and Dying

### Cultural Attitudes and Beliefs

As a largely Christian society (Episcopalian and Catholic), except for Hindus or Muslims of East Indian heritage, West Indians view death as terminal or the end stage of life. There is no belief in an "afterlife" in the sense that people do not believe that the dead person will return to earth in the form of an animal or as a newborn child.

At the time of death, it is believed that all physical life ceases, but the spirit or soul continues. The souls of those individuals who have lived a "good" life on earth are said to go to heaven for their reward. Conversely, the souls of those having lived a "bad" or "evil" life, referred to as **duppies** or **jumbies,** are thought to roam about the earth, with the ability to negatively affect the living.

### Rites and Rituals

Sadness, grief, and public displays of mourning that may last for several months surround death and accompanying burial rituals. Customarily, the body of the deceased is treated and handled with a great deal of respect. Traditionally, the body was retained at the family's residence for the ceremonial wake to be followed by the funeral service the next day. Today, the use of funeral homes is very much the norm. Cremation of the body, for most West Indians, is unacceptable. The exception is certain East Indian groups whose religious beliefs and practices call for cremation of the body soon after death.

### Mourning

**Cultural Expectations.** Mourning the dead lasts for an average period of 9 days. On the ninth day, a so-called "nine-night" reception is held. The "nine-night" reception is essentially a gathering of family and friends to pray for the departed soul. Although food and drinks, including alcoholic beverages, are served, this reception is usually a somber occasion. The surviving spouse and family members are expected to wear black, purple, or white clothing during the period of mourning. Wearing red or other bright-colored clothing at this time is considered disrespectful. It is also customary for the maternal grandmother or members of the extended family to care for young or minor children of a deceased mother.

**Coping.** Spirituality (especially prayers), frequent visits to the burial site, and faith in God (believing that it is God's will) are the means of coping most frequently used by the surviving family members.

---

**NOTE TO THE HEALTH CARE PROVIDER**

The mourning period and observance may appear prolonged and even pathologic by North American standards. Providers must respect and support a client's need to mourn. They should not attempt to minimize or hasten the mourning period. The client may benefit from referral to a grief support group.

---

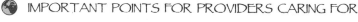

# IMPORTANT POINTS FOR PROVIDERS CARING FOR WEST INDIAN WOMEN

## The Medical Intake

### Literacy and English Proficiency

English is the primary language in most of the West Indian islands. Many, but not all, residents of the Dutch and French West Indies are proficient in English. Additionally, individuals from this region have a high literacy rate, making it unlikely that they will need the assistance of translators or help in filling out required forms.

### Status of the Provider

Health care professionals are highly respected. Women tend to be shy and are not likely to be forthcoming with information unless specifically questioned.

### Communicating Illness and Symptoms

Women are unlikely to volunteer significant medical history, especially information of a sexual nature or related to a private body parts. Answers to questions will often be brief. The provider should ask a variety of questions, most of which can be answered with yes or no, to establish rapport. If a client believes that an illness is the result of a spiritual issue, it is unlikely that she will convey this to the provider. The woman's spouse usually will not accompany her, but a female family member may, who will actively participate in providing information.

---

**NOTE TO THE HEALTH CARE PROVIDER**
Providers must be particularly discreet when asking questions that women may consider offensive, especially those pertaining to her sexual behavior.

---

## The Physical Examination

### Modesty and Touching

West Indian women tend to be very modest. Providers should avoid unnecessary exposure of the naked body during examinations. Also a female provider is much preferred. These women will generally avoid being examined during the menstrual period, unless it is an emergency.

### Expressing Pain

There is a tendency for women to be stoic when dealing with pain. Often, they will not complain or request analgesics unless the pain is severe.

## Prescribing Medications

### Drug Interactions

Drug interactions and the potentiation of prescription drugs are issues of concern for the health provider because of the group's widespread use of herbal teas and roots.

### Medication Sharing

Sharing prescription medications is not uncommon among West Indians. Also, if the client is taking medications prescribed by another health provider, she is unlikely to reveal this information unless specifically asked.

### Compliance

Since many of these clients seek medical attention only after various home remedies fail to resolve the problem, they are likely to initially comply with the medication regimen. As signs and symptoms of the disease subside, however, they are likely to discontinue medication use. Noncompliance may also be a problem if the client does not see or feel improvement in her condition in a timely manner. The health care provider should give the client a realistic time frame in which to expect results. Also, he or she should emphasize the importance of completing the full course of all prescription medications.

## Follow-up Appointments

Depending on the perceived severity of the illness, a client may or may not view follow-up visits as necessary. A reminder call the day before the appointment may help ensure patient compliance with follow-up visits.

### Orientation to Time

This group is oriented to social time; however, if the client recognizes the importance of seeing the provider, she is punctual. To increase follow-up care, the provider should inform the client of the need for a follow-up appointment during the initial visit.

## Prevalent Diseases

The diseases most prevalent within this group are hypertension and diabetes, for which genetics and dietary practices are believed to be the common causes. Coconut oil, which is high in saturated fats, is used regularly in the preparation of most meals. Likewise, salt fish, a food high in sodium, is a traditional dish savored throughout the Caribbean.

## Health-Seeking Behaviors

Medical attention may be sought at a more advanced stage of the disease process because many West Indians still rely heavily on herbs and home remedies to cure illnesses. Thus, they will seek medical help only when home remedies fail to correct the problem.

 BIBLIOGRAPHY

Ford, K. (1986). The Diverse Fertility of Caribbean, Central and South American Immigrants in the United States. *Sociology and Social Research*, 70(4), 281–283.

MacCormack, C. P. (1985). Lay Concepts Affecting Utilization of Family Planning Services in Jamaica. *Journal of Tropical Medicine and Hygiene*, 88, 281–285.

St. Hill, P. (1996). West Indian Immigrants *in* J. Lipson, L. Dibble & P. Minarik (Eds). *Culture & nursing care: A pocket guide*. San Francisco: UCSF Press.

1998 Statistical Yearbook of the Immigration and Naturalization Service (November, 2000). U.S. Department of Justice, Washington DC

# RESOURCES FOR WOMEN

## In the United States

### Women's Commission for Refugee Women and Children

122 East 42nd Street
New York, NY 10168-1289

Tel: 212-551-3111 or 3088
Fax: 212-551-3180
Internet: *www.womenscommission.org*

An independent organization formed with the assistance of the International Rescue Committee to advocate for the solution of problems affecting refugee women and children. The Commission works with a wide range of non-governmental organizations, United Nations agencies, governments, and individuals.

### The Hesperian Foundation

1919 Addison Street, Suite 304
Berkeley, CA 94704

Tel: 510-845-1447
Fax: 510-845-9141
Internet: *www.hesperian.org*

A nonprofit organization committed to improving the health of people in poor communities throughout the world by providing tools and resources for health education and informed self-care. The books use simple language and excellent line drawings, and many are translated into multiple languages.

*Women's Health Exchange: A Resource for Training and Education* is an information-packed, theme-based newsletter that comes out sporadically. E-mail: *whx@hesperian.org*

### International Council on Women's Health Issues (ICOWHI)

1111 Middle Drive, NU451
Indianapolis, IN 46202

Fax: 317-274-2996
E-mail: swilkers@indyvax.iupui.edu

An international, nonprofit organization dedicated to the goal of promoting the health, health care, and well-being of women throughout the world through participation, empowerment, advocacy, education, and research. The multidisciplinary membership includes women's health providers, planners, and advocates throughout the globe. The organization holds biennial international congresses and publishes the bimonthly journal, *Health Care for Women International*.

### National Women's Health Information Center (NWHIC)

8550 Arlington Boulevard, Suite 300
Fairfax, VA 22031

Tel: 1-800-994-9662
TDD: 1-888-220-5446
E-mail: 4woman@soza.com
Internet: *www.4woman.gov*

This nonprofit organization, sponsored by the U.S. Public Health Service Office on Women's Health, is dedicated to improving the health of women by providing *free* information and resource service on women's health issues to consumers, health care professionals, researchers, educators, and students. Acting somewhat like a Federal "Women's Health Central," this organization does not provide clinical advice but can link you directly to thousands of fact sheets, brochures, reports, and other important health information.

**Violence Against Women Office**
810 7th Street, NW                    Tel: 202-307-6026
Washington, DC 20531                  Fax: 202-307-3911

Committed to defending and seeking justice for women who are victims of violence, this office, in addition to its many other tasks, works with victim advocates and law enforcement in developing grant programs that support a wide range of services for victims of domestic violence, sexual assault, and stalking. Additionally, it is leading the effort nationally and abroad to intervene in and prosecute crimes of trafficking in women and children and is addressing domestic violence issues in international fora.

**Breast Health Access for Women with Disabilities (BHAWD)**
Alta Bates Medical Center              Tel: 510-204-4866
2001 Dwight Way, 2nd Floor             TDD: 510-204 4574
Herrick Campus Rehabilitation Services Fax: 510-204-5892
Berkeley, CA 94704                     Internet: *http://www.bhawd.org*

A clinic-based program dedicated to improving access to breast health care for women with disabilities. BHAWD, in collaboration with community agencies such as Center for Independent Living, United Cerebral Palsy of the Golden Gate, Community Resources for Independent Living, and Alta Bates Summit Medical Center (Rehabilitative Services and Comprehensive Breast Center), provides women with disabilities, 20 years and older free clinical breast examinations, self-breast examination education and training, and referral for a mammogram, if deemed appropriate. This program will also provide, *free of charge*, a trained presenter to talk to groups about breast health issues and concerns and mammography for women with disabilities.

**Caribbean Women's Health Association (CWHA)**
2725 Church Avenue                     Tel: 718-826-2942
Brooklyn, N.Y. 11226                   Fax: 718-826-2948
                                       Internet: *http://www.aidsnyc.org/cwha/*
                                                 *center.html*

Staffed with multilingual professionals, this nonprofit organization (with four offices in the Greater New York City area) is dedicated to assisting members of the Caribbean-American community to adjust and become self-sufficient, productive members in their host communities. Among the many assistance programs and services offered by the CWHA are low-cost legal services, immigration counseling and assistance, family and social support referral services, health care referral services, nutrition referral services, and substance abuse referral services.

## Migration and Refugee Services (MRS)

1900 South Acadian Thruway (physical address)
P.O. Box 4213 (mailing address)
Baton Rouge, LA 70821-4213

Tel: 225-346-0660
Fax: 225-346-0220

A member of the Louisiana State Refugee Advisory Council, MRS of the Catholic Community Charity Services is a program committed to developing and providing resettlement opportunities to incoming refugees and immigrants. Among the many services offered to immigrant and refugee families, the program assists immigrants and refugees toward self-sufficiency by providing social services, including English as a Second Language classes and employment services, as well as immigration, counseling, family reunification, and sponsorship development services.

## American Indian Community House (AICH)

404 Lafayette Street
New York, New York

Tel: 212-420-0879
Internet: *http://www.aich.org/services/ services.htm*

A not-for-profit organization serving the health, social service, and cultural needs of Native Americans residing in New York City. Among the many programs and services offered by this organization are job training and placement; free legal services; health services referral, including human immunodeficiency virus (HIV) referral and case management services; and counseling programs for alcoholism and substance abuse. AICH also publishes a quarterly bulletin—**AICH *Community Bulletin*,** maintains a video library, pow-wow listings, and an event listing, all available to scholars, students and educators at minimal or no charge. Subsumed under the health services division, the "Women's Wellness Circle Project" addresses barriers to health care for Native American women by providing a variety of accessible health and supportive services. Eligibility requirements for accessing AICH services, other than being Native American, vary depending on the service being accessed. Additionally, there are some programs available to anyone, regardless of eligibility.

## Hispanic Women's Network of Texas (HWNT)

Dallas Chapter
P.O. Box 516411
Dallas, TX 75251-6411

A nonprofit, state-wide organization of individuals from diverse backgrounds who are committed to promoting the participation of Hispanic women in public, corporate, and civic arenas. HWNT, with chapters in Austin, Corpus Christi, Dallas, El Paso, Fort Worth, Rio Grande Valley, and San Antonio, has become the premier Hispanic women's organization in Texas. The organization seeks to advance the education, cultural, social, legal, and economic well-being of all women through the broader awareness of their role in society, business, and family.

## In Canada

**Immigrant and Visible Minority Women Against Abuse**
P.O. Box 3188                                      Tel: 613-729-3145
Station "C"
Ottawa, Ontario K1Y4J4
Canada

A project in Ottawa, Canada, developed and staffed by immigrant and racial minority women to provide crisis service to help racial minority women who are abused and to enable the women access to the full range of services available for abused women. In addition to the crisis service provided, the project, through public education and outreach, also aims to sensitize social agency and community workers to existing cultural and racial discrimination and to raise the awareness among immigrant and racial minority women about wife abuse and violence against women and encourages them to break out of their isolation.

**Canadian Council for Refugees (CCR)**
6839 Drolet #320                          Tel: 514-277-7223
Montreal, Quebec, H2S2T1                   Fax: 514-277-1447
Canada                                    E-mail: ccr@web.net
                                          Internet: *www.web/~ccr/whowe.htm*

A nonprofit umbrella organization committed to the rights and protection of refugees in Canada and around the world and to the settlement of refugees and immigrants in Canada. Working at both the national and international levels, CCR works in cooperation with other networks to strengthen the defense of refugee rights. It advocates for the rights of refugees and immigrants through media and government relations, research, and public education. It also provides opportunities for networking and professional development through conferences, working groups, publications, and meetings.

**Ottawa Chinese Community Service Center**
391 Bank Street, 2nd floor                Tel: 613-232-2877 or 235-4873
Ottawa, Ontario K2P1Y3                    Internet: *http:infoweb.magi.com/~occsc/*
Canada                                    *history.htm*

A nonprofit, nonpartisan, community-based charitable organization initially established in response to the unmet social service and integration needs of the many non-English speaking Chinese immigrants in the Ottawa-Carleton Region. Later incorporated in Ontario, the organization remains committed to advancing the full social and economic integration and participation of newcomers, immigrants, and refugees in their host country. Among the many services offered by the organization are individual and family counseling for low-income individuals and families, English as a Second Language classes for middle-aged and older new immigrants and refugees, and a Support Group for people with mental illness. For the immigrant woman, the center offers, in collaboration with the Regional Health Department, a prenatal course for first time mothers and Well-Baby Drop-In, among other women's health services.

# BIBLIOGRAPHY ON IMMIGRANT AND REFUGEE WOMEN'S HEALTH

**Note: This is a selection, not a complete listing, of literature concerning women who have immigrated to the United States and Canada. Selected general books and articles are included because they provide a context for understanding the lives of immigrant and refugee women.**

 DEVELOPMENT

## Children

Aronowitz, M. (1984). The social and emotional adjustment of immigrant children: a review of the literature. *International Migration Review*, 18(2), 237–257.

Ajdukovic, M., & Ajdukovic, D. (1993). Psychological well-being of refugee children. *Child Abuse and Neglect*, 17, 843–845.

American Academy of Pediatrics. (1998). Committee on Bioethics (1998). Female genital mutilation. *Pediatrics*, 102 (Pt 1), 53–56.

DeSantis, L., & Thomas, J. (1994). Childhood independence: views of Cuban and Haitian immigrant mothers. *Journal of Pediatric Nursing*, 9, 258–267.

Fox, P. G., Cowell, J. M., & Montgomery, A. (1999). Southeast Asian refugee children: violence experience and depression. *International Journal of Psychiatric Nursing Research*, 5, 589–600.

Fox, P. G., Cowell, J., & Montgomery, A. (1994). The effects of violence on health and adjustment of Southeast Asian refugee children: an integrative review. *Public Health Nursing*, 11, 195–201.

Garbarino, J., Dubrow, N., Kostelny, K. & Prado, C. (1992). *Children in Danger*. San Francisco: Jossey-Bass Publishers.

May, K. (1992). Middle-Eastern immigrant parents' social networks and help-seeking for child health care. *Journal of Advanced Nursing*, 17, 905–912.

Mendoza, F., Ventura, S., Burciaga-Valdez, R., Castillo, R., Escoto Saldiva, L., Baisden, K., & Martorell, R. (1991). Selected measures of health status for Mexican-American, Puerto Rican, and Cuban-American children. JAMA, 265, 227–232.

Pickwell, S. (1981). School health screening of Indochinese refugee children. *The Journal of School Health*, 51, 102–105.

Pickwell, S. (1982). Primary health care for Indochinese refugee children. *Pediatric Nursing*, 8(2), 104–107.

Thomas, J., & DeSantis, L. (1995). Feeding and weaning practices of Cuban and Haitian immigrant mothers. *Journal of Transcultural Nursing*, 6, 34–42.

Zahr, L., & Hattar-Pollara, M. (1999). Nursing care of Arab American children: consideration of basic cultural factors. *Journal of Pediatric Nursing*, 13(6), 349–355.

## Adolescence

Frye, B., & McGill, D. (1993). Cambodian refugee adolescents: cultural factors and mental health nursing. *Journal of Child and Adolescent Psychiatric and Mental Health Nursing*, 6(4), 24–31.

Hattar-Pollara, M., & Meleis, A. (1995). Parenting their adolescents: the experiences of Jordanian immigrant women in California. *Health Care for Women International*, 16, 195–211.

Muecke, M., & Sassi, L. (1992). Anxiety among Cambodian refugee adolescents in transit and in re-settlement. *Western Journal of Nursing Research*, 14, 267–285; discussion 286–291.

Otero-Sabogal, R., Sabogal, F., & Perez-Stable E. J. (1995). Psychosocial correlates of smoking among immigrant Latina adolescents. *Journal of the National Cancer Institute. Monographs*, 18, 65–71.

## Adulthood

Anderson, J. M. (1985). Perspectives on the health of immigrant women: a feminist analysis. *Advances in Nursing Science*, 8(1), 61–71.

DeVoe, P. A. (1992). The silent majority: women as refugees. In R. Gallin, A. Ferguson, & J. Harper (Eds.). *The women and international development annual*, 3. Boulder, CO: Westview Press, pp. 19–49.

Martin, S. F. (1991). *Refugee Women*. London and New Jersey: Zed Books Ltd.

Mayotte, J. (1992). Refugee Women. In J. Mayotte (ed.) *Disposable people? The plight of refugees*. New York: Orbis Books.

Meadows, L., Thurston, W., & Melton, C. (2001). Immigrant women's health. *Social Science and Medicine*, 52, 1451–1458.

Messias, D. K. H., Hall, J. M., & Meleis, A. I. (1996). Voices of impoverished Brazilian women: health implications of roles and resources. *Women and Health*, 24, 1–20.

## Fertility/Prenatal Care

Ashford, L. (2001). New population policies: advancing women's health and rights. *Population Bulletin*, 56(1), Washington, DC: Population Reference Bureau.

Chamnivickorn, S. (1988). Fertility, labor supply and investment in child quality among Asian American immigrant women. *Pacific Asian American Mental Health Research Review*, 6, 28–29.

Hyman, I., & Dussault, G. (2000). Negative consequences of acculturation on health behaviour, social support and stress among pregnant Southeast Asian immigrant women in Montreal: an exploratory study. *Canadian Journal of Public Health*. Revue Canadienne de Sante Publique, 91, 57–60.

Kulig, J. (1995). Cambodian refugees' family planning knowledge and use. *Journal of Advanced Nursing*, 22, 150–157.

Kulig, J. (1994). Sexuality beliefs among Cambodians: implications for health care professionals. *Health Care for Women International*, 15, 69–76.

Kulig, J. (1990). Childbearing beliefs among Cambodian refugee women. *Western Journal of Nursing Research*, 12, 108–118.

Kulig, J. (1988). Conception and birth control use: Cambodian refugee women's beliefs and practices. *Journal of Community Health Nursing*, 5, 235–246.

Lindenberg, C., Strickland, O., Solorzano, R., Galvis, C. Dreher, M., & Darrow, V. (1999). Correlates of alcohol and drug use among low-income Hispanic immigrant childbearing women living in the USA. *International Journal of Nursing Studies*, 36, 3–11.

Mattson, S., & Lew, L. (1992). Culturally sensitive prenatal care for Southeast Asians. *Journal of Obstetric, Gynecologic, and Neonatal Nursing*, 21, 48–54.

Pritham, U., & Sammons, L. (1993). Korean women's attitudes toward pregnancy and prenatal care. *Health Care for Women International*, 14(2), 145–153.

Spring, M., Ross, P., Etkin, N., & Deinard, A. (1995). Sociocultural factors in the use of prenatal care by Hmong women, Minneapolis. *American Journal of Public Health*, 85, 1015–1017.

Vega, W., Kolody, B., Hwang, J., Noble, A., & Porter, P. (1997). Perinatal drug use among immigrant and native-born Latinas. *Substance Use and Misuse*, 32, 43–62.

Wright, R. E., & Madan, A. K. (1988). Union instability and fertility in three Caribbean societies. *Journal of Biosocial Sciences*, 20, 37–43.

Zambrana, R., Scrimshaw, S., Collins, N., & Dunkel-Schetter, C. (1997). Prenatal health behaviors and psychosocial risk factors in pregnant women of Mexican origin: the role of acculturation. *American Journal of Public Health*, 87, 1022–1026.

# Birth/Postpartum

Alexander, G., Mor, J., Kogan, M., Leland, N., & Kieffer, E. (1996). Pregnancy outcomes of US-born and foreign-born Japanese Americans. *American Journal of Public Health*, 86, 820–824.

Cervantes, A., Keith, L., & Wyshak G. (1999). Adverse birth outcomes among native-born and immigrant women: replicating national evidence regarding Mexicans at the local level. *Maternal and Child Health Journal*, 3(2), 99–109.

Choi, E. (1995). A contrast of mothering behaviors in women from Korea and the United States. *Journal of Obstetric, Gynecologic, and Neonatal Nursing*, 24, 363–369.

Choi, E. (1986). Unique aspects of Korean-American mothers. *Journal of Obstetrical Gynecological Neonatal Nursing*, 15, 394–400.

Cobas, J., Balcazar, H., Benin, M., Keith, V., & Chong, Y. (1996). Acculturation and low-birth weight infants among Latino {sic} women: a reanalysis of HHANES data with structural equation models. *American Journal of Public Health*, 86, 394–396.

Edwards, N., & Boivin, J. (1997). Ethnocultural predictors of postpartum infant-care behaviours among immigrants in Canada. *Ethnicity and Health*, 2, 63–76.

Faller, H. (1985). Perinatal needs of immigrant Hmong women: Surveys of women and health care providers. *Public Health Reports*, 100, 340–343.

Jones, M., & Bond, M. (1999). Predictors of birth outcome among Hispanic immigrant women. *Journal of Nursing Care Quality*, 14, 56–62.

Kulig, J. (1990). Childbearing beliefs among Cambodian refugee women. *Western Journal of Nursing Research*, 12, 108–118.

Meleis, A. I., & Sorrell, L. (1981). Arab American women and their birth experiences. *American Journal of Maternal Child Nursing*, 6, 171–176.

Minkler, D. (1983). The role of a community-based satellite clinic in the perinatal care of non-English speaking immigrants. *The Western Journal of Medicine*, 139, 905–909.

Muecke, M., & Hahn, R. (1987). Ethnic variation in birth outcomes: implications for obstetrical practice. *Current Problems in Obstetrics, Gynecology and Fertility*, 10, 133–171.

Park, K. J., & Peterson, L. M. (1991). Beliefs, practices and experiences of Korean women in relation to childbirth. *Health Care for Women International*, 12(2), 261–269.

Scribner, R., & Dwyer, J. (1989). Acculturation and low birth weight among Latinos in the Hispanic HANES. *American Journal of Public Health*, 79, 1263–1267.

# Menopause/Midlife

Berg, J. (1999) The perimenopausal transition of Filipino American midlife women: biopsychosocialcultural dimensions. *Nursing Research*, 48(2), 71–77.

Berg, J., & Lipson, J. (1999). Information sources, menopause beliefs, and health complaints of midlife Filipinas. *Women's Health Care International*, 20, 81–92.

Berg, J., & Taylor, D. (1999). Symptom responses of midlife Filipinas. *Menopause: Journal of the North American Menopause Society*, 6(2), 115–121.

Brown, A., Perez-Stable, E., Whitaker, E., Posner, S., Alexander, M., Gathe, J., & Washington, A. (1999). Ethnic differences in hormone replacement prescribing patterns. *Journal of General Internal Medicine*, 14, 663–669.

Im, E. O., & Lipson, J. (1997). Menopausal transition of Korean immigrant women: a literature review. *Women's Health Care International*, 18, 507–520.

Im, E. O., & Meleis, A. I. (2000). Meanings of menopause: low income Korean immigrant women. *Western Journal of Nursing Research*, 22, 84–102.

Im, E. O., & Meleis, A. I. (1999). A situation-specific theory of Korean immigrant women's menopausal transition. *Image—the Journal of Nursing Scholarship*, 31, 333–338.

Im, E. O., Meleis, A. I., & Lee, K. (1999). Symptom experience during menopausal transition: low income Korean immigrant women. *Women and Health*, 29(2), 53–67.

Im, E. O., Meleis, A. I., & Park, Y. S. (1999). A feminist critique of the research on menopausal experience of Korean women. *Research in Nursing and Health*, 22, 410–420.

Meadows, L., Thurston, W., & Melton, C. (2001). Immigrant women's health. *Social Science and Medicine*, 52, 1451–1458.

# Elderly

Ailinger, R., & Causey, M. (1995). Health concept of older Hispanic immigrants. *Western Journal of Nursing Research*, 17, 605–613.

Black, S., Markides, K., & Miller, T. (1998). Correlates of depressive symptomatology among older community-dwelling Mexican Americans: the Hispanic EPESE. *Journals of Gerontology. Series B, Psychological Sciences and Social Sciences*, 53, S198–208.

Boyd, M. (1991). Immigration and living arrangements: Elderly women in Canada. *International Migration Review*, 25(1), 4–27.

Kim, O. (1999). Predictors of loneliness in elderly Korean immigrant women living in the United States of America. *Journal of Advanced Nursing*, 29, 1082–1088.

Meleis, A. I., & Im, E. O. (2002). Grandmothers and women's health: for integrative and coherent models of women's health. *Health Care for Women International*, 23, 207–224.

Moon, J. H., & Pearl, J. H. (1991). Alienation of elderly Korean American immigrants as related to place of residence, gender, age, years of education, time in the U.S., living with or without children, and living with or without a spouse. *International Journal of Aging and Human Development*, 32(2), 115–124.

Omidian, P., & Lipson, J. G. (1992). Elderly Afghan refugees: Tradition and transition in northern California. In *Refugee Issues Papers*. Arlington, VA: American Anthropological Association, 1, 27–39.

Pang, K. Y. C. (1990). Hwabyung: the construction of a Korean popular illness among Korean elderly immigrant women in the United States. *Culture, Medicine and Psychiatry*, 14, 495–512.

Yee, B. W. K. (1992). Markers of successful aging among Vietnamese refugee women. In E. Cole, O. Espin, & E. Rothblum (Eds.) *Refugee women and their mental health: Shattered societies, shattered lives*. New York: Haworth Press, pp. 221–238.

# 🌐 ROLES, WORK, PARENTING

## Work

Amott, T., & Matthaei, J. (1991). Climbing gold mountain: Asian American women. In *Race gender, and work*. Boston: South End Press, pp. 193–256.

Boyd, M. (1984). At a disadvantage: the occupational attainments of foreign born women in Canada. *International Migration Review*, 18, 1091–1119.

Brown, D., & James, G. (2000). Physiological stress responses in Filipino-American immigrant nurses: the effects of residence time, life-style, and job strain. *Psychosomatic Medicine*, 62, 394–400.

Dallalfar, A. (1994). Iranian women as immigrant entrepreneurs. *Gender and Society*, 8, 541–561.

Gannage C. M. (1999). The health and safety concerns of immigrant women workers in the Toronto sportswear industry. *International Journal of Health Services*, 29, 409–429.

Im, E. O., & Meleis, A. I. (2001). Women's work and symptoms during midlife: Korean immigrant women. *Women and Health*, 33,(1/2), 83–103.

Kelly, G. P. (1994). To become an American woman: Education and sex role socialization of the Vietnamese immigrant woman. In L. Vicki et al (Eds.). *Unequal Sisters: A multicultural reader in U.S. women's history*. New York: Routledge, pp. 497–507.

Meleis, A. I., Douglas, M., Eribes, C., Shih, F., & Messias, D. (1996). Employed Mexican women as mothers and partners: valued, empowered and overloaded. *Journal of Advanced Nursing*, 23, 82–90.

National Council for Research on Women. (1995). The Lucy Parsons' initiative: laying the groundwork for contingent women workers. 1(3), 22–23.

Pessar, P. R. (1984). The linkage between the household and workplace of Dominican women in the United States. *International Migration Review*, 18, 1188–1211.

Repak, T. A. (1994). Labor recruitment and the lure of the capital: Central American migrants in Washington, DC. *Gender & Society*, 8, 507–524.

Stevens, P., Hall, J., & Meleis, A. (1992). Examining vulnerability of women clerical workers from five ethnic/racial groups. *Western Journal of Nursing Research* 14, 754–774.

Stier, H. (1991). Immigrant women go to work: analysis of immigrant wives' labor supply for six Asian groups. *Social Science Quarterly*, 72, 67–82.

Tienda, M., Jensen, L., & Bach, R. L. (1984). Immigration, gender and the process of occupational change in the United States, 1970–80. *International Migration Review*, 18, 1021–1044.

Weitzman, B. C., & Berry, C. A. (1992). Health status and health care utilization among New York City home attendants: an illustration of needs of working poor, immigrant women. *Women and Health*, 19, 87–105.

Zsembik, B. A., & Peek, C. W. (1994). The effect of economic restructuring on Puerto Rican women's labor force participation in the formal sector. *Gender & Society*, 8, 525–540.

## Spousal/Family Roles

Aroian, K., Spitzer, A., & Bell, M. (1996). Family stress and support among former Soviet immigrants. *Western Journal of Nursing Research*, 18, 655–674.

Fox, P. G., Cowell, J. M., & Johnson, M. (1995). The effects of family disruption on Southeast Asian refugee women: implications for international nursing. *International Nursing Review*, 42, 27–30.

Kim, B.-L. C. (1977). Asian wives of U.S. servicemen: women in shadows, *Amereia*, 4, 91–115.

Kulig, J. (1994). "Those with unheard voices": the plight of a Cambodian refugee woman. *Journal of Community Health Nursing*, 11, 99–107.

Lee, D. B. (1997). Korean women married to servicemen. In Y.I. Song and A. Moon (Eds.). *Korean American Women Living in Two Cultures*. Los Angeles: Keimyung-Baylor University Press, pp. 96–97.

Lipson, J. & Miller, S. (1994). Changing roles of Afghan refugee women in the U.S. *Health Care for Women International* 14, 171–180.

Ng, R., & Ramirez, J. (1981). *Immigrant housewives in Canada*. Toronto: The Immigrant Women's Center.

Rosenthal, D. A., & Feldman, S. S. (1990). The acculturation of Chinese immigrants: perceived effects on family functioning of length of residence in two cultural contexts. *Journal of Genetic Psychology*, 151, 495–514.

## 🌐 TRANSITIONS, IMMIGRATION, ASSIMILATION, AND ACCULTURATION

Anderson, J. M. (1987). Migration and health: perspectives on immigrant women. *Sociology of Health & Illness*, 9, 410–438.

Hattar-Pollara, M., & Meleis, A. (1995). The stress of immigration and the daily lived experiences of Jordanian immigrant women in the United States. *Western Journal of Nursing Research*, 17, 521–539.

Hongdagneu-Sotelo, P. (1994). *Gendered transitions: Mexican experiences of immigration*. Berkeley: University of California Press.

Kim, Y. & Grant D. (1997). Immigration patterns, social support, and adaptation among Korean immigrant women and Korean American women. *Cultural Diversity and Mental Health*, 3, 235–245.

Krulfeld, R. M. (1994). Buddhism, maintenance and change: reinterpreting gender in a Lao refugee community. In L. Camino & R. Krulfeld (Eds.). *Reconstructing lives, recapturing meaning* (pp. 97–127). Basel: Gordon and Breach.

Kulig, J. (1994). Old traditions in a new world: Changing gender relations among Cambodian refugees. In L. Camino & R. Krulfeld (Eds.), *Reconstructing Lives, Recapturing Meaning*. Basel: Gordon and Breach, pp. 129–146.

Lalonde, R. N., Taylor, D. M., & Moghaddam, F. M. (1992). The process of social identification for visible immigrant women in a multicultural context. *Journal of Cross-Cultural Psychology*, 23, 25–39.

Lynam, M. J. (1985). Support networks developed by immigrant women. *Social Science and Medicine*, 31, 327–333.

Meleis, A. (1995). Immigrant women in borderless societies: marginalised and empowered. *Asian Journal of Nursing Studies*, 2(4), 39–47.

Meleis, A. (1991). Between two cultures: identity, roles and health. *Health Care for Women International*. 12, 365–377.

Meleis, A. I., & Rogers, S. (1987). Women in transition: being versus becoming or being and becoming. *Health Care for Women International*, 8, 199–217.

Muecke, M. (1987). Resettled refugees' reconstruction of identity: Lao in Seattle. *Urban Anthropology and Studies of Cultural Systems and World Economic Development*, 16, 273–289.

Parvanta, S. (1992). The balancing act: plight of Afghan women refugees: the challenges and rewards. In E. Cole, O. Espin, & E. Rothblum (Eds.). *Refugee Women and Their Mental Health: Shattered Societies, Shattered Lives*. New York: Haworth Press, pp. 113–128.

Shin, K. R., Shin C. (1999). The lived experience of Korean immigrant women acculturating into the United States. *Health Care for Women International*, 20(6), 603–617.

Siegel, R. J. (1992). Fifty years later: am I still an immigrant? In E. Cole, O. Espin, & E. Rothblum (Eds.). *Refugee Women and Their Mental Health: Shattered Societies, Shattered Lives*. New York: Haworth Press, pp. 105–111.

# 🌐 HEALTH AND ILLNESS

## Cultural Health and Illness Beliefs

Calhoun, M. (1985). The Vietnamese woman: Health/illness attitudes and behaviors. *Health Care for Women International*, 6, 61–72.

Chin, S. Y. (1992). This, that and the other managing illness in a first-generation Korean-American family. *Western Journal of Medicine*, 157, 305–309.

Eyega, Z., & Conneely, E. (1997). Facts and fiction regarding female circumcision/female genital mutilation: a pilot study in New York City. *Journal of the American Medical Womens Association*, 52, 74–78, 187.

Frye, B., & D'Avanzo, C. D. (1994). Themes in managing culturally defined illness in the Cambodian refugee family. *Journal of Community Health Nursing*, 11, 89–98.

Miller, J. (1990). Use of traditional Korean health care by Korean immigrants to the United States. *Sociology and Social Research*, 75(1), 38–48.

Pang, K. Y. (1990). Hwabyung: the construction of a Korean popular illness among Korean elderly immigrant women in the United States. *Cultural Medicine and Psychiatry*, 14, 495–512.

Pang, K. Y. (1989). The practice of traditional Korean medicine in Washington, DC. *Social Science and Medicine*, 28, 875–884.

## General Health Issues

Anderson, J. M. (1985). Perspectives on the health of immigrant women: a feminist analysis. *Advances in Nursing Science*, 8, 61–76.

Anderson, J. (1991). Immigrant women speak of chronic illness: the social construction of the devalued self. *Journal of Advanced Nursing*, 16, 710–717.

Fruchter, R. G., Remy, J. C., Boyce, J. G., & Burnett, W. S. (1986). Cervical cancer in immigrant women. *American Journal of Public Health*, 76, 797–799.

Juarbe, T. (1995). Access to health care for Hispanic women: a primary health care perspective. *Nursing Outlook*, 43, 23–28.

Kulig, J. (1990). A review of the health status of Southeast Asian refugee women. *Health Care for Women International*, 11, 49–63.

Lipson, J. G., Hosseini, T. Kabir, S., Omidian, P., & Edmonston, F. (1995). Health issues among Afghan women in California. *Health Care for Women International*, 16, 279–286.

Meleis, A. I., & Aly, F. (1994). Women's health: a global perspective. In J. McCloskey & H. Grace (Eds.). *Current Issues in Nursing*, 4th Ed. St. Louis: Mosby–Year Book, 692–700.

Peragallo, N., Fox, P., & Alba, M. (1998). Breast care among Latino immigrant women in the U.S. *Health Care for Women International*, 19(2):165–172.

Reizian, A., & Meleis, A. I. (1987). Symptoms reported by Arab-American patients on the Cornell Medical Index (CMI). *Western Journal of Nursing Research*, 9, 368–385.

Sawyers, J. E., & Eaton, L. (1992). Gastric cancer in the Korean-American: cultural implications. *Oncology Nursing Forum*, 19(4), 619–623.

## Risk Factors, Screening, and Prevention

Cavan, K., Gibson, B., Cole, D., & Riedel, D. (1996). Fish consumption by Vietnamese women immigrants: a comparison of methods. *Archives of Environmental Health*, 51(6): 452–457.

Chen, Y., Dales, R., Krewski, D., & Breithaupt, K. (1999). Increased effects of smoking and obesity on asthma among female Canadians: the National Population Health Survey, 1994–1995. *American Journal of Epidemiology*, 150, 255–262.

Enas, E., Garg, A., Davidson, M., Nair, V., Huet, B., & Yusuf, S. (1996). Coronary heart disease and its risk factors in first-generation immigrant Asian Indians to the United States of America. *Indian Heart Journal*, 48, 343–353.

Juarbe, T. (1998). Cardiovascular disease-related diet and exercise experiences of immigrant Mexican women. *Western Journal of Nursing Research*, 20, 765–782.

Juarbe, T. (1998). Risk factors for cardiovascular disease in Latina women. *Progress in Cardiovascular Nursing*, 13(2), 7–27.

Martinez, R., Chavez, L., & Hubbell, F. (1997). Purity and passion: risk and mortality in Latina immigrants' and physicians' beliefs about cervical cancer. *Medical Anthropology*, 17, 337–362.

Maxwell, A., Bastani, R., & Warda, U. S. (1998). Mammography utilization and related attitudes among Korean-American women. *Women and Health*, 27(3), 89–107.

McPhee, S., Stewart, S., Brock, K., Bird, J., Jenkins, C., & Pham, G. (1997). Factors associated with breast and cervical cancer screening practices among Vietnamese American women. *Cancer Detection and Prevention*, 21, 510–521.

Mahloch, J, Jackson, J., Chitnarong, K., Sam, R., Ngo, L., & Taylor V. M. (1999). Bridging cultures through the development of a cervical cancer screening video for Cambodian women in the United States. *Journal of Cancer Education*, 14, 9–14.

Peragallo, N., Fox, P., & Alba, M. (2000). Acculturation and breast self-examination among immigrant Latina women in the USA. *International Nursing Review*, 47(1), 38–45.

Rajaram, S., & Rashidi, A. (1999). Asian-Islamic women and breast cancer screening: a socio-cultural analysis. *Women and Health*, 28(3), 45–58.

Rashidi, A., & Rajaram, S. (2000). Middle Eastern Asian Islamic women and breast self-examination. Needs assessment. *Cancer Nursing*, 23, 64–70.

Salgado de Snyder, V., Diaz Perez, M., & Maldonado, M. (1996). AIDS: risk behaviors among rural Mexican women married to migrant workers in the United States. *AIDS Education and Prevention*, 8, 134–142.

Shankar, S., & Figueroa-Valles, N. (1999). Cancer knowledge and misconceptions: a survey of immigrant Salvadorean women. *Ethnicity and Disease*, 9, 201–211.

Shankar, S., Gutierrez-Mohamed, M., & Alberg, A. (2000). Cigarette smoking among immigrant Salvadoreans in Washington, DC: behaviors, attitudes, and beliefs. *Addictive Behaviors*, 25, 275–281.

Suarez, L., Roche, R., Pulley, L., Weiss, N., Goldman D., & Simpson, D. (1997). Why a peer intervention program for Mexican-American women failed to modify the secular trend in cancer screening. *American Journal of Preventive Medicine*, 13, 411–417.

Taylor, V., Schwartz, S., Jackson, J., Kuniyuki, A., Fischer, M., Yasui, Y., Tu, S., & Thompson, B. (1999). Cervical cancer screening among Cambodian-American women. *Cancer Epidemiology, Biomarkers and Prevention*, 8, 541–546.

# Mental Health

Boone, M. S. (1994). Thirty-year retrospective on the adjustment of Cuban refugee women. In L. Camino & R. Krulfeld (Eds.). *Reconstructing Lives, Recapturing Meaning*. Basel: Gordon and Breach, pp. 179–201.

Canadian Task Force on Mental Health Issues Affecting Immigrants and Refugees (1988). In *After the Door Has Been Opened*. Health and Welfare Canada.

Cole, E., Espin, O., & Rothblum E. (Eds.) (1992). *Refugee Women and Their Mental Health: Shattered Societies, Shattered Lives*. New York: Haworth Press.

Fox, P. G., Cowell, J. M., Montgomery, A. C., & Willgerodt, M. A. (1998). Southeast Asian refugee women and depression: a nursing intervention. *International Journal of Psychiatric Nursing Research*, 4, 423–432.

Franks, F., & Faux, S. (1990). Depression, stress, mastery and social resources in four ethnocultural women's groups. *Research in Nursing and Health*, 13, 283–292.

Furnham, A., & Sheikh, S. (1993). Gender, generational and social support correlates of mental health in Asian immigrants. *The International Journal of Social Psychiatry*, 56, 22–33.

Kim, S., & Rew, L. (1994). Ethnic identity, role integration, quality of life and depression in Korean-American women. *Archives of Psychiatric Nursing*, 8, 348–356.

Lipson, J. G. (1993). Afghan refugees in California: mental health issues. *Issues in Mental Health Nursing*, 14, 411–423.

Meleis, A. I., & Silver, C. W. (1984). The Arab-American and psychiatric care. *Perspectives in Psychiatric Care*, 22, 72–76, 85–86.

Patel, S., & Gaw, A. (1996). Suicide among immigrants from the Indian subcontinent: a review. *Psychiatric Services*, 47, 517–521.

Saldaña, D. H. (1992). Coping with stress: a refugee's story. In E. Cole, O. Espin, & E. Rothblum (Eds.). *Refugee Women and Their Mental Health: Shattered Societies, Shattered Lives*. New York: Haworth Press, pp. 21–33.

Shin, K. R. (1993). Factors predicting depression among Korean-American women in New York. *International Journal of Nursing Studies*, 30, 415–423.

Tabora, B., & Flaskerud, J. (1997). Mental health beliefs, practices, and knowledge of Chinese American immigrant women. *Issues in Mental Health Nursing*, 18, 173–189.

Um, C., & Dancy, B. (1999). Relationship between coping strategies and depression among employed Korean immigrant wives. *Issues in Mental Health Nursing*, 20(5), 485–494.

Vega, W., Kolody, B., Valle, R., & Weir, J. (1991). Social networks, social support, and their relationship to depression among immigrant Mexican women. *Human Organization*, 50, 154–162.

Vega, W., Kolody, B., & Valle, R. (1987). Migration and mental health: An empirical test of depression risk factors among immigrant Mexican women. *International Migration Review*, 21, 512–530.

Vega, W., Kolody, B., Valle, R., & Hough, R. (1986). Depressive symptoms and their correlates among immigrant Mexican women in the United States. *Social Science and Medicine*, 22, 645–652.

Ying, Y. (1990). Explanatory models of major depression and implications for help-seeking among immigrant Chinese-American women. *Culture, Medicine and Psychiatry*, 14, 393–408.

# 🌐 VIOLENCE AGAINST WOMEN

## Domestic Violence/Rape

Bauer, H. M., Rodriguez, M. A., Quiroga, S. S., & Flores-Ortiz, Y. G. (2000). Barriers to health care for abused Latina and Asian immigrant women. *Journal of Health Care for the Poor and Underserved*, 11, 33–44.

Fontes, L. A. (Ed.) (1995). *Sexual Abuse in Nine North American Cultures*. Thousand Oaks, CA: Sage Publications.

Fontes, L. A. (1993). Disclosures of sexual abuse by Puerto Rican children: oppression and cultural barriers. *Journal of Child Sexual Abuse*, 2, 21–35.

Frye, B. A., & D'Avanzo, C. D. (1994). Cultural themes in family stress and violence among Cambodian refugee women in the inner city. *Advances in Nursing Science*, 16, 64–77.

National Council for Research on Women. (1995). Intervening: immigrant women and domestic violence. *Issues Quarterly*, 1, 12–13.

Rodriguez, M. A., Bauer, H. M., Flores-Ortiz, Y., & Szkupinski-Quiroga, S. (1998). Factors affecting patient-physician communication for abused Latina and Asian immigrant women. *Journal of Family Practice*, 47, 309–311.

## War/Torture

Herbst, P. K. R. (1992). From helpless victim to empowered survivor: oral history as a treatment for survivors of torture. In E. Cole, O. Espin, & E. Rothblum (Eds.). *Refugee Women and Their Mental Health: Shattered Societies, Shattered Lives*. New York: Haworth Press, pp. 141–154.

Locke, C. J., Southwick, K., McCloskey, L. A., & Fernandez-Esquer, M. E. (1996). The psychological and medical sequelae of war in Central American refugee mothers and children. *Archives of Pediatrics and Adolescent Medicine*, 150, 822–828.

Shepard, J., & Faust, S. (1993). Refugee health care and the problem of suffering. *Bioethics Forum* 9(3), 3–7.

#  CULTURALLY COMPETENT CARE

## Community Assessment

Laffrey, S., Meleis, A., Lipson, J., Solomon, M., & Omidian, P. (1989). Assessing health care needs of Arab immigrants. *Social Science in Medicine*, 29, 877–883.

Lipson, J. G., Omidian, P., & Paul, S. (1995). Afghan health education project: A community survey. *Public Health Nursing*, 12(3), 143–150.

Urrutia-Rojas, X., & Aday, L. A. (1991). A framework for community assessment: designing and conducting a survey in a Hispanic immigrant and refugee community. *Public Health Nursing*, 8, 20–26.

## Health Education/Health Promotion

Burns, A., Lovich, R., Maxwell, J., & Shapiro, K. (1997). *Where Women Have No Doctor*. Berkeley, CA: The Hesperian Foundation.

Choudhry, U. (1998). Health promotion among immigrant women from India living in Canada. *Image—the Journal of Nursing Scholarship*, 30, 269–274.

DeSantis, L., & Thomas, J. (1992). Health education and the immigrant Haitian mother: cultural insights for community health nurses. *Public Health Nursing*, 9, 87–96.

Gomez, C., Hernandez, M., & Faigeles, B. (1999). Sex in the New World: an empowerment model for HIV prevention in Latina immigrant women. *Health Education and Behavior*, 26, 200–212.

Im, E. O., & Choe, M. A. (2001). Physical activity of Korean immigrant women in the U.S.: needs and attitudes. *International Journal of Nursing Studies*, 38(5), 567–577.

Murty, M. (1998). Healthy living for immigrant women: a health education community outreach program. *Cmaj*, 159, 385–387.

Sanders-Phillips, K. (1994). Health promotion behavior in low income black and Latino women. *Women & Health*, 21, 71–83.

## Culturally Appropriate Interventions

Downs, K., Bernstein, J., & Marchese, T. (1997). Providing culturally competent primary care for immigrant and refugee women. A Cambodian case study. *Journal of Nurse-Midwifery*, 42, 499–508.

Gany, F., & Thiel de Bocanegra, H. (1996). Overcoming barriers to improving the health of immigrant women. *Journal of the American Medical Womens Association*, 51, 155–160.

Hatton, D. C. (1992). Information transmission in bilingual, bicultural contexts. *Journal of Community Health Nursing*, 9, 53–59.

Ivey, S., & Kramer, E. (1998). Immigrant women and the emergency department: the juncture with welfare and immigration reform. *Journal of the American Medical Womens Association*, 53(2), 94–95, 107.

Lipson, J. G., & Meleis, A. I. (1985). Culturally appropriate care: The case of immigrants. *Topics in Clinical Nursing*, 7, 48–56.

Lipson, J. G., & Meleis, A. I. (1983). Issues in health care of Middle Eastern patients. *Western Journal of Medicine*, 139, 854–861.

Luna, L. (1994). Care and cultural context of Lebanese Muslim immigrants: using Leininger's theory. *Journal of Transcultural Nursing*, 5, 12–20.

Marsella, A. J. (1993). Counseling and psychotherapy with Japanese Americans: cross-cultural considerations, *American Journal of Orthopsychiatry*, 63, 200–208.

Mahon, J., McFarlane, J., & Golden, K. (1991). De madres a madres: A community partnership for health. *Public Health Nursing*, 8, 15–19.

Maltby, H. (1999). Interpreters: a double-edged sword in nursing practice. *Journal of Transcultural Nursing*, 10, 248–254.

Meleis, A. I. (1997). Immigrant transitions and health care: an action plan. *Nursing Outlook*, 45, 42.

Meleis, A. I. & Lipson, J. G. (1993). Mideast S.I.H.A.: a primary health care center. In M. J. Kim (Ed.). *Primary Health Care: Nurses Lead the Way—A Global Perspective*. Washington, DC: American Association of Colleges of Nursing, pp. 19–23.

Meleis, A. I., Omidian, P. A., & Lipson, J. G. (1993). Women's health status in the United States: an immigrant women's project. In B. J. McElmurry (Ed), *Women's Health and Development: A Global Challenge*, Sudbury, MA: Jones & Bartlett, Publishers, pp 163–181.

Muecke, M. (1995). Trust, abuse of trust, and mistrust among refugee women from Cambodia: a cultural interpretation. In J. C. Knudsen & E. V. Daniel, (Eds.), *Mistrusting Refugees*. Berkeley: University of California Press, pp. 36–55.

Muecke, M. (1983). In search of healing: Southeast Asian refugees in the American health care system. *Western Journal of Medicine*, 139, 835–840.

Ong, A. (1995). Making the biopolitical subject: Cambodian immigrants, refugee medicine and cultural citizenship. *Social Science & Medicine*, 40, 1243–1257.

Vu, H. (1996). Cultural barriers between obstetrician-gynecologists and Vietnamese/Chinese immigrant women. *Texas Medicine*, 92(10), 47–52.

## 🌐 RESEARCH ISSUES

DeSantis, L. (1990). Fieldwork with undocumented aliens and other populations at risk. *Western Journal of Nursing Research*, 12, 359–372.

Im, E. O., Meleis, A., & Lee, K. (1999). Cultural competence of measurement scales of menopausal symptoms: use in research among Korean women. *International Journal of Nursing Studies*, 36, 455–463.

Lipson, J. G. (1997). The politics of publishing: Protecting participants' confidentiality. In J. Morse (Ed.). *Completing a Qualitative Project*. Thousand Oaks, CA. Sage Publications, pp. 39–58.

Lipson, J. G., & Meleis, A. I. (1989). Methodological issues in research with immigrants. *Medical Anthropology*, 12, 103–115.

Lynam, M., & Anderson, J. (1986). Generating knowledge for nursing practice: methodological issues in studying immigrant women. In P. Chinn (Ed.). *Nursing Research Methodology: Issues and Implementation*. Rockville, MD: Aspen, pp. 259–274.

Muecke, M. A. (1992). New paradigms for refugee health problems. *Social Science and Medicine*, 35, 515–523.

Sawyer, L., Regev, H., Proctor, S., Nelson, M., Messias, D., Barnes, D., & Meleis, A. I. (1995). Matching versus cultural competence in research: methodological considerations. *Research in Nursing and Health*, 18, 557–567.

Thompson, J. L. (1991). Exploring gender and culture with Khmer refugee women: reflections on participatory feminist research. *Advances in Nursing Science*, 13, 30–48.

##  LITERATURE REVIEWS AND BOOKS COVERING MULTIPLE CULTURAL GROUPS

Centre for Documentation on Refugees (CDR). (1989). *Refugee women: Selected and annotated bibliography*. Geneva: United Nations High Commissioner for Refugees.

Giger, J., & Davidhizar, R. (1999). *Transcultural Nursing: Assessment and Intervention*. St. Louis: Mosby.

Levinson, D., & Ember, M. (1997). *American Immigrant Cultures*, Vols I & II. New York: Simon & Schuster Macmillan.

Lipson, J. G., Dibble, S., & Minarik, P. (Eds.) (1996). *Culture and Nursing Care: A Pocket Guide*. San Francisco: UCSF Nursing Press.

Lipson, J. G., & Meleis, A. I. (1999). Immigrants and refugees. In A.S. Hinshaw, Feetham, S., & Shaver, J. (Eds.). *Handbook of Clinical Nursing Research*. Thousand Oaks, CA. Sage Publications, pp. 87–105.

Meleis, A., Lipson, J., Muecke, M., & Smith, G. (1998). *Immigrant Women and their Health: An Olive Paper*. Indianapolis: Nursing Press of Sigma Theta Tau.

Meleis, A. I., & Lipson, J. G. (1999). Research on immigrant women. In J. Fitzpatrick (Ed.). *Encyclopedia of Nursing Research*. New York: Springer, pp 266–267.

Muecke, M. (1992). Nursing research with refugees: A guide and review. *Western Journal of Nursing Research* 14, 703–720.

Obermeyer, C. (1999). Female genital surgeries: the known, the unknown, and the unknowable. *Medical Anthropology Quarterly*, 13, 79–106.

Purnell, L., & Paulanka, B. (1998). *Transcultural Health Care: A Culturally Competent Approach*, Philadelphia: F. A. Davis.

# INDEX

follow-up appointments for, 140
health-seeking behaviors of, 141
infertility in, 131–132
literacy of, 137–138
medical intake for, 137–138
menopause in, 134–135
menstruation in, 126–127
middle age of, 134–135
miscarriage in, 131
modesty of, 127
newborn care by, 133–134
in North America, 123–124
pain in, 139
physical examination for, 139
postpartum period of, 133
pregnancy in, 132
psychosexual development of, 125–126
pubescence of, 125–127
rape among, 129
self-care by, 141
son preference among, 124
teen sexuality among, 126
union formation among, 128
El Arbeen, 136
El Sanaweya, 136
Ethiopians and Eritreans, 142–155
abortion in, 148
adulthood of, 146–150
aging in, 150–151
at birth, 143
birthing process in, 149
care provision to, 152–155
childhood of, 144
communication with, 153
contraception in, 148
death/dying in, 151–152
definition of, 142
diseases in, 155
divorce among, 147
domestic violence among, 146–147
drug prescribing for, 154
dysmenorrhea in, 145
education of, 144
female, 143–152
female birth among, 143
fertility in, 147–148
follow-up appointments for, 154
health-seeking behaviors of, 155
in North America, 142–143
infertility in, 148
literacy of, 152
medical intake for, 152–153
menopause in, 151
menstruation in, 145
middle age of, 150–151
miscarriage in, 148
modesty of, 146
old age of, 151
physical examination for, 153–154
postpartum period of, 149–150
pregnancy in, 148–149

psychosexual development of, 145
pubescence of, 144–146
rape among, 147
son preference of, 143
teen sexuality of, 145
union formation among, 146

Familismo, 218, 224
Fertility
in African Americans, 18–19
in American Indians/Alaska Natives, 35
in Arab Americans, 51–52
in Brazilians, 69–70
in Cambodians, 83–84
in Chinese, 98–99
in Colombians, 114
in Egyptians, 130
in Ethiopians and Eritreans, 147–148
in Filipinos, 162
in Haitians, 178–179
in Japanese, 194
in Koreans, 207–208
in Mexican Americans, 225
in Puerto Ricans, 241
in Russians, 254
in South Asians, 273
in Vietnamese, 293
in West Indians, 312
Filipinos, 156–171
abortion in, 163
adulthood of, 160–165
aging in, 165–167
at birth, 157–158
birthing process in, 164–165
care provision by, 168–171
child custody practices of, 162
childbearing in, 162
childhood of, 158
communication with, 169
contraceptive practices of, 162
death/dying in, 167–168
definition of, 156
developmental stages of, 159
diseases of, 170–171
divorce among, 161–162
domestic violence among, 161
drug prescribing for, 169–170
dysmenorrhea in, 160
education of, 159
elderly housing in, 167
family expectations for, 159
female birth among, 157–158
female role in, 157–168
fertility of, 162
follow-up appointments for, 170
health-seeking behaviors of, 171
infertility in, 163
literacy of, 168
medical intake for, 168–169
menstruation in, 159–160
middle age of, 165–166